Professional Practice in Health, Education and the Creative Arts

Joy Higgs
Angie Titchen

b

Blackwell
Science

© 2001 by
Blackwell Science Ltd
© Joy Higgs and Angie Titchen Chapters 1, 21, 22
© Joy Higgs Chapter 3
© Emma Coats Chapter 20

Editorial Offices:
Osney Mead, Oxford OX2 0EL
25 John Street, London WC1N 2BS
23 Ainslie Place, Edinburgh EH3 6AJ
350 Main Street, Malden
  MA 02148 5018, USA
54 University Street, Carlton
  Victoria 3053, Australia
10, rue Casimir Delavigne
  75006 Paris, France

Other Editorial Offices:

Blackwell Wissenschafts-Verlag GmbH
Kurfürstendamm 57
10707 Berlin, Germany

Blackwell Science KK
MG Kodenmacho Building
7–10 Kodenmacho Nihombashi
Chuo-ku, Tokyo 104, Japan

Iowa State University Press
A Blackwell Science Company
2121 S. State Avenue
Ames, Iowa 50014-8300, USA

First published 2001

Set in 10/13 pt Times Roman
by DP Photosetting, Aylesbury, Bucks
Printed and bound in Great Britain by
MPG Books Ltd, Bodmin, Cornwall

The Blackwell Science logo is a trade mark of
Blackwell Science Ltd, registered at the United
Kingdom Trade Marks Registry

DISTRIBUTORS

Marston Book Services Ltd
PO Box 269
Abingdon
Oxon OX14 4YN
(*Orders:* Tel: 01235 465500
         Fax: 01235 465555)

USA
Blackwell Science, Inc.
Commerce Place
350 Main Street
Malden, MA 02148 5018
(*Orders:* Tel: 800 759 6102
              781 388 8250
         Fax: 781 388 8255)

Canada
Login Brothers Book Company
324 Salteaux Crescent
Winnipeg, Manitoba R3J 3T2
(*Orders:* Tel: 204 837-2987
         Fax: 204 837-3116)

Australia
Blackwell Science Pty Ltd
54 University Street
Carlton, Victoria 3053
(*Orders:* Tel: 03 9347 0300
         Fax: 03 9347 5001)

A catalogue record for this title
is available from the British Library

ISBN 0-632-059338

Library of Congress
Cataloging-in-Publication Data
is available

For further information on
Blackwell Science, visit our website:
www.blackwell-science.com

Contents

List of Contributors

Lee W. Andresen BSc, DipEd, PhD   Retired, previously Senior Lecturer, Professional Development Centre, The University of New South Wales, Sydney, Australia. Currently freelance consultant in Higher Education and Academic Development and affiliate of the Centre for Professional Education Advancement (CPEA) at the University of Sydney, Australia.

Hilary Byrne-Armstrong DipPhys, Grad Dip Soc Ec, MSc (Hons) PhD Lecturer, Centre for Critical Psychology, School of Psychology, Faculty of Social Inquiry, University of Western Sydney, Australia.

Dawn Best Dip Physio, MEd, MAPA   Senior Lecturer, School of Physiotherapy, La Trobe University, Bundoora, Australia.

Jim Butler BSc, PhD   Associate Professor, Graduate School of Education, The University of Queensland, Australia.

Dr Rosemary Cant MEd, PhD   Senior Lecturer, School of Behavioural and Community Health Sciences, Faculty of Health Sciences, The University of Sydney, Australia.

Dr Cathy Charles BA, MA MPhil PhD   Associate Professor, Clinical Epidemiology and Biostatistics, Faculty of Health Sciences, McMaster University, Canada.

Emma Coats   Independent Consultant and Creative Arts Facilitator, Alchemy Consulting, London.

Ann Cusick BAppSc (OT), MA (Psych), MA (Interdisc Stud), PhD   Associate Professor, Faculty of Health, University of Western Sydney, Macarthur, Campbelltown, New South Wales, Australia and Hon. Research Associate, School of Physiotherapy, Faculty of Health Sciences, University of Sydney.

Sally Denshire Dip OT (NZ) MAppSc(OT)   Lecturer, School of Community Health, Charles Sturt University, Albury, Australia.

Fran Everingham BA, MHPEd, Grad Dip Ed (Hlth Stud), DipEd   School of Behavioural and Community Health Sciences, Faculty of Health Sciences, The University of Sydney, Australia.

Robyn Ewing BEd (Hons), PhD   Senior Lecturer, School of Policy and Practice, Education Faculty, The University of Sydney, Australia.

Dawn Fredericks RN, Grad.Dip.Ed (TESOL)   Formerly Project Officer, Helping Early Leavers Program, Department of Education and Training, Sydney. Affiliate of CPEA at the University of Sydney, Australia.

Ian Fredericks Eng.   Affiliate of CPEA at the University of Sydney, Lidcombe, Australia.

Joy Goodfellow Dip SKTC, BA, MEd, PhD   Co-ordinator of Early Childhood Professional Experience, School of Learning, Development and Early Education, University of Western Sydney, Australia.

Charles Higgs BSurv, MSocEcol   Key Performance Consulting, Centre for Professional Education Advancement, Faculty of Health Sciences, The University of Sydney, Australia.

Professor Joy Higgs BSc, GradDipPhty, MPHEd, PhD   Director, Centre for Professional Education Advancement, Faculty of Health Sciences, The University of Sydney, Australia.

Debbie Horsfall BEd, MA, PhD   Senior Lecturer, School of Sociology and Justice Studies, University of Western Sydney, Australia.

Jude Irwin BSW, MA, MASSW   Associate Professor, Department of Social Work, Social Policy and Sociology, The University of Sydney, Australia.

Robert Kay BAppSc (Hons), PhD   Lecturer, School of Construction and Building Sciences, University of Western Sydney, Sydney, Australia.

Ian Maxwell BA (Hons) PhD DipArts (Dram Arts)   Centre for Performance Studies, The University of Sydney, Australia.

Lindy McAllister MA (SpPath) (Hons), BSpThy   Head of Program and Senior Lecturer in Speech Pathology, School of Community Health, Charles Sturt University, Australia.

Colleen Mullavey-O'Byrne MA (Hons)(Macq), DipOT   Director Intercultural Interactions, Honorary Associate Professor, School of Occupational and Leisure Sciences, The University of Sydney, Affiliate, CPEA, Australia.

Sue Radovich BAppSc (Sp Path)   Consultant, Educational Speech Pathology, Research Officer, CPEA, The University of Sydney, Australia.

Roderick Rothwell MA (Psych)(Syd), MA (Phil)(Syd), PhD (Syd)   School of Behavioural and Community Health Sciences, The University of Sydney, Australia.

Susan Ryan MSc, BappSc (OT)   Reader in Educational Development in the Health Sciences, University of East London, UK.

Dorothy Scott (BA (Hons), DipSocStud, MSW, PhD   Associate Professor, School of Social Work, University of Melbourne, Australia.

David L. Smith BA (Hons), PhD   Senior Lecturer, School of Policy and Practice, Education Faculty, The University of Sydney, Australia.

Lyn Spence BSc (Hons), BA   Centre for Professional Education Advancement, Faculty of Health Sciences, The University of Sydney, Australia.

Angie Titchen DPhil (Oxon), MSc   R&PD Fellow and Lead, Clinical Supervision Developments, RCN Institute, Oxford, England.

Gillian Webb Dip Physio, Grad Dip Ex for Rehab, MClin Ed   Senior Lecturer, School of Physiotherapy, The University of Melbourne, Parkville, Australia.

Sandra West BSc, PhD (Macq), RN, CM, IntCare Cert   Senior Lecturer, Department of Life Science in Nursing, Faculty of Nursing, University of Sydney, Australia.

Preface

This book invites you to explore a multidimensional and multiprofessional view of professional practice. The authors have explored four key dimensions of professional practice: 'doing', 'knowing', 'being' and 'becoming'. These concepts have been chosen to represent professional practice as being much more than applying learned knowledge in practice situations. Instead, professionals bring much of themselves to their work. They engage with others who are also *being* and *becoming* people, they generate as well as refine their knowledge and understanding of their role and of the broader people-centred context of professional practice, and they incorporate all of these understandings, skills and learnings into their actions. For this reason, we present professional practice as a lived experience, a service for (and with) others and a way of being and behaving. Further, we view professional practice as a team activity involving our clients, their caregivers and other team members. (The term client is used throughout the book to refer to all categories of people who seek the benefit of professional practice, including patients, customers, clients, students, family, caregivers and other relevant members of the community.)

The multidisciplinary focus of the book is reflected in the participating authors and our intended audience. Our audience broadly encompasses professional people engaged or interested in practice, and members of the community interested in the way professionals practise and frame their practice. The authors are professionals currently engaged in practice, the study of practice and/or teaching about professional practice. The authors were drawn from the fields of education, the health sciences and the creative arts. In our writing the rich and diverse mix of these backgrounds is harnessed; and while addressing these groups specifically in our examples and experiences, we consider our deliberations and findings relevant to other professional fields.

This book resulted from a collaborative research inquiry and writing project (see Chapter 3 for details of this writing process and experience). The project involved 29 people who participated directly in a writing retreat and another three who were invited to contribute chapters during the inquiry process. Each chapter has been peer reviewed. We retreated from our immersion in our professional roles to interact with creative arts media and nature and to engage in reflection, discourse, inquiry and debate about the nature of professional practice and to explore this topic through interaction with creative arts media and our natural surroundings. Our goals during this week-long retreat were to commence the inquiry process, to construct a conceptual and operational framework for a collaborative writing project (with the aim of producing a book on professional practice) and to identify areas of further inquiry needed. With these goals achieved, the process of inquiry and writing continued over the following 18 months. This book is the product of this research and writing collaboration.

The book explores the essential unity of knowledge and practice through discourse, narrative, imagery and critical debate. It is located in the human sciences, with interactions between people at the core and the human services professions as the broad focus. It is a book for all those willing or seeking to learn and to improve practice, including practitioners, students, teachers, researchers, practice developers, consumers, managers and reviewers.

One of the challenges we faced in preparing for this project and engaging in the inquiry and writing activities was to confront the questions: What is a profession? What is professional practice? We chose a broad definition of profession to encompass occupations where practice is underpinned by a body of discipline-specific (as well as generalist) knowledge and where principles of professionalism, including ethical behaviour and a service orientation, provide the foundation for professional practice. In this context we identified a number of similarities as well as differences between the creative arts professions, education and the health professions in relation to their use of different forms of knowledge in practice and ways of being and becoming in these professions. Therefore, we invited people from these three professional areas to participate in this project, as is reflected in the chapters in the book. In addition, we used creative arts during the retreat to break down barriers between word knowledge and wordless knowing, to explore our ideas through creative media and to produce images (in art, poetry and music) to express emerging ideas and visions arising from our exploration of professional practice. The colour plates and chapter title images in the book contain some of this artwork.

By examining issues and themes in this multidimensional topic area, the book seeks to be:

- *Transformative of practice*, encouraging more thoughtful and reflexive practice, and the extension or removal of practice boundaries
- *Transcendental of concepts*, moving decisively beyond the artificial divide often placed between knowledge and practice
- *Liberating of arguments on knowledge*, firmly acknowledging different ways of knowing, particularly the credibility of practice–generated knowledge
- *Stimulating of further insight and exploration into knowledge and practice*, through practice, education and research.

In exploring knowledge and professional practice we recognised the value of different forms of knowledge, including knowledge gained from research and theory (propositional knowledge), knowledge emerging from professional experience (professional craft knowledge) and knowledge derived from personal experience (personal knowledge). Professionals who engage with people and who use evidence from each of these knowledge sources as a foundation for their practice will find much of relevance within this book. For those who adopt a more traditional approach, immersed in professional mystique and 'the knowledge of the discipline', we hope this book will challenge you to extend your horizons.

The book is divided into four sections. In section one we introduce the concepts of doing, knowing, being and becoming, and present the inquiry process involved in producing the book. Section two deals with dimensions of professional practice, examining issues such as uncertainty, artistry, embodiment of knowledge, relationships, technology and practice research. Section three presents a variety of professional practice journeys considering personal-professional links, learning relationships, transformation of self and practice, developing creative expertise and using creativity in practice development. Section four reflects on being and becoming in practice.

We invite you to explore the products of our inquiry and to consider their relevance and application to your experiences and situation. We hope that you will find, as we have, questions as well as relevant insights and ideas in this book and that this will result in further questioning and reflections about professional practice.

Joy Higgs and Angie Titchen

Acknowledgements

The authors in this book participated in a research inquiry funded by the School of Physiotherapy and the Centre for Professional Education Advancement (CPEA) of the Faculty of Health Sciences, The University of Sydney. The research project and writers' retreat was organised by CPEA. CPEA promotes the advancement of research and scholarly activities in the area of professional development and education in the health sciences, in a multidisciplinary and human interaction context.

We wish to acknowledge the outstanding contribution made by Joan Rosenthal to the implementation and production of this volume. We express our grateful appreciation to Charles Higgs for his magical contribution to our graphics production.

Dedication

This book is dedicated to one of our group of authors, Ian Fredericks, who epitomised the spirit of the group and the search for humanity, creativity and knowledge that is embedded in us all.

Part One
Introduction

Chapter 1
Framing Professional Practice: Knowing and Doing in Context

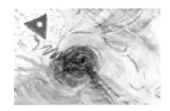

Joy Higgs and Angie Titchen

'Most practitioners today ... would agree that they act under conditions that are almost exactly the reverse of pre-defined, unilaterally controlled (and hence uninterrupted) experimental conditions. Consequently, the conditions under which knowledge is gained when following the canons of rigorous experimental research are simply not generalizable to the conditions practitioners face. Practitioners are generally attempting to act well in situations which they do not fundamentally comprehend, in pursuit of purposes which are not initially fully explicit and to which their commitment is initially ambivalent, *and* they are being interrupted all the while by other claims on their attention. Of course, it is not altogether pleasant and reassuring to acknowledge the degree of uncertainty and discontinuity to which (this) ... points, ... what practitioners really require is a kind of knowledge that they can apply to *their own behaviour* in the midst of ongoing events, in order to help them *inquire* more effectively with others about their common purposes, about how to produce outcomes congruent with such purposes.'

(Torbert 1981, p. 143)

This argument was presented by William Torbert in support of the need for a new paradigm of research in which collaborative inquiry and a search for knowledge address the real-world needs and situations of practice. His argument is reflected in the goals and mode of inquiry we adopted in the research which produced this book. In addition, Torbert's points illustrate the focus we are selecting to frame this book: 'doing', 'knowing', 'being' and 'becoming' in the context of professional practice.

This chapter explores the knowing and doing dimensions of our framework for professional practice. It provides the landscape upon which the subsequent chapters are enacted. As the book progresses, this focus on the more concrete and immediate dimensions of practice is transformed into a greater emphasis on the future and more ephemeral dimensions of being and becoming. The last two chapters explore these two issues respectively, reflecting the image of professional practice as a process of dynamic professional socialisation.

The context of professional practice is of major importance to the shaping and structure of this practice. As Fig. 1.1 illustrates, the knowing and doing of professional practice (or the knowledge-in-action which comprises practice) are influenced by many factors. Some factors, such as the culture, personal frame of reference and life history, are particular and internal to the practitioner. Other factors, including the practice situation, other people and other cultures, occur in the practice environment and influence directly or indirectly the practice design, process and outcomes.

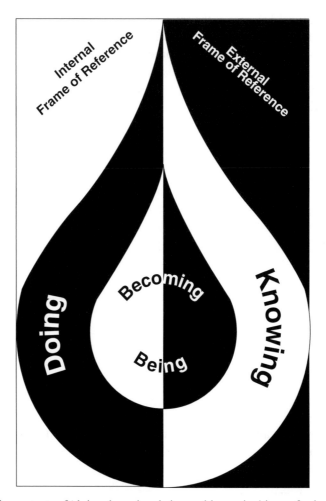

Fig. 1.1   The contexts of 'doing, knowing, being and becoming' in professional practice.

This book challenges traditional notions of what it means to be a professional. We propose a valuing of propositional knowledge (research-based and theoretical knowledge), professional craft knowledge (gained from professional experience) and personal knowledge (derived from personal experience) as credible evidence for professional practice. At the same time, we set high expectations for professionals, namely, that their knowledge claims are well tested and that knowledge is communicated in substantiation of practice. The authors in various chapters examine the dances and tensions which occur in professional practice between practice and research, between rational, intuitive and creative thinking, and between art, craft and science. In this way we seek to bridge the theory–practice gap. We extend professional practice discourse through consideration of emerging types of partnerships (in place of dominant roles for the professional, and more passive 'receiver' roles) and through exploration of the use of the creative arts to generate professional knowledge and expand practice horizons. Professional practice, we contend, is a rare blend of people-centred and interactive processes, accountability and professional standards, practice wisdom, professional artistry, openness to knowledge growth and practice development and engagement in professional journeys towards expertise.

Our conceptual framework

The cooperative inquiry (see Chapter 3) which generated this book resulted in the development of a conceptual framework which represents a vision of people-centred, accountable, context-relevant professional practice suitable for the demanding world of human services which we are facing today and tomorrow. This framework draws on a number of the practice dimensions above and seeks to interpret the elements and wholeness of this proposed approach to professional practice. The framework is structured around the following themes and sub-themes that we overview here and explore in more depth in the subsequent chapters.

Practice which is people-centred

- Aesthetic dimensions of practice – creating a form that is satisfying
- The nature and importance of people-centred practice
- Personal and public discourse and stories, knowledge and voices in practice.

Practice which is context-relevant

- Culture and context as they apply to practice, and the obstacles and opportunities they create
- The need for, and influence of, flexibility, uncertainty, ambiguity and boundaries in professional practice
- Practice in relation to individual and collective considerations.

Practice which is authentic

- Issues of authenticity, credibility, valuing, power, and authority in professional practice
- Ethics, morality and professional practice
- Professional practice and philosophy – how we view truth, reality/realities, perceptions.

Practice which is wise

- Practice as a process of transformation of actions, knowledge and people
- Practice as a process of awareness – attending to the unspoken needs and edges as well as the obvious
- Practice wisdom – considering wise practice, not best practice.

These themes are integrated in Fig. 1.2. We have chosen an Aztec drawing to reflect the integration of elements from everyday and spiritual life, the mundane as well as the aesthetic, the people and things in the context of our lives and well-being, the symbols of learning, wisdom and philosophy, as well as the stories which comprise our lives, cultures and histories. This drawing symbolises the complexity, the humanity, the practical and the mystical which is professional practice. The need for flexibility, boundaries, awareness and authenticity in professional practice is represented by the snake, an image of the healing arts. The choice of an ancient artistic symbol prompts our discussion in this book of the value of investigating ways of knowing, doing, being and becoming through an exploration of our creativity and the wisdom of other cultures, both past and present.

Practice which is people-centred

The participants in our cooperative inquiry strongly supported a model of professional practice which highly valued working with and for people. Whatever the profession, we saw the goal of professional service being primarily concerned with the enhancement, empowerment and development of people, their lives or environments. The three sub-themes illustrate this contention.

Aesthetic dimensions of practice – creating a form that is satisfying

One of the firm points of agreement which arose in our inquiry was the support for the artistic as well as the technical/craft and science dimensions of professional practice. In supporting the aesthetic/artistic side of professional practice we are espousing recognition of and preparation for the human interactions which lie at the centre of the professional's service role, whether this be in the health, education, law, creative arts or other professions. The quality of this

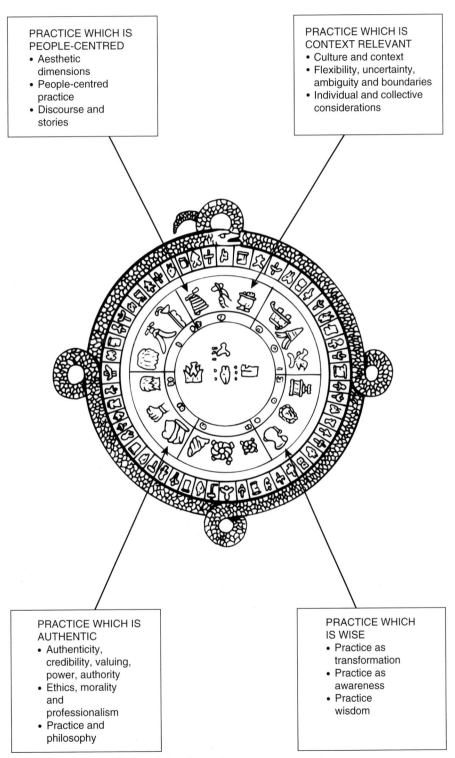

PRACTICE WHICH IS
PEOPLE-CENTRED
• Aesthetic
  dimensions
• People-centred
  practice
• Discourse and
  stories

PRACTICE WHICH IS
CONTEXT RELEVANT
• Culture and context
• Flexibility, uncertainty,
  ambiguity and boundaries
• Individual and collective
  considerations

PRACTICE WHICH IS
AUTHENTIC
• Authenticity,
  credibility, valuing,
  power, authority
• Ethics, morality
  and
  professionalism
• Practice and
  philosophy

PRACTICE WHICH
IS WISE
• Practice as
  transformation
• Practice as
  awareness
• Practice
  wisdom

Fig. 1.2 Dimensions in professional practice.

human interaction is a significant topic today. On the one hand, the pressures of globalisation, consumerism and economic rationalism are promoting market economies and 'service contexts' where professional services are commodified, where profit margins rather than professional standards are paramount, and where consumer satisfaction represents a willingness to re-purchase, rather than a feeling that the professional service received was personally satisfying. On the other hand, with an increasingly well-educated society and a greater under-standing of the 'purchased' and 'purchasable' product alternatives, the recipient of professional services is increasingly expecting, and indeed demanding, a form of service that is both professional and relevant.

Aesthetics in health care is illustrated by Titchen (2000) who speaks of 'graceful care'. Graceful care is realised through presence, comportment, use of body, touch and humour, through valuing, creating a caring climate, balancing therapeutic closeness and professional distance and through moderated love to promote personal and professional growth.

The nature and importance of people-centred practice

People-centred practice is an approach to professional practice which is gaining growing support among professionals and clients alike. This approach reflects a return to the traditional valuing of the client as the focus and centre of pro-fessional service (as opposed to organisational goals, outcomes and procedures), with an emphasis on humanistic values and the empowerment goals of the critical social sciences. It recognises and seeks to avoid the problems which can arise from the depersonalisation of professional practice. People-centred practice is also, increasingly, an expectation of clients who expect the high standards of the best that science and technology have to offer, but who want to relate to people and be treated like people. In addition, there is a growing number of professional practitioners who aspire to base their services not on technical rationality, but on practice wisdom based on their humanity and life learnings and a desire to provide quality services for and with the people who are their clients.

We live in an age of change and globalisation. To be competent is no longer enough, and to work, even with very high levels of competence, in the absence of effective interaction with others and the environment is to limit the quality of professional services and contribution to society. In the model of the *interactional professional*, the beginning practitioner attains the traditional abilities of com-petence and professionalism and a new vision of professional accountability and interaction with consumers and society in both local and global contexts (Higgs & Hunt 1999).

This new vision of person-centred, interactional practice requires a capacity to understand the concerns and lived experiences of clients who seek or receive professional services, not only from the professional's perspective, but also from the client's. The balancing of the two perspectives in designing, implementing and evaluating the particular service offered, is more likely to result in a personalised interaction which is mutually satisfying and in a service that benefits the environments of which each is a part.

Personal and public discourses and stories, knowledge and voices in practice

People often communicate via stories. The histories and lives of individuals, societies and nations are embedded in personal and public discourses. To understand the roles, needs and realities of participants in professional practice we need to hear their voices, their knowings and their stories. Sometimes these voices are silenced by unequal power differentials, so singing up these voices requires critical approaches in education, practice, research and practice development.

Practice which is context-relevant

Professional practice needs to be suited to the context of practice on many levels: the international and national as well as local environments which shape and challenge practice, the context of the specific profession, and the real world of particular clients and their families, friends and so on.

Culture and context as they apply to practice, and the obstacles and opportunities they create

Professionals cannot be insensitive to or independent of the culture and context in which they work. Since they provide services to the community they need to understand and work within the obstacles, constraints and opportunities that these community contexts provide.

Current and future graduating professionals will work in a society that is culturally and linguistically diverse, technologically oriented and increasingly international in its outlook and interactions. Some of the most pressing challenges for educators in professional entry programmes that have been created by these developments, are the need to prepare students to work in a global community, the range of ways of viewing the world, the cultural diversity inherent in cultural groups and multicultural multiethnic society, the need to understand and value diversity, and the need to confront one's own cultural orientations (Mullavey-O'Byrne 1999).

The need for, and influence of, flexibility, uncertainty, ambiguity and boundaries in professional practice

In today's rapidly evolving, globalising and unpredictable working worlds, the decision we need to make is how to live with change, rather than whether or not to change. In addition, professionals commonly work in social arenas, or at least in consideration of the needs of the social world. Therefore, we are choosing to live and work in contexts where uncertainty and ambiguity are prevalent and where there is a need to set some boundaries to facilitate practice implementation, as well as to restrict possible chaos and burnout from working in potentially limitless jobs. To say we need effective survival skills, as well as flexibility, tolerance of ambiguity and a strong capacity for perspective transformation, is an understatement.

Practice in relation to individual and collective considerations

Professional practice in health, education and the creative arts professions involves service to individuals and groups. This raises a number of issues in professional practice: establishing priorities in relation to services that address the needs of the individual client versus the group; providing services (e.g. classes, performances, creative products) which build on expectations and anticipated characteristics of the group, but which also serve the interests of the individual providing the service; addressing the needs of individuals who are culturally different from the rest of the population (e.g. minorities), whilst balancing the need of the collective.

Practice which is authentic

Authentic practice is compatible with the professional role and standards, as well as the individual values of the practitioner. To be authentic, professionals need to understand the role and influence they have and the expectations (quality, ethics, accountability) which clients and society can reasonably expect of them. And this authenticity requires self-knowledge.

Issues of authenticity, credibility, valuing, power, and authority in professional practice

Membership of professions brings status, power and authority. The inquiry linked to this book examined issues related to the question of the relevance and place of professional mystique and authority today. Terms like 'clinical', 'academic', and even 'professional' have understandably acquired connotations of distance, reserve and dominance, through such factors as exclusive education, privileged knowledge bases and technical expertise. But these connotations are also attributable to professional socialisation programmes which result in adopted and learned modes of professional conduct, and which commonly encourage maintaining professional distance, and also to professional bodies which promote the respect, status and market share of their professions. This is illustrated by Richardson (2001) who presents the following arguments.

Professions are structures of privilege and market place dominance. They are socially sanctioned and are regarded as a special kind of occupation which embodies a promise of service to the community. Changes in the operation and roles of the professions are reflecting changes in society. Definitions of health care have changed with a move to primary care which is offering significant changes in the role and dominance of health care professions. These changes reflect a growing influence of women and consumer groups who recognise the more humane issues of nurture, care and support (Sidell 1995). However, the challenge is now to consider the ethics of professional practice and the need to engage in moral and civic purposes (Sullivan 1994) as befits mature professions.

Ethics, morality and professional practice

One of the changes facing society is changing patterns of ethics, morality and professional standards. The world of professionalism is facing unsettling times in relation to balancing its ethical responsibilities with the need to deal with issues and practices of market competitiveness. One of the challenges faced by the professions is to re-create and regulate the ethical and professional standards of their members and to seek forms of accountability which consider the growing role of the community as participant stakeholders, not just recipients of pre-scribed or profession-determined services. One option being proposed is demo-cratic stakeholder regulation in which professions would work with those who have a stake in the service they offer. This would mean that professionals' voices in the debate would neither be totally controlling or totally controlled (Davies 2000).

Professional practice and philosophy – how we view truth, reality/realities, perceptions

Professions have a tradition of 'learning the rules' – the ground rules, the rules of thumb and the legal and ethical rules of operation. There is perhaps less attention being paid to understanding the truth, realities and perceptions which underlie these rules. Curricula commonly focus strongly on technical/professional skills and knowledge acquisition. Some level of research skills is included in most professional curricula; minimally, learning to critically appraise and utilise published research. More recently, skills of interpersonal interaction have received increasing attention. However, few curricula explicitly include practice epistemology in their requirements. Students learn to learn, and learn to practice. But they learn less about how knowledge is generated, understood and critiqued in their professional context. To be competent authentic practitioners, we argue, professionals need to understand the philosophy, the knowledge generation paradigms and the truths, realities and perceptions which ground, frame and define their professions.

Practice which is wise

The wise practitioner brings to practice a higher level of knowing; a capacity to see bigger pictures and creative, meaningful possibilities, not just solutions. Practice wisdom considers not just the best of what is, but the broader possibi-lities of what could be.

Practice as a process of transformation of practice, knowledge and people

For everyday practice to be effective, creative and responsive to clients' needs, it has to be imbued with evaluative processes, otherwise it cannot be called professional. In addition, professionals have a responsibility to contribute to the knowledge bases of their professions. Increasingly, professionals meet these dual responsibilities by using a critical social science approach to transform themselves, their practices and their cultures, at the same time as generating new knowledge. This approach emphasises the enlightenment (perspective transformation), empowerment and emancipation of oppressed people and silenced voices.

Knowledge is generated through using the research process in collaboration with others, but there is a special emphasis on knowledge creation through critique, contestation and debate (Carr & Kemmis 1986; Titchen & Ersser, 2001). It is proposed that all the stakeholders involved in a particular professional practice under consideration should be involved in this knowledge creation. If practitioners thereby create new knowledge about their current practices and the historico-social, cultural and political contexts that shape them, they can use these new theoretical understandings and insights to inform the actions they undertake to change practices and to counter inhibiting contexts and factors. New knowledge can then be generated about the change process itself, the transformed practices and their effectiveness in achieving what they set out to achieve. Thus critical social science offers a way of illuminating and transforming practice simultaneously.

Practice as a process of awareness – attending to the unspoken needs and edges as well as the obvious

Expertise in health, education and the creative arts involves high degrees of self-awareness, attunement and creativity. Earlier, in our consideration of the aesthetic dimensions of practice, we mentioned graceful care. This process is an integral part of Titchen's (2001) conceptualisation of person-centred health care as skilled companionship. Skilled companions take themselves as people, as well as professionals, into their relationships with others. They must, therefore, be highly aware of all aspects of their humanness, their bodies, comportment, emotions and so on in order to use themselves therapeutically and so transform the experiences of their patients. In bringing their emotions into their care, for example, they have not only to be fully aware of these emotions, they also have to be attuned to the needs of others and the ways in which this can be done therapeutically. At the same time, they have to protect themselves and their patients from over involvement that fosters dependency, neediness or inappropriate interactions. Skilled companions are aware of the uncertainties in their work with others and are prepared to take risks in order to meet their patients' needs. This often requires creative and unique practices. Skilled companions' attunement also enables them to anticipate patients' needs and to help them to empower themselves. Thus they engage in critical practices.

As they develop expertise and expand the edges of their practice, skilled companions aspire to articulating their tacit, as well as explicit, knowledge bases, making them available to public scrutiny and verification. Critical awareness also marks the ways that a facilitator of person-centred practice works with others to transform practice, knowledge, people and organisations. Critical companionship, described by Titchen (2000), parallels the awareness of skilled companionship through the facilitative use of self.

The importance of critical awareness in learning and knowledge generation is emphasised by Torbert (1978, pp. 109–10), who contends that liberation in learning and knowing involves 'a higher quality of attention than we ordinarily bring to bear on our affairs' and that this high level of attention is necessary for the search for shared purpose, self-direction and quality work which 'create the possibility for adult relatedness, integrity, and generativity'. Given the goals of our collaborative inquiry, this framework for operation was clearly a desirable choice.

Practice wisdom – considering wise practice, not best practice

Best practice is loudly advocated in many professional practice arenas. But best practice is frequently interpreted as merely the best of what currently exists. It guarantees neither the most ideal practice experience, process or outcomes for the individual client, nor the best practice that can be imagined or created. Rather, we should aspire to wise practice or practice based on a depth of propositional knowledge as well as non-propositional knowledge (based on experience); practice based on wise action informed by sound professional judgment, imagination and caring to provide what is best for the individual.

> 'Knowledge is still defined according to the criteria of the research community alone – as codified, published and public ... a much broader framework is needed for studying the creation of professional knowledge, and the situation looks very different if we move the academic research from the centre of the universe. First we notice that new knowledge is created also by professionals in practice ... (second) knowledge use and knowledge creation cannot be easily separated ... Finally we should not underestimate the degree to which unsystematized personal experience affects the knowledge creation process.'
>
> (Eraut 1994, pp. 54–5)

An integrative factor – creativity

In this book we recognise and value the uniqueness and individuality of people as both recipients and providers of professional services, or more desirably, as partners in professional practice. To achieve this outcome requires professional artistry, or creativity and expertise in *doing*, *knowing*, *being* and *becoming*. This is the topic and vision of this book. Our *doing* or practice role and intervention need to be individually tailored to the client's (or group's) needs, building on credible, defensible knowledge from our professional field and own experience. *Knowledge*, apart from being creatively used in practice situations, needs to be created through research, theory and experience to meet practice demands. Our *being*, the self we bring to professional practice, is a creative entity, meeting individual needs with individual solutions. Our *becoming* is a creative process and outcome, responding to our needs for growth and to our practice needs for development.

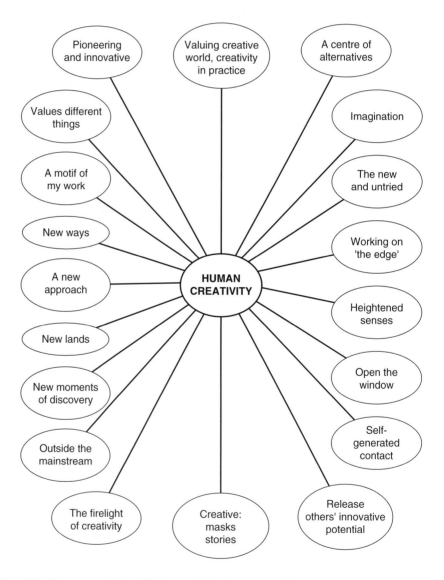

Fig. 1.3   Human creativity. With permission from Denshire (2000).

And, finally, creativity is a medium for facilitating the processes of practice as well as the raised awareness and transformation which enables professional artistry to be realised. Figure 1.3 was designed by one of our authors to represent creativity in professional practice.

References

Carr, W. & Kemmis, S. (1986) *Becoming Critical: Education, Knowledge and Action Research*, Falmer Press, London.

Davies, C. (2000) *Stakeholder Regulation: A Discussion Paper*, Royal College of Nursing, London.

Denshire, S. (2000) *Imagination, occupation, reflection: Ways of coming to understand practice*. Masters thesis, The University of Sydney.

Eraut, M. (1994) *Developing Professional Knowledge and Competence*, Falmer Press, London.

Higgs, J. & Hunt, A. (1999) Rethinking the beginning practitioner: 'the Interactional Professional', in *Educating Beginning Practitioners: Challenges for Health Professional Education* (eds J. Higgs & H. Edwards), Butterworth-Heinemann, Oxford, pp. 10–18.

Mullavey-O'Byrne, C. (1999) Issues in intercultural and international learning in health science curricula, in *Educating Beginning Practitioners: Challenges for Health Professional Education* (eds J. Higgs & H. Edwards), Butterworth-Heinemann, Oxford, pp. 143–9.

Richardson, B. (2001) Professionalisation and professional craft knowledge, in *Practice Knowledge and Expertise in the Health Professions* (eds J. Higgs & A. Titchen), Butterworth-Heinemann, Oxford, pp. 42–47.

Sidell, M. (1995) *Health in Old Age*, Open University Press, Buckingham, Philadelphia.

Sullivan, W.M. (1994) *Work and Integrity*, Harper Business, New York, pp. 159–90.

Titchen, A. (2000) *Professional Craft Knowledge in Patient-Centred Nursing and the Facilitation of its Development*, University of Oxford DPhil thesis, Ashdale Press, Oxford.

Titchen, A. (2001) Skilled companionship in professional practice, in *Practice Knowledge and Expertise in the Health Professions* (eds J. Higgs & A. Titchen), Butterworth-Heinemann, Oxford, pp. 69–79.

Titchen, A. & Ersser, S. (in press) Explicating, creating and validating professional craft knowledge, in *Practice Knowledge and Expertise in the Health Professions* (eds J. Higgs & A. Titchen), Butterworth-Heinemann, Oxford, pp. 35–41.

Torbert, W.R. (1978) Educating toward shared purpose, self-direction and quality work – the theory and practice of liberating structure, *Journal of Higher Education*, **49**, pp. 109–35.

Torbert, W.R. (1981) Why educational research has been so uneducational: The case for a new model of social science based on collaborative inquiry, in *Human Inquiry: A Sourcebook of New Paradigm Research* (eds P. Reason & J. Rowan), John Wiley and Sons, Chichester, pp. 141–51.

Chapter 2
Doing, Knowing, Being and Becoming: the Nature of Professional Practice

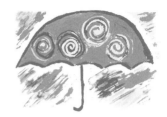

Robyn Ewing and David Smith

In this chapter we argue that professional practice is about doing, knowing, being and becoming. Our practice is about doing things with and for other people within a purposeful, informed, ethical and aesthetic framework. As practitioners or people who are exploring practice, it is impossible for us to separate out who we are from what we do: we bring our beliefs and our already acquired knowing and understanding to our practice. Being is embedded in our practice of doing and, through the doing, as practitioners we continue to become who we are. Through doing, including the opportunity to deliberately reflect, we have the potential to develop new ideas, understandings and skills, thus learning more about our practice and ourselves.

In attempting to illustrate the intimate connection between doing, knowing, being and becoming, this chapter begins with three cameos of professional practice. These cameos are deliberately drawn from the work of a wide spectrum of practitioners. We assert that all arenas of professional practice have a number of elements in common, to a varying extent. While any example of practice is complex and multilayered, it is argued that there are at least five interrelated distinguishable features of all professional work. Professional practice is:

- People-centred
- Purposeful
- Based on informed action
- Individual
- Located in a specific context which is itself embedded in wider historical, sociopolitical and economic cultures.

A number of ideas, themes and issues introduced in this chapter are further discussed and elaborated in the chapters following.

Cameo I

The ambulance siren screams to a standstill as the paramedics rush the gurney with the seriously injured motorcyclist into the emergency ward of the large regional hospital. Already doctors and nurses in the emergency team are assessing the state of the patient's vital signs and injuries and making decisions about the life supports that may be necessary to stabilise the patient's condition. It never ceases to amaze Karl how the team's responses seem to occur spontaneously and seemingly without thinking.

Cameo 2

Greg wearily locks the classroom door and walks slowly towards the school staff-room as he has done every day during this first term of his first year of teaching. The thought of two hours of professional development this afternoon daunts him, given the hours of programming he sees ahead of him tonight. How can he meet the learning needs of such a diverse group of kindergarten children, let alone the expectations their parents have already implied? He feels that, even with all the knowledge from his degree, he has a long way to go.

Cameo 3

Samantha puts her pen down and sighs. Her eyes focus on the detailed drawings she has been working on for weeks. In her mind she can see the completed structure of the bridge. It arches against the sky joining the two promontories of land and facilitating the transport of people from one side of the harbour to the other. The many stress and load calculations associated with her design lie beside her drawings. 'I suppose I should run these through once more to be sure,' she sighs.

These three brief cameos illustrate a number of important features of professional practice. They are each about people. The professional's actions are purposeful, based on professional judgments. These are built on a knowledge base derived from a diverse range of sources. The cameos are individual, in that it is the practitioner's processing of the situation, which cannot be separated from the practitioner, that leads to the subsequent actions with others. Most important, they all occur within or have implications for a specific context in which the practice began and in which the resultant effects of the practice will be implemented. Each of these characteristics is important in defining the nature of professional practice.

Practice is people-centred

One of the most important characteristics of professional practice is that it usually concerns people. First, practice is always construed, directed and implemented by an individual or by a team of people working together. In the latter situation, obviously interpersonal skills and the ability to cooperate are central to the effectiveness of the result.

The task is often one of challenge and excitement for the practitioner because of the degree of uncertainty in seeking the most appropriate way forward. Thus, all professional practice relies on value-based perceptions, interpretations and judgements. Indeed, some definitions of 'professional' specifically include such a notion: professionalism is characterised as acting based on informed judgement (Beare 1992). There are many aspects of professional practice for which there are no set rules or procedures, where practitioners bring all their experience and knowledge to bear on a completely new situation, procedure or treatment.

More important, however, is that practice is directed to one or more individuals. The notion of altruistic service to others, the concept of a 'calling' is certainly central to much of the early writing and history of professional practice (Dingwell & Lewis 1983). It was the case in the above scenarios. Sometimes the people who are affected by the practice are immediately present, as in cameos 1 and 2. Sometimes, however, they are distant, implied and may never come into contact with the practitioner, as may be the case in Cameo 3. Nevertheless, it is this person-centred nature of practice that raises the important moral obligations of the practitioner and thus the many issues of ethical responsibility.

Ethics, power and authority

Ethical responsibilities of professionals are directly related to the fact that professional practice is about doing things with and for people: it is social. In turn, this means that there are important issues of high levels of communication and interpersonal skills and often an asymmetry of power and authority which raises serious questions of accountability and the demand that practice is ethical. The ethical responsibilities of professionals (Berg 1987) include the following:

- To maintain the dignity of the human person
- To recognise and protect the interests of the client (Berg 1987; Beare 1992)
- To respect the well-being and rights of clients and not take advantage of them. This includes protection of the client against any form of physical, sexual, emotional or psychological abuse by the practitioner.
- To respect the client's confidentiality and privacy
- To recognise the asymmetrical balance of power and authority which the professional person holds and to use this power in the interests of the client. Similarly, abuses of power should be avoided.

Beyond what is required by law or by professional codes of conduct where legal or practice sanctions may be imposed for transgressions, the essential ethical practice of the professional person relies on professional integrity and professional judgement. Knowledge born of the wisdom of experience, precedent and eldership may be important in such judgements and in accountability for them.

Communication

Professional practice concerns relationships between people. Professional relationships and responsibilities require clear and effective communication between practitioner and client. If practitioners are to act in the interests of the client, they must be able to explain clearly the key issues of the problem or situation, the alternatives available, the likely consequences of choosing a particular alternative recommended by the practitioner, and reasons for it. Such matters return us to the centrality of the professional judgement of the practitioner. More important than explaining and talking, however, may well be actively listening to the underlying feelings, fears, excitements and anxieties of the client. Thus, much of professional practice is about the negotiation of meanings and understandings through effective and empathic communication.

The development and effective use of a range of interpersonal and communication skills is difficult enough to maintain in the complex and busy life of practice when the cultural backgrounds of practitioner and client are similar. Sustaining effective communication becomes increasingly difficult with increasing distance between the practitioner's and client's language, background, age and cultural experience (including ethnicity, sex, race and life experience). It is, however, in the maintenance of effective communication that the accountability of the practitioner can be established.

Accountability

Professional practice is based on professional judgement as well as various forms of scientifically established knowledge theories, technical procedures and knowledge gained from experience. In addition, professionals' decisions involve their perceptions, interpretations and values. Professionals work in indeterminate practice arenas (Schön 1983) where there are many possibilities/alternatives available and many choices to be made from among them. For instance, there are often no right or wrong decisions in teaching, only judgements that this knowledge or this learning strategy is more or less appropriate in this context with these learners (Lovat & Smith 1995; Groundwater-Smith *et al.* 1998).

Given the reliance on professional judgement in practice, it follows that the decisions and actions taken by professionals, which can significantly affect the lives of their clients, must be accountable. Broadly, accountability underlies all actions and decisions on the part of the professional. This includes actions such as keeping up to date with the latest professional knowledge and procedures, participating in the development of the profession (e.g. through research), and critical self-evaluation, as well as actions taken on behalf of individual clients (e.g. seeking help from colleagues, taking responsibility for one's action). Accountability also includes explaining to the client issues and reasons behind decisions made on behalf of the client, and engaging the client in the decisions to be made.

Practice is purposeful

Any professional act has a deliberate purpose which, as has been argued above, should work towards the interests of the client. Generally the objective of professional practice is to make some aspect(s) of the life of the individual or collective client better, easier or of a higher quality. This is clearly reflected in all the cameos above. Such purposes relate directly to the notions of service and altruism that have been identified with concepts of the authentic professional (Gyarmati 1975).

Often the purposes of a professional act or series of decisions can be specifically and explicitly defined. Thus, a lawyer engaged in developing documents for a will, a doctor performing minor surgery and a teacher explaining to a parent the outcomes their daughter has achieved during the year are all undertaking professional acts that, while still requiring aspects of professional judgement and effective interpersonal skills, may be seen as being within the bounds of relatively routine and uncomplicated practice. However, because they are based on human interaction, even straightforward professional acts may quickly become more problematic because of some reaction or concern of either party.

There are, however, other more complex situations of professional practice where the purposes are not so clearly definable, where the purposes evolve or change as the practice itself evolves or where achievement of desired outcomes is hindered by resource constraints or work overload. Much professional practice occurs within hazy, ill-defined boundaries where there is ambiguity and uncertainty, and the risk-taking and value-based judgement nature of professional practice is highlighted. Such a complex environment is clearly recognised as one of the central issues in education. In the development of effective organisational practices to achieve quality learning, one of the key obstacles is the abstract and ambiguous nature of both the purposes and practices of schooling (Turney *et al.* 1992). On the other hand, we could also argue that the central need for professionals and for professional judgement and decision-making is to cope with just such complexities and uncertainty. These dimensions of our work settings bring richness and challenge to our professional roles.

Practice involves informed action

Practice requires action informed by sound knowledge and by competent professional judgement, including assessment and interpretation of relevant phenomena concerning the client's situation, in order to be accountable and responsible. There are different sources for knowledge and different ways of knowing (Belenky *et al.* 1986). Knowledge may originate in experience, particularly experience that has been processed and reflected on. This can be termed reflexive knowing derived from praxis (Habermas 1972). Other knowledge may be tacit (Polanyi 1966) or implicit, sometimes intuitive (Scott 1990).

It is the essential and longitudinal intensive study of an established knowledge base that is central to many definitions of 'profession' and is used as the rationale for extended professional preservice and inservice education (Gyarmati 1975; Eraut 1994). Thus most professions are based on three (or more) years of pre-service university education. Indeed, it is the acquisition of this specialised knowledge base that is often the rationale for professionals being remunerated more highly and having greater status in society (Dingwell & Lewis 1983). Such arguments were probably more easily accepted when the knowledge bases of the professions and the roles of professionals themselves were considered to be more clearly defined and explicit. Increasingly it can be argued that this is no longer the case. However, the sources and nature of the claimed knowledge bases have always been problematic and contested (Marginson 1987).

It can be argued that the knowledge base of all professions is a mixture of knowledge gained in preservice education as well as knowledge gained from the experience of the job, and there have been strong arguments relating to which of these is more important and useful (Turney 1993). The exact mix of these two broad knowledge sources will vary from one profession to another and from one point in time to another. Within preservice education for nurses, doctors, dentists, lawyers, surveyors and engineers there may be a number of what might be described as technical procedures which do not vary significantly across clients or contexts. In the preservice education of teachers, on the other hand, it could be argued that there may be fewer of these generalisable technical procedures.

Preservice knowledge includes knowledge which is derived from traditional propositional or scientific paradigms (Higgs & Titchen 1995). Within the uncertain and ambiguous context of much of professional practice it is likely that much of this theoretical knowledge base will be reformed and reframed to make it useful in its application in the contexts in which it will be used. Thus theoretical or principled knowledge becomes more applied (Eraut 1994).

The knowledge that is central to the practice of a number of professions is knowledge that is derived from an intelligent and sensitive understanding of a specific context and the application of theoretical and applied knowledge reformed or modified for that context (Eraut 1994). Such a concept of the professional's knowledge base has been characterised in different ways at different times. It has been called 'practical knowledge' (Clandinin & Connelly 1987), 'practice wisdom' (Scott 1990), 'professional artistry' (Schön 1983) or 'craft knowledge' (Calderhead 1987). Although there are important differences in the characteristics of each of these concepts, they all differentiate the knowledge used by practitioners from theoretical knowledge as it is defined and used by physical scientists. Each concept seeks to convey the notion that the knowledge used by professionals in their practice includes knowledge born of reflective experience as well as the application of principled knowledge to a specific context (i.e. contextualised science-based action similar to the practices of skilled artisans). Professional practice needs a complex mixture of knowledge based on scientific principles and theory and practice knowledge applied in a particular context with aesthetic judgment born of the experience of the craft.

In writing of this knowledge base in relation to teaching, Grimmett and MacKinnon (1992, p. 396) characterise the knowledge that teachers as professionals use in their practice in the following manner:

> 'Thus craft knowledge of teaching is not substantive subject matter knowledge, nor is it syntactical knowledge (procedural inquiry knowledge) from the disciplines; rather it is a particular form of morally appropriate and sensible know-how that is constructed by teachers … in the context of their lived experiences.'

Similarly, Kennedy (1987, in Grimmett & MacKinnon 1992, p. 399) suggests that the craft knowledge of teachers concerns itself:

> '… both with teachers' representations of knowledge contained in subject matter content and with teachers' tacit instantiations of procedural ways of dealing rigorously and supportively with learners. As a form of professional expertise, craft knowledge is neither technical skill, the application of theory or general principles to practice, nor critical analysis; rather it represents the construction of situated, learner focused, procedural and content-related pedagogical knowledge through deliberate action.'

While these quotes deal with the professional knowledge base of teachers, arguably the key concepts in these statements apply in different degrees to the knowledge base of all professions. These concepts can be described as follows:

- The sum of professional knowledge is not just theoretical or technical knowledge, neither is it necessarily generalisable. It comprises scientific, experiential and personal knowledge which is applied through sensitive interpretation and understanding of a specific context.
- It is the readying, the reframing, the modification of knowledge gained from principle or experience to suit judgements that makes theoretical knowledge useful in a given context.
- The most important knowledge that appears to be used in practice is not principled or paradigmatic knowledge. This critical knowledge is developed through increasing opportunities to practise but more importantly to deliberately reflect on the practice in ways that facilitate deeper understanding and alternative possibilities (Hatton & Smith 1995). It is through the increasing experience of practice that practitioners are provided with the potential to learn and develop as professionals and to steadily increase the knowledge base on which they base their judgements and actions.
- Quality practice requires knowledge gained from experience of instances,

which is shaped to fit the current context and instance through value-based judgement. Thus, practice knowledge is contextualised knowledge.

- Practice knowledge is also ethical knowledge, since it is directed to form decisions and actions that are judged to be morally appropriate in relation to clients.
- Professional practice requires personal knowledge. Practice is inherently based in personal (individual) value-based interpretations and judgements. The practice cannot be separated from the person. It is always embodied and embedded in the actions of the practitioner.

Practice is individual

Professionals face a particular challenge when they endeavour to match the dual demands of external accountability and being consistent with their personal frame of reference and judgement. External accountability, in an age of evidence-based practice, is frequently interpreted in a science-valuing society as being able to justify professional actions with scientific knowledge. To deal with the grey areas of practice uncertainty and the variabilities and preferences inherent in dealing with people, practice validation needs to consider evidence or knowledge derived from accepted forms of practice and from the judgement of experienced professionals. The latter needs to be sustained by articulated professional craft knowledge and demonstration of its links with theoretical or research knowledge.

Beyond knowledge of the field which can inform practice, the professional's actions are individual (in that decisions and actions are individually created by the professional for the particular client and situation) and personal (i.e. it is not possible to separate the practitioner's or the client's actions and self). Professional practice is intricately connected with the histories, the biographies, the life experiences of practitioners and clients and the stage in the biographies where the particular practice is occurring. Thus increasingly the search to understand how practitioners work and how their beliefs and perceptions influence their work has employed strategies such as narrative inquiry, storying and oral history (Clandinin & Connelly 1987).

Beliefs and perceptions

Professional practice is based on value-based perceptions and judgements, the predispositions (Rokeach 1970) of practitioners. As Beattie (1997, p. 155) writes of teaching:

'When we learn to teach we bring our life histories to the learning situation and enact our beliefs, values and understandings in our behaviour and in our practices. The same assertions could arguably be applied to each of the professions and their practitioners.'

While actions of practitioners are based on an important knowledge/experiential base, the knowledge base and the perceptions of the context and the client are still filtered through the beliefs of the practitioner (Calderhead 1987). Sometimes the belief filters of the practitioner are explicit. More often they are implicit. It is often difficult to be aware of the beliefs and interests that are central to our decisions and actions because of the saturation of our consciousness (Apple 1992) by our everyday experience. It is for these latter reasons that strategies to facilitate critical reflection (Schön 1983; Hatton & Smith 1995) and the employment of 'critical friends' (Smith 1996; Titchen 1998) are essential to help us understand our underlying beliefs and interests.

Decision-making space

Research (e.g. Lovat & Smith 1995) on decision-making space and belief systems of teachers and health professionals clearly reflects the importance of practitioners' beliefs and suggests that each practitioner constructs a personal decision-making space. This space identifies prior practice decisions which define the parameters of the practice, and decisions which have not yet been made and are open to choice by the practitioner. For example, in teaching, the decision-making space defines those decisions related to how and what to teach. In nursing or medicine this space can include accepted options for treatment based on patient data, available resources and local policies.

Some of the factors defining decision-making space will be external to the practitioner (e.g. government and system decisions, practice norms) while some are directly related to the practitioner, such as levels of self-efficacy (Bandura 1986). What is most important, however, is that the decision-making space and the factors that influence it are perceptual, not absolute. They are filtered through the beliefs and perceptions of the practitioner. Thus the manner in which the context is perceived and the available options for practice are directly related to the person who is the practitioner, and that person's beliefs, attitudes, cultural heritage and biography.

Self-efficacy

The range of options for practice are to some degree dependent on the practitioner's perceived level of self-efficacy (Bandura 1986; Labone 1994; Lovat & Smith 1995). Self-efficacy describes the number of different options of practice that the practitioner feels confident and competent to perform. Self-efficacy in part relates to levels of self-concept and self-confidence. It also relates to the level of experience of a practitioner. The greater the experience, the more likely that a higher level of self-efficacy exists.

Professional growth

Being a practitioner provides enormous potential for learning and growing. In our experience, practitioners who do not grow in and through their practice generally demonstrate low morale and limited self-concept and self-efficacy. As professionals dealing constantly with other people, we are always on view and are constantly receiving feedback about ourselves and our competency through verbal and nonverbal interaction and the impacts and effects of our actions. Critical self-evaluation and ongoing professional development are clear expectations of professionals.

In our development as professional practitioners we must continue to reconcile our ideal professional self and our actual professional self (Labone 1994). This means that through our growth we gradually bring together our ideals of practice with what we perceive we are doing. Failure to reconcile these differences often leads to disillusionment and low morale. We can work towards congruence by increasing our levels of self-efficacy towards our ideals or by adjusting our practice, or both. Either way, the congruence of ideals and actuality is important to professional growth.

There are a number of models dealing with the development of professional practice (e.g. Fuller 1969). A common notion in these models is that professionals begin their career with a stage of *self-focused survival*. The concern at this point is, 'Am I able to do the job I am being asked to do?'. The second stage deals with *self-centred concerns* about levels of competency in specific skills and about ways of enhancing these. The third stage is an *other centred* stage and represents concerns about 'What impact is my practice having and with what results for the client?'. The length of each of these stages will differ according to practitioner and context. Movement through them is again linked to increasing levels of self-concept and self-efficacy. Thus, practice is an individual and personal affair. We cannot escape ourselves in our practice, and our perceptions and beliefs are central to everything we do. We constantly receive feedback and we have to learn to deal with it as we grow and continue to become who we are. Both deliberate strategies and experience which increase our levels of self-efficacy are important in this growth.

Practice occurs in context

Professional practice occurs in a specific context and our doing, knowing, being and becoming as professionals is influenced by the way we make sense of as well as shape this context. For instance, practice takes place in a specific person/space/time setting; the characteristics of the people, who they are and where they are in their biographies all affect how they make sense of and respond to the situation. For this reason it is necessary for the professional to be able to reframe, modify and make ready professional knowledge to suit the specifically perceived conditions of the particular context and instance.

Context also relates to the different types of professional practice, such as social work, legal work, physiotherapy, nursing, engineering, teaching, architecture and performance. For each of these different professions the nature of the interactions between practitioner and client, the use of interpersonal and communication skills, the ethical issues and the location, physical space and resources will also be different.

Thirdly, context includes the wider historical, political, social and economic situation in which the practice instance occurs. The economic and political contexts in which a practice occurs may have significant implications for the manner in which that practice is undertaken and the nature of the interaction between practitioner and client. It is the economic context, for instance, that is likely to determine the resource base that is available. The social and cultural contexts in which a practice is located often influence the nature of the beliefs and mores of practitioner and client, and thus often affect the nature of their interaction and expectations.

Socialising institutions in our cultures shape our perceptions and beliefs. In many respects, it is these beliefs and perceptions that help to establish the parameters of our practice and define our decision options. Thus while practice occurs in a specific time/space context, it is the wider contexts in which we are socialised, educated and then practise that are significant in helping to define the nature and characteristics of a specific practice.

Conclusion

A number of important elements help to define and characterise the nature of professional practice. Professional practice is about people, their beliefs, their perceptions and their biographies. Because practice is social and undertaken in social contexts, effective communication and interpersonal skills are vital and there are important ethical and legal responsibilities for every practitioner. Practice draws upon a complex and interrelated web of professional knowledge which includes propositional knowledge, experience-based knowledge and personal knowledge. Knowledge needs to be prepared and related for use in the specific context and with the particular people engaged in the practice. The contextual nature of practice is of particular importance and in addition to the specific instance context, practice occurs within a wider set of historical, politico-economic and socio-cultural contexts.

Professional practice is a complex and demanding interactive social human activity. It relies on a complex mix of previously acquired knowledge and a pool of increasingly diverse experience. Practice cannot be divorced from the practitioner as a person with life experience: the doing is the being. Practising provides powerful opportunities for learning, and in doing and reflecting is the seed for becoming. In this way then doing, knowing, being and becoming are inextricably linked in a perpetual cycle that provides the potential for the essential growth of the professional.

References

Apple, M. (1992) *Ideology and Curriculum*, 2nd edn, Routledge, New York.

Bandura, A. (1986) *Social Foundations of Thought and Action: A Social Cognitive Theory*, Prentice Hall, New Jersey.

Beare, H. (1992) 'A national professional body: Will teachers control it?', *Newsletter of the Australian College of Education*, **11**(1).

Beattie, M. (1997) Collaboration in the construction of professional knowledge, in *Recreating Relationships: Collaboration and Education Reform* (ed. H. Christiansen), SUNY Press, New York, pp. 153–76.

Belenky, M., Clinchy, B., Goldberger, N. & Tarule, J. (1986) *Women's Ways of Knowing: The Development of Self, Voice and Mind*, Basic Books, New York.

Berg, G. (1987) Developing the teaching profession, *Australian Journal of Education*, **27**(2), 37–45.

Calderhead, J. (1987) *Exploring Teachers' Thinking*, Cassell, London.

Clandinin, D. & Connelly, F. (1987) Teachers' knowledge: What counts as personal in studies of the personal, *Journal of Curriculum Studies*, **19**(6), 487–550.

Dingwell, R. & Lewis, P. (1983) *The Sociology of the Professions*, Macmillan, London.

Eraut, M. (1994) *Developing Professional Knowledge and Competence*, Falmer Press, London.

Fuller, F. (1969) Concerns for teachers: A developmental conceptualisation. *American Educational Research Journal*, **6**, pp. 207–26.

Grimmett, P. & MacKinnon, A. (1992) Craft knowledge and the education of teachers, in *Review of Research in Education 18* (ed. G. Grant), American Education Research Association, Washington, pp. 385–456.

Groundwater-Smith, S., Cusworth, R. & Dobbins, R. (1998) *Teaching: Challenges and Dilemmas*, Harcourt Brace, Sydney.

Gyarmati, K. (1975) Doctrine of the professions: Basis of a power structure, *International Social Science Journal*, **10**, pp. 21–34.

Habermas, J. (1972) *Knowledge and Human Interests* (translated by J. Shapiro), Heinemann, London.

Hatton, N. & Smith, D. (1995) Reflection in teacher education: Towards definition and implementation, *Teaching and Teacher Education*, **11**, pp. 36–51.

Higgs, J. & Titchen, A. (1995) The nature, generation and verification of knowledge, *Physiotherapy*, **81**(9), 521–30.

Labone, E. (1994) *Teacher burnout: Towards preventative strategies.* Paper presented at Australian Association for Research in Education Annual Conference, Newcastle, NSW, November.

Lovat, T. & Smith, D. (1995) *Curriculum: Action on Reflection Revisited*, Social Science Press, Wentworth Falls, NSW.

Marginson, S. (1987) *Some Aspects of Teacher Professionalism*, Australian Teachers Federation, Canberra.

Polanyi, M. (1966) *The Tacit Dimension*, Doubleday, Garden City, New York.

Rokeach, M. (1970) *Beliefs, Attitudes and Values*, Jossey, California.

Schön, D. (1983) *The Reflective Practitioner*, Basic Books, New York.

Scott, D. (1990) Practice wisdom: The neglected source of practice research, *Social Work*, **35**(6), 564–7.

Smith, D. (1996) *Facilitating reflection in teacher education: Revisiting some sacred cows.* Paper presented to European Research Association Conference, Seville, Spain, September.

Titchen, A. (1998) *A conceptual framework for facilitating learning in clinical practice*, Occasional Paper No. 2, Centre for Professional Educational Advancement, Faculty of Health Sciences, University of Sydney.

Turney, C. (1993) *Where the Buck Stops*, Sydmac, Sydney.

Turney, C., Hatton, N., Laws, K., Sinclair, K. & Smith, D. (1992) *Educational Management Project: The School Manager*, Allen and Unwin, Sydney.

Chapter 3
Our Collaborative Inquiry

Joy Higgs

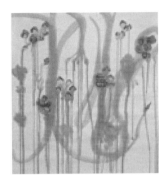

This chapter portrays the collaborative inquiry process which created this book. To introduce this process I present three stories of events which occurred around the time of the genesis of our collaborative journey.

The editors and project leaders

Angie Titchen and I have collaborated on a number of projects over the years in the areas of practice, education and research in the health sciences. Many of these projects have been multidisciplinary, both within and beyond the health professions, particularly involving educators and creative artists. Our interests include:

(1) The nature of practice knowledge (especially the value of professional craft knowledge as an important dimension of practice wisdom)
(2) The use of knowledge-in-action and a variety of ways of knowing which inform practice
(3) The nature of professions and professionalism
(4) Modes of inquiry which illuminate the human face of professional practice with its many voices, stories and challenges.

About two years before the publication of this book we were planning projects for the future. Our professional and research journeys at that time had led us to a fascination with the knowledges embedded in professional practice, or rather the dynamics between knowledge and practice and the practitioners themselves. A key interest was the impact of the way in which formal (propositional) knowledge is commonly privileged in society over both practice and other forms of knowledge (especially professional craft knowledge or knowledge resulting from professional experience). Secondly, our experience with health science curricula had resulted in the observation that practice is often regarded as the application of learning and as a venue for students or graduates to 'practise' knowledge and skills learned elsewhere. In our practice and research we have seen the rich opportunities for deep learning which touched both personal and professional spheres of individuals. We have also observed the power of practice both as a source for learning and as a partner with knowledge in the role and growth of professionals. We decided to explore this synergy between knowledge and practice. Knowing of other practitioners, researchers and educators who, through their experience, teaching and writing, could contribute to this exploration, we determined on a collaborative research approach.

Participants at a university training programme

Several participants attended a staff development programme in the year prior to this project. Our conversations at these sessions often drifted towards the need we all shared to relate self to work, rather than allowing work to dominate self. We found, for instance, that attending the weekly programme sessions of two hours over thirteen weeks presented a major organisational challenge, particularly where travel and heavy workloads were a problem. We shared a concern at the rapid pace of work and change we daily encountered, which made time for personal and professional development a luxury often not attainable. We recognised the predominance of task and deadlines in our work and rewards, and we knew the pressures and sacrifices generated in our selves and our lives 'beyond' work with families and friends. We saw the finance-restricted, pressured directions of our professional lives shutting out the personal needs and strengths we brought with us to the workplace. We appreciated the time we were allocating to professional development which encompassed self, as well as work capacity, and talked about the value of some quality and extended 'time-out' for reflection and regeneration.

Where art and scholarship collide – or perhaps collude

In planning the inquiry/writers' retreat we needed to explore options for audience and process. Our consideration included the following discussion:

'You want to bring a group of academics and practitioners together and ask them to explore the topic through finger painting?!'
    'For sure, any sort of painting, drawing or art – crayons, newsprint, creative art, nature sculptures. I'd like to try dancing and music, perhaps poetry and song.'
'Some of them will run a mile, or clam up probably.'
    'Let's think about it – we want people to open up – to "unfreeze" from their habits and usual way of thinking and looking at things. Exploring our creative side helps to do this, I've found.'
'OK, preparing for change and different viewpoints is good, but what about inhibitions and lack of cooperation?'
    'Partly we're talking about creating a climate of trust, of allowing options and providing opportunities. I'd like to go further as well – we should mix the groups –

creative artists and academics, practitioners and researchers, and take the opportunity to use creative arts as well as scholarly discussion to explore our topic, not just for warming the group up.'

The collaborative inquiry process

Thus our journey of collaborative inquiry began. When inviting participants to join the project we defined collaborative inquiry as:

> 'a group of people who set out to explore a topic or phenomenon. This research process involves participants in discussing the topic, examining different viewpoints, setting up strategies to investigate the topic further and drawing the findings of all of these deliberations together. The goal is to develop a greater understanding of the phenomenon/topic in question.'
>
> (Invitation letter)

Collaborative inquiry is described by Torbert (1981, p. 145) as:

> 'a new model of social science inquiry. The model of collaborative inquiry begins from the assumption that research and actions, even though analytically distinguishable, are inextricably intertwined in practice.'

The goal of such inquiry is not to develop knowledge about action, but to generate knowledge for action and develop genuinely well-informed action:

> 'Research, as understood in the model of collaborative inquiry, is an actual experiential process.'

Reason (1991) describes the way that collaborative inquiries change the pattern of interaction between research participants. Collaborative inquiries move away from the traditional mutually exclusive roles of researcher and subject, where the thinking is contributed by the researcher and the action being studied is contributed by the subject. In cooperative or collaborative inquiries, this pattern is replaced by 'a relationship based on bilateral initiative and control, so that all those involved work together as co-researchers and co-subjects' (Reason 1991, p. 2) in framing the research questions and methods and making sense of their experiences. They engage in cycles of action and reflection:

> 'Ideally in co-operative inquiry there is full reciprocity, with each person's agency, their potential to act as self-directing persons fundamentally honoured both in the exchange of ideas and in the action.'
>
> (Reason 1991)

According to Titchen (1994, p. 15) 'collaborative research is rooted in the experience of the people it seeks to understand ... (in) the shift away from the natural science approach ... (of) studying people.' She argues that *philosophically*, there is an expanding view in the scientific community that legitimates different approaches to knowledge generation. These approaches can include the natural science approach (which generates technical knowledge in search of prediction and control), the interpretive approach (which develops practical knowledge and seeks understanding and meaning in the world of human interactions) and the critical approach (which produces emancipatory knowledge and seeks illumination of how situations can be improved). Collaborative research is usually undertaken through interpretive and critical approaches. *Politically*, there is increasing recognition that knowledge generation is not the sole prerogative of academics and that practitioners can and do generate knowledge from their experience.

Based upon these outlines of collaborative research, the following dimensions were identified as guidelines for our inquiry:

- The researchers would simultaneously be participants in the inquiry.
- The researchers' knowledge gained from prior learning and experience would be an important input into the inquiry process. There would be a high level of commitment and endeavour on behalf of all participants to welcome, honour and utilise the contributions of all participants throughout the project. The project leaders would act predominantly as facilitators of the process.
- The researcher-participants' actions during the inquiry process would be included in the field observations. Similarly, the outcomes of inquiry, dialogue and reflection by the participants (building on and enhancing their entry experience) would provide data or findings to inform the inquiry. The process employed in this project reflects Torbert's (1981, pp. 148–9) analysis of the four research media used in collaborative inquiry, i.e.:

(1) 'an attention capable of interpenetrating, of vivifying, and of apprehending simultaneously its own ongoing dynamics and the ongoing theorizing, sensing, and external "event-ualizing"'

(2) 'symbolic, ironic, diabolic thinking and feeling capable of vivifying and apprehending the significant issues at stake, the value-assumptions in actors' behaviour, the degree of congruity or incongruity between purposes and effects, and the efficient paths for common effort'

(3) 'action – movements, tones, words, and silences ... such disciplined research action does not screen out strangeness and disconfirmation, but rather invites tests of its own and others' sincerity and effectiveness'

(4) 'collection, analysis, and feedback on data collected, where data arises from actions and the quality of experiences'.

The framework for the inquiry would be a liberating programme system. Such systems incorporate three key concepts: shared responsibility for both process and outcomes, with participants being co-managers of the programme; adapting task expectations to participants' readiness to perform and expertise in particular tasks; and creating an environment of *controlled freedom* (Higgs 1993). Controlled freedom requires a context that generates freedom and increased consciousness through the provision of relevant structure.

The primary goal of the inquiry was to inform debate on the topic of professional practice. Our findings represent the sum of the products of our individual experiences and collective synergy and collaboration. The outcome of the research is a collection of these findings and a contribution to professional practice discourse. It seeks to inform and make available the practice wisdom we generated, but not to generalise. The secondary goal, through contributing to discourse, was to provide a revised view of practice that challenged traditional hegemonies of propositional knowledge over other knowledges, of empirico-analytical research over other ways of knowing, of professional separation over engagement of the whole person in professional practice and of knowledge over practice. Through this revised view we are seeking to influence future directions in professional education, practice and research.

The key criterion for ensuring quality of the research process and of the principal product (the book) would be credibility. To seek this outcome, we worked as critical companions during the inquiry process and as critical reviewers during the writing process. Each chapter was reviewed by a minimum of three members of the team in addition to the authors. The long-term effects on practice, research and education will be an issue of credibility and relevance for those who would use our findings and contributions.

Preparing for the collaborative inquiry

Four main activities occurred in preparation for the collaborative inquiry: decisions about the nature of the inquiry and programme, determination of the research group, organisational preparation and individual preparation.

Deciding on the nature of the inquiry and programme

In keeping with the perceived need to take a period of concentrated 'time-out' to reflect on and discuss our topic, and building on previous experiences of writing retreats, we determined on a 'writers' retreat' as the main interactive focus of the collaborative research and agreed that the principal collaborative product would be a book on the research topic.

The retreat was five days in duration. It was conducted during university non-teaching time and school holidays, for the benefit of project participants who worked in universities and/or those who with school age children. To enhance participation, collaboration, and a general 'time-out' from busy lives, a regional venue (Leura in the Blue Mountains of Australia) was selected. A number of the participants travelled from Sydney, some from further afield (interstate and overseas), to attend the retreat. The tranquillity and beauty of the setting, space to meet and explore in harmonious surroundings, room to be creative, and distance from faxes and telephones created a highly suitable environment for collaboration and immersion in our inquiry.

The programme is outlined in Table 3.1. The project leaders developed themes for the week and goals for each day to provide a structure for the process, to reflect the creative nature of the process of bringing together the three participant groups (education, health sciences, creative arts) and to interweave the symbolism of creative arts, both in the labelling and the processes of the programme.

Table 3.1   The retreat programme.

Tuesday	*Theme:* Painting the broad canvas – form, structure and perspective *Goal:* Producing the book outline – content, structure, audience, style
Wednesday	*Theme:* Adding depth and texture – themes, ideas, nuances *Goals:* Clarifying issues, themes, exploring content
Thursday	*Theme:* Adding features – roles, synchronicity and interplay *Goals:* Negotiating tasks, identifying names and topics within themes
Friday	*Theme:* Fine touches *Goals:* Clarification of individual roles/tasks, production of chapter outlines
Saturday	*Theme:* Taking another look *Goals:* Finalising contracts, reflection on inquiry and book

The process of interaction was framed around the goal of providing a liberating structure for participants to engage in cycles of action and reflection to generate understanding and knowledge, as well as being a framework which facilitated effective group processes. The retreat became a process of 'conversations with' each other, in the large group and in sub-groups, and periods of awareness-raising through creative arts sessions and personal or group reflection. In this way, we endeavoured to model the notion of crystallisation of knowledge as a reflection of creative qualitative research. We sought to foster interaction through a variety of group facilitation processes (e.g. brainstorming, activities to help people get to know each other, small groups) and social activities (e.g. bush-walking, bike riding and social events such as musical evenings). These activities served to acknowledge the creative artists among the group. For instance, a composer played recordings of his compositions, some people led singing sessions and others read poetry, including poems created during the retreat itself. These activities were invaluable in facilitating group formation and the depth of knowing and understanding of each other that the participants needed to enhance their exploration of the inquiry topic. These activities were particularly important given the large group size (29) and the limited time for whole group interaction.

Creative arts sessions became an integral and fundamental part of the programme process and success. Initially we had planned that they would be largely optional, with alternative discussion sessions being available for those who chose not to participate. The group's first 'storming' or 'revolt' focused on the identified need and wish (indeed 'demand') for all the group to experience all that the programme had to offer, rather than to separate into different group work modes. The creative arts sessions of music making, painting, creative dance and enjoying the natural surroundings served several purposes. They provided valuable opportunities for group development and small group formation, time to unwind and open our minds to broader issues and an avenue for wordless expression of our developing insights and understandings of the synergy between self, knowledge and practice. Indeed, the creative artistry aspect of the programme became so indivisible from the knowledge creation process that our identity as a group and the expression of our findings became connected closely with our artistic products.

Participants' comments on the creative arts role in the programme included the following:

'At this retreat I recognised the power and effectiveness of combining creative arts and recreation in an inquiry process. The combination was productive, stimulating and thought-provoking.'
'It has been an interesting process to be part of, and I have been fascinated and excited about what can emerge when a group of people gather to explore a topic which touches their intellectual, creative and personal passions.'
'Through this retreat I learned how creative activities can enhance the inquiry and writing processes.'
'The creative process was integral to drawing the programme and people together.'
'I was really glad that the programme engaged the whole person.'

Determination of the research group

In this chapter I use 'we' to indicate the collective researchers more than myself as a singular author, since this chapter represents the product of joint effort, and the voices of the research collective are both implicit and evident in the discussion. At times 'we' more precisely refers to Angie Titchen and myself as the programme leaders, and at times to the team of Angie, myself, Charles Higgs and Sue Radovich who were the organisers. However, since very rapidly, even before the retreat, the distinction between these smaller groups and the larger group disappeared, it seems fitting to use 'we' to encompass all three groupings.

Initially we had planned to invite approximately 15 people to participate in the collaborative inquiry and writing project. A number of the original invitees accepted the invitation with alacrity and also identified other colleagues who 'we *definitely* needed to invite', due to their particular expertise or experience which would be invaluable to the inquiry and writing process. A larger participant group emerged. Some people invited were unable to attend the retreat. This led to replacement invitations and to two invited chapters (Chapters 19 and 20) from people who were unable to attend.

Those who participated in the inquiry project are included in the list of contributors at the front of the book. The backgrounds of these participants were rich and varied. As already stated, the group included people with health, education and creative arts backgrounds. These three professional areas were chosen since our experience had identified multiple connections and overlaps in practice among them as well as some natural differences. Other professions were the subject of discussions. Practical considerations of numbers and spread of interests precluded broader participation. Those attending included practitioners, educators in academic and practice settings and researchers. Some were experienced researchers and authors, while some were 'tenderfoots'. Our group differed considerably in age and life experiences. Each person brought a wealth of different experiences: professional practice, parenting, career beginnings and retirement, personal life challenges and many questions about where lives and careers were taking us. Many of the participants wore several 'hats' including educator/researcher, practitioner/educator, health professional/creative artist, educator/dramatist, health practitioner/clinical educator and so on. Together, they shared attributes of curiosity, people-orientation and a willingness to push the boundaries, particularly in the case of exploring the nature, depths, potential directions and possibilities of creative, rewarding and people-centred professional practice.

Organisational preparation

The Centre for Professional Education Advancement at the Faculty of Health Sciences of the University of Sydney provided administrative support in the organisation of the programme, venue and list of participants, as well as financial support for participants and technical expertise. Technical expertise was required to facilitate electronic as well as more standard means of communication throughout the project, (tape-recording of group discussions for later follow-up of ideas and tasks), and for the book: photographing, scanning and processing of artwork, production of graphics, and administrative management and copy-editing. Further, a detailed authors' guide was produced to provide directions for writing and presentation of manuscripts.

Individual preparation

For each individual as well as for the group, this collaborative inquiry and writing project was a journey. Preparation for participation in the process involved, firstly, a choice to be involved in the project. For some, this was an enthusiastic and immediate 'yes' when they were approached, based on their interest in the topic and/or a desire to work with the group. For some, it was a welcome opportunity to take 'time-out' from busy working lives to contemplate and seek development in their personal or professional lives or to engage deeply with a topic of considerable importance to their work or career. Others were tantalised by the rare opportunity this project provided to work across disciplines and professional areas in order to examine and learn from the similarities and differences in professional practice within the health, education and creative arts professions. Some were tentative, fearing their personal readiness or professional journeys were too junior or premature to participate in what they saw as a challenging project. For these people, especially, the journey of growth we all experienced to a greater or lesser extent began with the empowerment they experienced through individual preparation and the courage they found to decide to attend the retreat.

Participants were informed of the nature of the planned retreat programme and the intended ongoing inquiry activities and were asked to commit themselves to participation in the inquiry and to the production of a chapter for the proposed research outcome, a book on professional practice (see Table 3.2). All but one of the 29 participants completed these commitments.

The inquiry process

The (overlapping) phases of group development have been described as forming, norming, storming and performing (Tuckman 1965). Forming of the group began at the birth of the idea to investigate this topic, continued through the generation of a collaborative model, the retreat group inquiry and writing group investigations, and culminated in performing and celebrating the finished product. Norming involved generating expectations, the determination of participants, the negotiation of the contract and the process of interaction and inquiry, and setting standards during the retreat and in the review and editing process.

Our discussions in the forming and norming stages of the enquiry process modelled our topic discussions on the deconstruction and reconstruction of our knowledges of professional practice and the received truths which embed the professional literature (e.g. the argument that propositional/established knowledge drives professional practice rather than practice being, in any valid way, a source of real knowledge). We spent some time as a group 'unfreezing', along the lines of a change model described by Lewin (1958). We actively left our work responsibilities and our preconceptions behind us, and we explored our understandings of professional practice in an open and supportive way that challenged

Table 3.2   The participants' contract.

Prior to the retreat participants are asked to:

- Provide a brief introduction of yourself for other participants
- Think deeply about the topic of knowledge in practice – what does it mean?
- Gather together useful references and bring a copy of articles and books to the retreat for others to look at
- Read articles we will send you (see list in Table 3.3)
- Consider what topic areas you could write about in the book

During the retreat participants will contribute to achieving the following goals:

- To explore the nature of professional knowledge and practice, particularly in relation to the fields of education, health sciences and creative arts
- To develop a framework for the book we will produce, i.e. a conceptual framework, key issues and topics to be addressed and organising elements (e.g. themes) which will hold together a book written by a collection of different people and produce a 'whole' as well as a vehicle for expressing different voices
- To develop a structure for the book (e.g. table of contents, listing chapters and authors)
- To achieve sufficient progress in the intense, creative five day interaction to provide a sound foundation for subsequent writing and investigation
- To identify areas for which the inquiry aspect of our collaborative research needs to continue post-retreat
- To contract together to produce an agreed strategy, format and timeline for further inquiry, writing individually or in teams, reviewing and editing the chapters/book
- To agree upon individual tasks and responsibilities to be completed
- To organise strategies for technical aspects of communicating and writing

After the retreat participants' roles will be to:

- Continue to discuss your ideas and writing projects with others most involved (e.g. co-author(s) of your chapter or authors of related chapters)
- Investigate your topic area further
- Write your paper by the agreed date
- Review other people's chapters as requested by the editors
- Make revisions as needed to your chapter

our ideas, while at the same time listening attentively and affirmingly to the ideas and experiences of fellow participants. The growth of our individual under-standings, as well as our collective reconstruction in the dynamic sense of evo-lution of knowledge, resulted in the development of a conceptual framework which contained the central directions and themes of our emerging knowledge (see Table 3.4). For individuals and the group a clear perspective transformation resulted as this knowledge and conceptual framework (as discussed in Chapter 1) emerged. Mezirow (1990, p. xvi) describes 'perspective transformation' or 'transformation learning' as 'the process of learning through critical self-reflection, which results in the reformulation of a meaning perspective to allow a

Table 3.3 Extracts from reading preparation for the writers' retreat.

Scott (1990)
'Practitioners continue to draw heavily on experiential knowledge, yet "practice wisdom" or clinical judgment, generally has been ignored in ... practice research.' Practice wisdom can be understood as a 'process of incipient induction' into the (relevant) profession (p. 564).

Higgs & Titchen (1995)
In order to provide a valid and functional basis for professional practice the knowledge base of the practitioner 'needs to comprise propositional, professional and personal knowledge' and needs to be continually tested and updated to enhance practice expertise (p. 528). We support Barnett's (1990) view that 'modern society is unreasonably dominated by the cognitive framework of science, to the extent that other potential forms of knowledge are downgraded and not even regarded as real forms of knowledge' (p. 526). 'Approaches to generating (and testing) knowledge include: working through research paradigms (such as the empirico-analytical, critical and interpretive paradigms) and also utilising different 'ways of knowing' (p. 521).

Manley (1991)
Many dimensions of professional knowledge need to be considered in understanding knowledge use in practice. These include the nature and processes of knowledge and knowing, and relationships between knowledge and philosophy, theory, practice, power, professionalism and accountability.

Eraut (1994)
Eraut discusses knowledge use in professional practice and issues concerning different types of professional knowledge, different modes of application of knowledge and the influence of context on learning.

Butler (1995)
'The qualities of the personal "self" within the professional ... are the key to excellence ... Professional development is radically centred in development of the "self" ... (on) personal being and becoming ... (a central issue) is the understanding of individual human agency in the realm of practical actions' (p. 153).

Fitzgerald, Mullavey-O'Byrne & Clemson (1997)
Within professional higher education 'increasing attention is being given to incorporating cultural content into curricula' (p. 1).

---

more inclusive, discriminating, and integrative understanding of one's experience' and a greater capacity to act on these insights.

Storming, as mentioned above, occurred during the planning (or rather re-planning) of the retreat programme, when the group strongly identified a preference to run counter to the proposed programme. Interestingly, through this storming process the cohesion of the large group was strongly cemented and a strong basis for collaboration arose through these shared experiences. Storming also occurred in several of the small writing groups when differences in expectations regarding participation arose and other life or work events interfered with the smooth implementation of the agreed roles and timetabled activities after the

Table 3.4   Writing matrix.

Content	Credible	Exploratory	Intellectually humble	Valuing own ignorance	Explain terms	Approach
Themes informing the whole book Exploring						Forms Different lenses, frames Examples from different professions
Aesthetic dimension to practice – form that is satisfying						Lived experiences – public histories, private domains
People centred						Narratives, case studies
Authenticity, credibility valuing, power, authority						Voices, giving voicies to issues Critical debate
Culture and context, climate – obstacles, opportunity						Being reflexive Dialogues, discourses
Flexibility, uncertainty, ambiguity, boundaries						Engaging readers in our book, relationship
Ethics, morality						Imagery, metaphors
Transformation – of practice, knowledge, people – attending to the edges						Vignettes e.g. biographical, personal stories and public faces Posing questions
Truth, reality/realities, perceptions						Dialectics – reflective narratives
Personal and public – stories, knowledge, voices						Exploring differences and synergies, unpacking intersections
Wisdom – wise practice, not best practice						Attending to the edges, our voices at the cutting edge
Individual and collective considerations						Inviting readers into the gaps in our knowledge
Content			Style			Approach

retreat. These 'storms' were dealt with through negotiation between the small group members generally. However, on occasion the group needed to refer to one of the project leaders for advice or assistance. This intervention helped to facilitate solution or reduction of the conflict by negotiation, 'permission' to change the contracted targets (e.g. division of one chapter into two, in two cases), rearrangement of writing teams and encouragement to persist or try different strategies in collaboration.

Strategies we adopted to deal with storming reflected the two group conflict strategies proposed by Reason (1991). Our attention to group processes and to choice and structuring of the operational setting recognised the differences inherent in the various groups we brought together (the *realistic* strategy). The *idealistic* strategy underpinned our belief in, and further search for, higher levels of integration and collaboration which delighted in and valued our differences. Thus, we searched for knowledge born from our synergies and from our choice of exploration strategies which awakened creative thinking and fostered open communication and relationships among the participant-researchers. As two participants commented:

'It has been a privilege to be part of a very supportive yet diverse group where members had a common goal and where the environment created by the organisers facilitated the achievement of that goal. In this collaborative group the tensions generated waxed and waned, provided energy and cohesion and enabled new learning to occur and challenges of the unknown to be met.'

'Through this process I discovered that there *are* academics who are not bound to their territory and a need to push their agenda competitively at all costs and on all occasions.'

Performing was achieved early in the retreat timetable. As a group, active performance was clearly in progress during the first day, building on the advance preparation of individuals and organisers. For some individuals, participation at an active level was somewhat slower than for others, linked to the overall natural dynamics of any group (particularly one of this size) and the spread in confidence and experience levels in the group. Soon, however, all participants were comfortably participating in the process within the overall group supportiveness, the facilitative programme framework and/or the support of mentors and friends.

Tasks accomplished in this performing stage during the retreat included: determining the task, understanding the interactions between the inquiry and writing processes, defining the audience of the book, framing the book in terms of content and scope, negotiating style and size of writing projects, planning collaboration groups and inquiry tasks, planning timelines and identifying post-retreat inquiry targets. After the retreat, the focus turned to further inquiry and writing. Over the months chapters were written, reviewed and edited, keeping in mind the collective vision, the conceptual framework and the issues of quality that formed an important part of our mutual commitment.

Mourning the end of the retreat and going through the stages of finalising our collaboration was a powerful experience for the participants. While recognising the strength of ongoing relationships which would endure, and feeling enthusiasm for the tasks ahead, there was a strong sense of mourning mixed with celebration of our achievements, as we came to the final day of the retreat. Participants honoured the Leura experience that day in many ways; for instance, creating a group body sculpture, doing a group painting and writing poems. At the time of writing we are planning a reunion to celebrate the completion of our project and launch of the book. Participants' feedback on the retreat and the whole inquiry programme reflects the dual inquiry and writing experiences:

> 'Working across disciplines was a positive and fruitful experience – not only did we learn a great deal from each other but the multidisciplinary grouping limited the posturing which sometimes arises in some professional groups and we were forced not to use jargon.'
> 'I'm feeling quite sad. It has been a wonderful journey for me – from doubt and uncertainty to a sense of belonging and being able to contribute.'
> 'Your vision and adaptability was invaluable in providing us with structure, direction and freedom to choose and bring ourselves richly into the process.'
> 'Thank you for your energy, caring and the wonderful opportunities for whole being experiences.'

Inquiry outcomes

Knowledge development

The other chapters in the book provide evidence and content of the knowledge developed through the inquiry. Here I present views of the participants about the knowledge development outcomes of the inquiry:

> 'This was an opportunity to argue the givens, to move beyond the standard arguments and norms.'
> 'The dialogue entered into within our chapter group did much to expand and make visible our understanding of the knowledge processes within the practice context.'
> 'People brought together in this way can create and realise the subtle connections between the aesthetic and the intellect. Knowledge was also generated through personal interactions, relationships and exploration of workload passions.'
> 'We learned much about the nature of professional practice across the disciplines – the diversities, similarities and complexities.'

Personal and professional development

The chance to explore the topic in a residential and natural setting of great beauty, away from the routine of our working lives, was unique. We had time to reflect and to learn about ourselves and others: our doing, knowing, being and becoming as professionals. Many participants talked about their personal and professional journeys arising from this collaboration:

'For me the project and the retreat was tremendously empowering. By confronting my own professional experience and engaging so intensively with the concepts of professionalism and what it meant to be a professional, I learned a great deal about myself as a professional and this helped me replan my career directions.'

'I have developed my awareness of so many aspects of my thinking.'

'This experience helped me re-evaluate my professional identity. For the first time I was content to see my real career as being an artist, to recognise my strengths as a professional.'

'I valued linking up with others. It helped me to more rapidly develop my own vague thoughts. I felt validated. I still feel anxious when I move out of my own world, but at least I have enough strength to do it now.'

Beattie (1995) reflects similar outcomes in a report on related research investigating professional knowledge. This is the story of a teacher's professional journey of growth and development through inquiry. The teacher developed a new unity of self within the professional context. The journey is described as 'making of music'.

Throughout this book we have presented the record of our collective inquiry, our group explorations, our personal explorations and our findings. This chapter has presented our collaborative inquiry as an evolving process. This process can also be viewed as a series of journeys of discovery, within our combined journey of a continuing exploration of a topic, which together, we found to be a fascinating living phenomenon. Figure 3.1 illustrates these intertwining journeys.

Chapters and a book (or two) – entering the public discourse

This book is a key outcome of the inquiry process. Even though many outcomes arose, some of them life-changing for the participants, the book and the community created by the participants are the joint enduring products of our inquiry. As we contribute this book to the discourse on professional practice, we believe that we have advanced debate on this important topic.

The collaboration process has also given rise to further collaborations. A number of potential participants who were unable to attend but who were interested in participating in this line of inquiry were invited to contribute to a

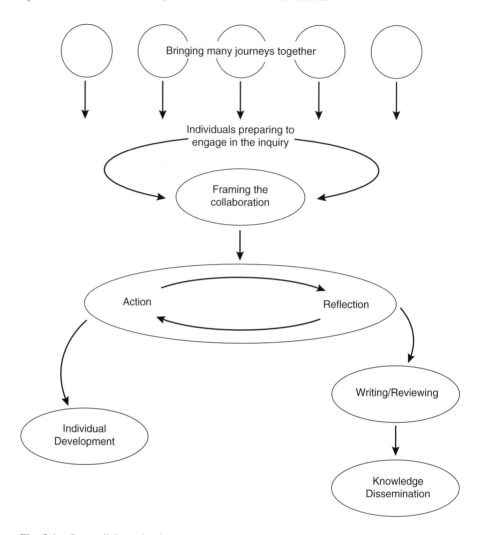

Fig. 3.1   Our collaborative journey.

companion volume on practice knowledge (Higgs & Titchen 2001). Other collaborative writing projects have been generated from the 'Leura process'. These other books deal with creative dimensions and challenges in qualitative research (Byrne-Armstrong *et al.*, in press), practice knowledge in education, relationships in clinical education and practice epistemology.

Conclusion: critiquing the process

We had determined that the key criterion for judging the quality of our inquiry and its products was credibility. For the participants, the process during and after the retreat was credible in terms of it being an effective collaborative inquiry and writing process and a process which modelled collaboration and critical companionship. It was also credible in the positive affirmation and development of individuals and enduring working partnerships. The product was deemed credible by the reviewers who commented and provided feedback with constructive comment on each chapter, and by the editors and reviewers who read the whole product and critiqued the product as a unit. The credibility of the product as perceived by our readers will be determined over time.

The success of the collaborative process as one of liberation and generation of understanding is evident in the discussions above on individual development. We end this chapter with further comments by participants:

'I discovered that collaborative inquiry has a gestalt effect and that taking time out serves as an antidote to economic rationalism.'
'I valued the special opportunity and encouragement to be creative and to push the boundaries. It was a liberating experience.'
'The process of the retreat was excellent, particularly the flexibility of the structure and the clarity of the structure, in combination with time for people and time to reflect.'

The design, goals and outcomes of this project place it within the critical and interpretive research paradigms. The project produced emancipatory knowledge for individuals and the group as a whole and contributed to a deeper understanding and interpretation of the phenomenon of professional practice.

References

Barnett, R. (1990) *The Idea of Higher Education*, The Society for Research into Higher Education and Open University Press, Buckingham.

Beattie, M. (1995) The making of a music: The construction and reconstruction of a teacher's personal practical knowledge during inquiry, *Curriculum Inquiry*, **25**(2), 133–50.

Butler, J. (1995) Designing for personal and professional excellence: The designer as life-long learner, in *The Experience of Quality in Higher Education* (eds J. Cachs, P. Ramsden & L. Phillips), Griffith University, Brisbane, pp. 153–74.

Byrne-Armstrong, H., Horsfall, D. & Higgs, J. (eds) (in press), *Critical Moments in Qualitative Research*, Butterworth-Heinemann, Oxford.

Eraut, M. (1994) *Developing Professional Knowledge and Competence*, Falmer Press, London.

Fitzgerald, M.H., Mullavey-O'Byrne, C. & Clemson, L. (1997) Cultural issues from practice, *Australian Occupational Therapy Journal*, **44**, pp. 1–21.

Higgs, J. (1993) The teacher in self-directed learning: Manager or co-manager? in *Learner Managed Learning: Practice, Theory and Policy* (ed. N. J. Graves), World Education Fellowship, London, pp. 122–31.

Higgs, J. & Titchen, A. (1995) The nature, generation and verification of knowledge, *Physiotherapy*, **81**, pp. 521–30.

Higgs, J., & Titchen, A. (eds) (2001) *Practice Knowledge and Expertise in the Health Professions*, Butterworth-Heinemann, Oxford.

Lewin, K. (1958) Group decision and social change, in *Readings in Social Psychology*, 3rd edn (eds E.E. Maccoby, T.M. Newcomb & E.L. Hartley), Methuen, London, pp. 197–211.

Manley, K. (1991) Knowledge for nursing practice, in *Nursing: A Knowledge Base for Practice* (eds A. Perry & M. Jolley), Edward Arnold, London, pp. 1–27.

Mezirow, J. (1990) Preface, in *Fostering Critical Reflection in Adulthood: A Guide to Transformative and Emancipatory Learning* (eds J. Mezirow and Associates), Jossey-Bass, San Francisco, pp. xiii–xxi.

Reason, P. (1991) *Power and conflict in multidisciplinary collaboration*, Research Report, Centre for the Study of Organisational Change and Development, The University of Bath, England.

Scott, D. (1990) Practice wisdom: The neglected source of practice research, *Social Work*, **35**(6), 564–8.

Titchen, A. (1994) Roles and relationships in collaborative research, *Surgical Nurse*, **7**(5), 15–19.

Torbert, W.R. (1981) Why educational research has been so uneducational: The case for a new model of social science based on collaborative inquiry, in *Human Inquiry: A Sourcebook of New Paradigm Research* (eds P. Reason & J. Rowan), John Wiley and Sons, Chichester, pp. 141–51.

Tuckman, B.W. (1965) Developmental sequence in small groups, *Psychological Bulletin*, **63**(6), 384–99.

Part Two
Dimensions of Professional Practice

Chapter 4
Practising Without Certainty: Providing Health Care in an Uncertain World

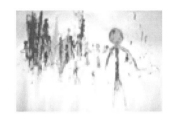

Colleen Mullavey-O'Byrne and Sandra West

An uncertain world

Today's society is characterised by 'shifting boundaries of identity and responsibility and ... constantly changing demands' (Zohar & Marshall 1994, p. 24). These dynamic forces are present in the systems that operate within a society, making dealing with change and indeterminacy unavoidable for both recipients and providers of human services such as education, welfare and health care. Burnet (1963, cited in Zohar & Marshall 1994, p. 24) captured the essential dynamism of these forces of change when he described the world as in a constant state of flux 'where nothing ever is, all is becoming'.

The ideas that 'things are always changing' and 'there are very few things that we can continue to be certain about' are not new. These are things that people have always known at some level of their being and have dealt with more or less successfully in various ways; for example, by resistance, denial, lamenting 'the good old days' but reluctantly accepting that things are different, and by actively participating in the change process. However, the extent of contemporary changes and the speed and relentlessness with which they appear to be taking place have been described by many as unprecedented, with far reaching consequences for reform in health and health care services currently and in the future.

Health care in an uncertain world

The health care system that has been evolving in Australia during the 1980s and 1990s serves to illustrate the impact of forces that have been driving health care reform in Western countries, such as increased demands, rising costs and government constraints on allocation of funding to health. Spending on health care in Australia continues to be described as adequate and reasonable at about 8% of the annual GDP. Bloom (2000, p. 4) suggests that recent reforms to the Australian health care system have been driven in part at least by a fear of rising costs and an attempt to preserve and increase equity in health and access to health care services. Other factors that are influencing change include the changing philosophies, sweeping reforms and restructuring activities that are characteristic of a health care system that is placing greater emphasis on prevention and public health issues than in the past. Still other equally influential factors that are driving changes in health care are related to the expanding role of technology, especially information technology and the information explosion in medical and health sciences.

At the service delivery level, the dynamics of change evident in the wider health care system add to the lack of predictability that is inherent in interactions between health professionals and the individuals and groups they serve. Moral codes together with legal and ethical requirements provide a stabilising base for practice, but even these 'givens' are subject to scrutiny, debate, question and possible change within evolving systems.

Certainty-uncertainty in health care

To become involved in health care as consumer, carer or practitioner inevitably means confronting the certainty-uncertainty problematic. The pressures towards certainty that are increasingly evident among practitioners in health care derive from multiple sources, including consumers, carers and practitioners themselves, professional bodies, health care systems and governments. Uncertainties emanating from or fuelled by these same sources are among the main driving forces behind the mounting quest for certainty that is evident among practitioners.

The certainty-uncertainty problematic and the reasons for our heightened awareness of its pervasive presence become clearer when viewed against a backdrop of the economically driven health care reforms that have been taking place in Australia and other western countries in recent years. These relatively rapid and sweeping reforms, the inevitable rounds of restructuring that accompany implementation, the often unclear realignments, adjustments and reallocation of resources all create an uncertain and ever-changing backdrop to practice in the current health care system.

In this chapter we explore the certainty-uncertainty problematic that presents for health professionals working in health and health care during a period of changing health philosophies and major reforms in the Australian health care system. Following this exploration we suggest ways in which health professionals might reframe their thinking and come to see uncertainty in the workplace not as a hindrance to effective practice but as a window of opportunity to seek out alternative and innovative ways of being a health professional in the health care system. Our understanding of the system includes the various settings (e.g. acute hospital care, community health, community mental health, outpatient services, specialist clinics) in which the certainty-uncertainty dilemma is experienced on a day-to-day basis by health practitioners and the consumers and carers who receive their services.

Main concepts

Three main concepts are woven into our discussions of the certainty-uncertainty problematic: expectation, knowledge and certainty.

> 'Expectation: a belief that something will happen or be the case.
> Expect: regard as likely to happen, do or be the case; suppose or assume; require as appropriately due.
> Expectancy: hope or anticipation that something, especially something pleasant, is about to happen; anticipating receiving something.'
>
> (The Concise Oxford Dictionary 1999)

Two sets of practitioner expectations are important to our discussions in this chapter:

- Practitioner expectations of themselves and about factors (human and non-human) that they encounter in the health care work environment
- Practitioner perceptions of expectations placed on them by professional associations, consumers and carers, the particular health care setting in which they work and the health care system in general.

Health professionals in a practice role in clinical settings have expectations of themselves in their particular clinical roles and of their clients in their roles as service recipients. The professional socialisation experience has led them to expect or assume that events and relationships in the clinical setting are likely to proceed according to a broad set of principles and practices that have come to be associated with providing their professional services in clinical settings. They also anticipate certain intrinsic and extrinsic benefits that will result from the work they do – benefits that are appropriately due to them. To the extent that they hold such expectancies, health professionals may be said to be in a state of expectancy with regard to roles, relationships, tasks they and others perform within the clinical setting, and rewards they are likely to receive. When change is introduced into the system and/or setting, the state of expectancy is likely to be disrupted; what people may have reasonably assumed is disconfirmed in the changed circumstances.

Expectations are related to assumptions we all make about people, situations, environments and systems, that we acquire through experiences in our sociocultural environment. While some have their origins in sociocultural norms (general expectancies), others are based on prior knowledge of ways in which individuals, groups and/or circumstances differ from the norm (particularised expectancies) (Burgoon 1993; Mullavey-O'Byrne & Fitzgerald 1995). During times of extensive and wide-ranging change people may find that the general and particularised expectancies they have depended upon in a range of situations and relationships in the past are not as useful or are no longer relevant.

> 'Knowledge: information and skills acquired through experience or education; justified belief, as opposed to opinion; awareness or familiarity gained by experience.
>
> Know: to be aware of through observation, inquiry or information; be absolutely sure of something; have personal experience of something.'
>
> (The Concise Oxford Dictionary 1999)

Philosophical analysis informs us that there are various types of knowledge, some of which are associated with knowledge that something is so (propositional knowledge), knowledge of something, knowledge about something (by experience, acquaintance or direct awareness) and knowledge of how to do something. Health professionals in clinical settings are versed in these various types of knowledge and draw on them in their daily practice. The drive towards evidence-based practice, a component of the change currently being experienced in health care settings, questions previously acceptable practices based solely on personal experience and clinical judgment in individual and/or cumulative instances, in the absence of systematic documented research into clinical interventions.

> 'Certainty: the quality or state of being certain; a true fact or event that is definitely going to take place.
>
> Certain: able to be firmly relied on to happen, to be the case; completely convinced of something; without doubt.'
>
> (The Concise Oxford Dictionary 1999)

Within the domain of philosophical inquiry, certainty is regarded either as a psychological property of persons or as an epistemic feature of beliefs, utterances and statements (Audi 1997).

Psychological certainty is a situation/state in which a person has no doubt about what they see, believe, feel or say; that is, they believe it to be true, regardless of the justification they have for the belief they hold. The presence of this state in the person in no way guarantees the truth of what the person feels certain about, only that the person feels certain about it. People hold strong feelings about the certainty of many propositions they have no evidence to support; this is especially so if they want to believe them or are in some way comforted or feel strengthened by believing them.

The widespread impact of forces for change evident in the health care system currently impacts on the psychological certainties that practitioners and consumers alike have about aspects such as what constitutes health, roles and relationships in health care, and the nature and scope, relevance and appropriateness of services. At the individual level it is not so much a question of whether the influences are positive or negative, but of being open to questioning previously held certainties and the sources that support them, and then finding new ways of working in the changed environment.

Backdrop: the Australian context

Statements announcing sweeping changes to health care along with descriptions of the benefits that will accrue from these changes have dominated the health-related literature over the past 5–10 years in Australia. Government policy documents (e.g. Health Ministers' Forum 1994; NSW Health Department 1992) and other related documents produced by government supported institutions (PHIAC 1998) are positive and optimistic about the changes that are taking place (while recognising that there is still room for improvement). In *Australia's Health 1998* (AIHW 1998) we are informed that 'Australia is one of the healthiest countries in the world and Australians are becoming even healthier'. In this same document we are also reminded that 'ready access to health care when needed is available to most people' but that 'good health is not enjoyed by all and the health of Aboriginal and Torres Strait Islander peoples is poor by any standard' (AIHW 1998, p. 1).

People at all levels in health care, such as health care providers, health administrators, health professionals, consumers and carers, are seeking new ways of managing old problems. Guidelines to ensure quality, consumer-focused service delivery are being drawn up, competency standards for practitioners are being developed and increasing emphasis is being placed on the role of continuing education in maintaining practice standards. Outcome measures have come to the fore as a means of gauging the effectiveness of treatments/interventions, and case management has taken over as the preferred method of providing services to consumers within the public health and rehabilitation systems.

The emphasis placed on consumer and carer involvement has resulted in a more vocal and active public. Consumers are invited to comment on services provided, and encouraged to register complaints when they encounter problems. Through elected or government-nominated representatives to various committees within the health care system the public is able to have a greater say in health policy development and health services management.

Concurrent with these developments, even precipitating them in some instances, are the very real issues of rising health care costs, the decreasing health dollar and the decrease in the number of people who hold private health cover. There is little doubt that in order to deal with these issues health care is being rationalised, commodified and corporatised. Incentives have even been set in place to encourage people to retain private health cover and there is evidence to indicate that the rate of decrease in private health membership has slowed

(PHIAC 1998). Many of the developments mentioned briefly in the previous paragraph fit well with this image of an emerging health care system that has a more business-like focus than in previous times. We are told we will have a better health service; indeed there are signs that in some areas at least this is happening.

Yet there are signs that all is not well with the system. At the macro level uncertainties have been expressed about whether the emerging system is adequate to meet (or has even been conceived as having the potential to meet) the ever-changing and expanding needs of the diverse population it is intended to serve. In a recent address to graduating health science students at the University of Sydney, Janet Kahler, Executive Director of the National Industry Association for Disability Services, located problems experienced by those involved in delivering disability services within the economic rationalist model that informs current government decision-making:

> 'The trouble we all face now is that society is dominated by economists and efficiency experts, tight-fisted individuals determined to make life difficult for those who need extra assistance and those whose job it is to supply that extra.'
>
> (Kahler 1999).

This statement can also be applied to health care, welfare and other areas of human service provision. Issues that frequently make headline news in the popular press include:

- Perceived imbalances in service provision
- The high cost of technology
- Rationalisation and/or downsizing of services
- Availability of services
- The quality and appropriateness of services
- Inadequacies and imbalances in the distribution of staffing resources.

The quest for certainty in health care in an uncertain world

Underpinning the identification of these issues is the quest for certainty. People want to feel certain that what they believe they need from a health care system will be available, accessible, appropriate to their needs, and delivered by quality staff in a timely manner and in the way they believe it should be delivered. That such an expectation is not the experience of many in the community is not surprising, given the issues that have been identified and if our belief that we are in a constantly emerging society.

Informal communication among health practitioners in association newsletters, at conferences and in interest group meetings suggests that the quest for certainty among health practitioners is associated with uncertainties which practitioners are experiencing on a number of fronts. Uncertainty in its various forms underpins the issues that are frequently raised by practitioners, for example:

- Insufficient funding to adequately maintain services
- Changing professional roles in the restructured system
- Increasing demands on practitioners in health care settings
- Demands and expectations of professional organisations
- Perceived continual restructuring in some areas leading to instability
- Redistribution of resources
- The virtual disappearance of professionally-based allied health departments in many institutions
- Changing structures and processes for service delivery.

These areas of uncertainty common to the working environments of health professionals frequently add to doubts they may have about the adequacy of their own work in the changing and complex health care environment.

The following quote from a mental health worker illustrates some of the effects that flow from uncertainty in the health practitioner's working environment:

'Well it is really hard to stay enthusiastic about the service when we are unsure if our funding will continue. I mean, I don't know whether I should be applying for other jobs or what. The whole team feels anxious; I'm sure our clients notice a difference in us. Rumour is that we may get partial funding to continue – that means some of us will have to move on. The biggest concern though is our client group. We have just got a really good service under way for them and now it looks like they will lose it. It's really discouraging when this happens.'

(pers. comm., March 1999)

Other issues associated with these tensions have their origins in the human desire and/or need for certainty. Uncertainty is perceived as undesirable in many situations, presenting concerns for those involved in the management and administration of health services, and health professionals involved in delivering particular services, as well as consumers and their carers. The desire/need for certainty is motivated by two sets of interacting forces: those that arise within the individual and those that are external to, but have an impact on, the individual, causing them to seek out a position of certainty in relation to the particular issue or matter.

The practitioner in the practice setting

The quest for certainty, or at least the deep-seated desire for such a state, is a silent partner in almost every encounter between a health care practitioner and a client. Put simply, the client has come to the health practitioner in the expectation that in the treatment/intervention that the practitioner will provide lies *the* answer to the particular health care problem or health issue that is troubling them. Similarly, the majority of practitioners desire, even expect, either consciously or unconsciously, that they will be able to provide *the* answer for the client from the armature of professional knowledge and skill that underpins their practice. The practitioner and the client enter into an unspoken conspiracy to maintain the illusion of certainty in the uncertain world of health care. In so doing they create a state of expectancy that may or may not be fulfilled or only partially fulfilled for one or both participants.

Writers who discuss the concept of expectancy in relation to interpersonal encounters also address potential personal responses to situations in which expectancies are not met, or are disconfirmed (Brislin *et al.* 1986; Bhawuk 1990; Burgoon 1993).

Expectancies are disconfirmed when what people anticipate will happen fails to occur or when things do not happen in quite the way they had anticipated, that is 'things are not how they were meant to be' (Mullavey-O'Byrne & Fitzgerald 1995). Responses to such situations are often charged with high levels of emotionality that may or may not be expressed; alternatively a disconfirmed expectancy may also lead to a positive emotional response.

Writing from a cross-cultural perspective, Brislin suggests that high level emotional responses associated with disconfirmed expectancies in intercultural communication occur in response to the contrast between peoples' expectations and the problem that prevents the achievement of the expectations, not in response to the unexpected which presents in the situation (Brislin *et al.* 1986). This has resonance for practitioner-client interactions in health care; for example, when cultural differences between the practitioner and the client create different expectancies for treatment and behaviour in the clinical setting (Mullavey-O'Byrne & Fitzgerald 1995). In this situation, certainty expectations may be shaken or disconfirmed.

The personal quest for certainty on the part of the practitioner and the client is further complicated by the interplay of many relatively local factors. These factors create, or are perceived as creating, external pressures for certainty that enter into and compound the individual states of expectancy created by the practitioner and client. Some of these factors are shown in Fig. 4.1. While the internal and external pressure-generating factors that fuel the quest for certainty may be different for each practitioner, the main domains (expectations of self, consumer-client expectations and expectations of the professional group/body) are seen as remaining relatively constant.

The diagrammatic representation of local factors in Fig. 4.1 illustrates some situations in which expectations and the desire for certainty (that the expectations will be fulfilled) are juxtaposed against current realities in the practice environment. For a variety of reasons the expectations may not be fulfilled at all, to quite the level anticipated, or in the way that was anticipated. This disconfirmation of

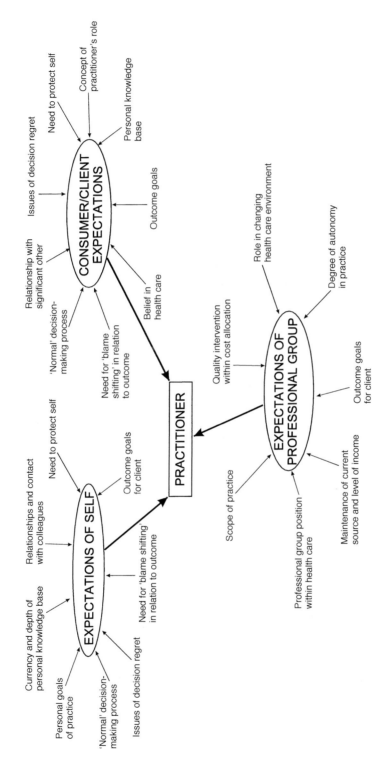

Fig. 4.1   The practitioner in the practice setting: realities and expectations.

the expectancies held by participants in the situation may evoke a high level of emotional response in one or both parties and can lead to negative outcomes for the intervention.

Findings from intercultural research in health care both support and illustrate the part played by 'disconfirmed certainty expectations' in many of the issues that have been identified with intra- and intercultural differences in health care and health care service provision. The following quote from data gathered for the Intercultural Interactions Project 1994 – ongoing) and cited in Mullavey-O'Byrne & Fitzgerald (1995) – illustrate this in relation to consumer–client expectations of the practitioner role (Fig. 4.1):

> 'but for occupational therapists and physiotherapists, you have to teach patients to do something. It's patients that get better by their own efforts, and when they don't try we think, why aren't they?'

Therapists, like other health professionals, expect to play a professional role that is consistent with the knowledge base they have acquired in their training. That professional role is based on assumptions about, for example, behaviours in the therapeutic encounter. Professional socialisation encourages practitioners to feel certain about specific dimensions of their role and the role of their clients/ patients: 'you have to teach patients to do something', 'it's patients who get better by their own efforts'.

When these certainties are disconfirmed, 'patients indicate to you, you're the one who is supposed to get me better, I don't do any of this, you get me better', the outcome may be unsatisfactory for both therapist and client:

> 'I discharged her from treatment because she was non-compliant. She is now wheelchair bound.'

Conclusion and a possible way forward

Practitioners experience both the pressures associated with uncertainty and the pressures of their own and others' quests for certainty. These pressures come from sources within themselves (intrapersonal), from relationships with clients and other health practitioners (interpersonal) and from factors in the practice environment (external). Underpinning all these local factors, more or less indirectly, are forces generated from the wider sociopolitical and economic factors operating on the national and international stages.

All these potential sources of pressures of uncertainty and pressures towards certainty are interconnected, deriving their identity and strength from that interconnectedness. An analogy can be seen in the concept of a nexus used by Zohar and Marshall (1994, p. 173) to discuss quantum reality:

'every system is entangled with every other and derives parts of its identity from that entanglement.'

Indeterminancy, uncertainty and the potential for the co-existence of multiple realities are characteristic of the way change occurs, or the way one system is transformed into another (Zohar & Marshall 1994). Where many systems are interconnected the potential for interdeterminancy, uncertainty and the coexistence of multiple realities is increased enormously.

A reality for health care practitioners is that, due to ongoing pressures to respond to the demands of a complex diverse society within prevailing economic constraints, the health care system will continue as an evolving system, even though the rate of change will slow when a new system settles. Another reality is the changing nature and volume of professional knowledge that may cause practitioners to feel uncertain about the extent and currency of their knowledge and feel pressured to update their professional knowledge base. A third reality lies within the inherent uncertainty present in professional relationships with clients.

These 'realities' produce pressures of uncertainty and pressures towards certainty that are not in themselves necessarily negative or detrimental to health practitioners or their practice; it depends on the way they are perceived and addressed in the evolving world of health care. Health professionals who are able to change their social perceptions, question their values and accommodate alternative views, and appreciate the latent possibilities in multiple realities will grasp the potential in uncertainty and use it creatively to counterbalance pressures towards certainty. For this to be the norm rather than the exception among health practitioners a major shift is required in the way they view their practice environment, the events and people that are a part of it, and themselves.

Some tentative principles that could inform a shift of this magnitude are:

(1) It is highly probable that the state of certainty sought by practitioners and clients alike is not achievable, but can exist only in part, under certain circumstances, in specific contexts and for indeterminable periods of time. It is also questionable whether absolute certainty in practice is desirable (beyond the conditions mentioned in the previous sentence). The potential that uncertainty in practice offers for seeking and identifying alternative/more appropriate and even better strategies for managing health related problems cannot be dismissed, given the changing and evolving nature of the world.

(2) It may be that the quest for certainty has become a quest for survival, a quest that individual practitioners, consumers and carers, professional bodies and health bureaucrats each perceive as critical to holding their position during a period of health care reform that is having unprecedented impact on people's expectancies about health care and the provision of health care services.

(3)   It is clear that the environment in which health practitioners provide care is uncertain. It is equally clear that health practitioners (like other participants in health care settings) bring personally, professionally and culturally derived expectancies to situations and relationships that provide them with a reference point for how the situation might unfold and how others are likely to behave.

(4)   Paradoxically, the very strategy adopted to provide this reference point can interfere with the person's (in this case the health practitioner's) ability to perceive and attend to persons and events in the immediate situation.

If health practitioners are able to view change within the health system and within the knowledge base of the professions as developmental and potentially growth-inducing, uncertainty and pressures for certainty take on new and positive meanings within health care settings. Similarly, if they are able to accept and learn to feel comfortable with uncertainty and pressures for certainty in inter-personal contacts with their clients, they will create opportunities to explore alternative ways of being with others in providing their services within the evolving system that is health care.

References

Audi, R. (ed.) (1997) *The Cambridge Dictionary of Philosophy*, Cambridge University Press, Cambridge.

AIHW (1988) *Australia's Health 1998*, Australian Institute of Health and Welfare, Canberra, Australia.

Bhawuk, R. (1990) Cross-cultural orientation programs, in *Applied Cross-Cultural Psychology* (ed. R. Brislin), Sage, Newbury Park, CA, pp. 248–52.

Bloom, A.L. (ed.) (2000) *Health Care Reform in Australia and New Zealand*, Oxford University Press, Oxford.

Brislin, R., Cushner, K., Cherrie, G. & Yong, M. (1986) *Intercultural Interactions: A Practical Guide*, Sage, Newbury Park, CA.

Burnet, J. (1963) *Early Greek Philosophy*, Meridian Books. Cleveland.

Burgoon, J. (1993) Interpersonal expectations, expectancy violations, and emotional communication, *Journal of Language and Social Psychology*, **12**, March, pp. 30–48.

Fitzgerald, M. H. & Mullavey-O'Byrne, C. (1994) *The Intercultural Interactions Project*, School of Occupational and Leisure Sciences, Faculty of Health Sciences, The University of Sydney.

Health Ministers' Forum (1994) *Towards a National Health Policy: A Discussion Paper*, State Health Publications, Sydney, Australia.

Kahler, J. (1999) Graduation address, Occupational therapy graduation, The University of Sydney, 20 April.

Mullavey-O'Byrne, C. & Fitzgerald, M. H. (1995) *Disconfirmed expectancies in intercultural interactions*. Paper read at 18th Federal and Inaugural Pacific Rim Conference, Australian Association of Occupational Therapists, Hobart, Australia, 12–15 July.

NSW Health Department (1992) *Leading the Way: A Framework for NSW Mental Health Services 1991–2001*, New South Wales Health Department, Sydney, Australia.

PHIAC (Private Health Insurance Administration Council) (1998) *Annual Report, 1997–98*, Commonwealth of Australia, Canberra, Australia.

Zohar, D. & Marshall, I. (1994) *The Quantum Society: Mind, Physics and the Quantum Self*, Flamingo, Harper Collins, London.

Chapter 5
The Meaning(s) of Uncertainty in Treatment Decision-making

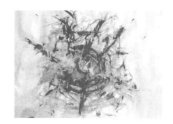

Cathy Charles

'...we need physicians who are able to acknowledge uncertainty. Doctors will be able to do this better if they recognize uncertainty to be not a technological failure caused by limitations in their knowledge or skill in applying it, but rather a ubiquitous element of the inherently interpersonal, context-specific, and judgement-dependent nature of the practice of medicine.'

(Beresford 1991, p. 11)

In the delivery of health care, providers face considerable pressure to achieve certainty in decision-making, that is, to correctly identify and classify illness problems and to administer the most appropriate treatment. The concept of *uncertainty* has been an important one in research and conceptual thinking on treatment decision-making (Fox 1957, 1980; Tversky & Kahneman 1974; Eddy 1984; Katz 1984; Anderson & Mooney 1990; Beresford 1991; Charles & DeMaio 1993; Chalmers & Thompson 1996). However, it has also taken on different meanings depending on the disciplinary and situational context. In this chapter I provide a selective overview of sociological perspectives on the meaning of uncertainty in the context of treatment decision-making. Next, I explore a more recent statistical approach to defining and reducing clinical uncertainty. The chapter concludes by identifying some of the limitations of using aggregate level research data as the basis for making individual treatment decisions.

Certainty is defined in the Concise Oxford Dictionary as an 'undoubted fact' and 'beyond the possibility of doubt'. Uncertainty has the opposite meaning: of questionable fact, doubtful, unconfirmed, unpredictable (Seaton *et al.* 1989). In the context of health care, the problem of uncertainty about the best treatment is important for both physicians and patients. First, for many serious illnesses such as cancer, there may not be one 'best' (i.e. most effective) treatment but rather alternative treatments that have both benefits and risks, and often the most effective treatment is also the one with the most serious side effects. In such situations, a trade-off must be made between the benefits and risks associated with the alternative treatments in order to determine which to implement. Since it is the patient who will live (or die) with the consequences of the decision, increasingly both physicians and patients believe that the latter should make such trade-offs taking into consideration their own values and lifestyle preferences (Charles *et al.* 1997a).

Second, many treatment decisions are viewed by patients as value-laden. If the treatment outcomes are positive, patients are likely to feel that they made the *right* decision. If outcomes are negative, patients may feel that they made the *wrong* decision and blame themselves for the bad outcomes. However, the 'right decision' is not knowable in advance; it will become evident only after the decision has been made, because there is no way to accurately predict which treatment will be better for an individual patient. Rather, clinical trials are used to identify whether patients, *on average*, do better with treatment A or B (Charles *et al.* 1998). The pressure to create certainty, on the other hand, comes from a desire to predict in advance, from all available treatment alternatives, the most appropriate intervention for a specific patient with a given set of clinical characteristics and social circumstances.

Finally, good health, however defined, often takes on a special meaning and importance to individuals because it is so closely tied to personal issues of self-identity and performance of a wide range of social and occupational roles. People generally value their health. When ill, they have a vested interest in choosing a treatment with positive outcomes and they subjectively assess for themselves whether the treatment worked. All of this puts pressure on the health care provider and the patient to make the *right* decision according to criteria used by each party (which may or may not be the same).

Sociological perspectives

The concept of uncertainty and a description of its key characteristics in the context of the diagnosis and treatment of disease were first discussed in the sociological literature by Renée Fox in her seminal article entitled 'Training for uncertainty' (Fox 1957). This paper was originally published in *The Student Physician*, edited by Merton, Reader and Kendall, two American sociologists and a physician. Merton and his colleagues took as a basic premise that the role of the physician in the USA has both technical and attitudinal components. The researchers wanted to explore the attitudes, values and expectations that medical students learned as they progressed through each year of medical school and the ways in which these attributes prepared students for careers as physicians.

Using predominantly qualitative research methods, Fox conducted a longitudinal study of medical students over four years in a single medical school in the USA. On the basis of her results Fox identified three types of knowledge uncertainty or gaps experienced by medical students. First, they came to recognise that there were vast amounts of knowledge to be learned and that they could not possibly master it all. Second, they learned that there were significant gaps in medical knowledge independent of their own limitations. When combined, these two problems gave rise to a third: uncertainty in distinguishing between personal ignorance on the one hand and limitations of existing medical knowledge on the other (Fox 1957; Rizzo 1993).

Fox contended that students gradually overcame these problems as they learned how to identify the different types of knowledge uncertainty and gained experience with and confidence in their clinical skills. Over time, the students came to see that they would never have as much knowledge as they would like, but that they had to make clinical decisions in spite of knowledge uncertainty. In this work, and in her later writings, Fox stressed the concept of uncertainty as a major aspect of medical culture which students were socialised into living with (rather than seeking to eliminate) in order to gain professional competence (Fox 1957, 1980; Atkinson 1984).

Over the years, sociologists have identified other dimensions of uncertainty that are important to treatment decision-making. Light (1979), for example, extended Fox's original typology to include, among other things, uncertainty in treatment outcomes for individual patients, and uncertainty in patient responses. As used by Light in this context, uncertainty seems to take on the meaning of unpredictability.

Other sociologists have been interested in the concept of uncertainty within the context of the patients' preferences for participation in treatment decision-making (Charles *et al.* 1998). When a patient consults a physician for the first time, the latter has no way of knowing or predicting the patient's preferences in this regard. Studies from different clinical contexts have shown marked variations in the extent to which patients want to be involved in this process. Not surprisingly, the sociodemographic factor most consistently associated with such preferences is age; that is, the older the patient, the less likely it is that (s)he will want to share the decision-making process (Sutherland *et al.* 1989; Beisecker & Beisecker 1990; Degner & Sloan 1992; Deber *et al.* 1996). Whether this finding reflects an ageing or a cohort effect is not known.

Uncertainty as to patients' understanding of treatment benefits and risks is another area of increasing interest to medical sociologists (Charles & DeMaio 1993; Lupton 1993; Gabe 1995; Adelswärd & Sachs 1996). This is an important issue because physicians typically use scientific language, e.g. probability statements, to explain to patients differences in the benefits and risks of relevant treatments. Studies have shown, however, that some patients may not understand or retain the concept of probability (Charles *et al.* 1998). Others may understand the concept but have difficulty making personally meaningful data on average treatment outcomes for groups of patients in randomised controlled trials. Faced with such information, patients want to know the significance of these findings for their own treatment decision-making process. Typically they will attempt to do this by interpreting the meaning of average outcomes in the context of the personal decision that they must make. When making such interpretations, patients use their own beliefs, values and everyday ways of knowing to filter the research information. As a result, the intended meaning which physicians hope to convey to patients about the research evidence may be changed or lost altogether (Parsons & Atkinson 1992; Charles *et al.* 1998).

Interestingly, the effect on patients of expressing provider uncertainty (meaning the expression of some doubt by a physician when making a specific therapeutic recommendation and then trying to resolve this doubt by accessing various types of information resources) has been found to cause anxiety in some patients (Curely *et al.* 1984; Johnson *et al.* 1988). Fear of creating patient anxiety has been cited as one reason that some health care providers have been reluctant to disclose uncertainty to patients regarding either diagnosis or treatment outcomes (Katz 1984).

Scientific approach to uncertainty in treatment decision-making

During the 1990s there has been a growing international movement within the medical profession to reduce uncertainty in clinical practice by developing and applying explicit decision rules to determine the 'best' (i.e. most effective) treatment to implement in a given clinical context. Over time, these rules have been formalised into a hierarchy of different levels of research evidence, differentiated by the rigour of the studies producing the evidence. The highest level of evidence is seen to derive from randomised, controlled clinical trials. Physicians practising evidence-based medicine (EBM) believe that research results from such studies should be used as the basis on which to determine treatments for individual patients. Many not only practise EBM, they also teach it in the hope of convincing others to do the same (Evidence-Based Medicine Working Group 1992; Kleijnen & Chalmers 1997).

The development and implementation of clinical practice guidelines is one manifestation of this research oriented (rather than clinical judgement-based) approach to treatment decision-making. Guidelines are generally developed from the results of systematic reviews of relevant and current research evidence in a particular medical area. The evidence-based approach to treatment decision-making is consistent with a positivistic world view in which reality is seen as objective and based on truths that are knowable, measurable and predictable (Pozatek 1994).

The argument that research evidence can be used to decrease uncertainty in treatment decision-making by identifying the 'best' treatment to implement in different clinical contexts is clearly important. Clinical uncertainty (meaning doubt about the most effective treatment to implement) has been implicated as a major factor accounting for variations in physician practice patterns that are unrelated to differences in patient health status within small geographic areas (Eddy 1984; Anderson & Mooney 1990; Iscoe *et al.* 1994). Reducing physician uncertainty should also reduce practice variations that are attributable to this factor. Put another way, reducing clinical uncertainty should enable physicians to improve the level of precision between health inputs (treatments) and health outcomes (health status) (Lomas & Contandriopoulos 1994).

Whether uncertainty in treatment decision-making can be eliminated altogether is an issue of some debate (Wennberg 1990; Beresford 1991; Pozatek 1994). Arguing against the case, Beresford, from the Hastings Institute in the USA, has noted that even in cases where research evidence and clinical guidelines point to the superior effectiveness of a particular treatment over others for a given clinical problem, physicians can still face uncertainty about whether the particular clinical situation and social characteristics of their patient match those of patients in the research studies from which the guidelines were developed. In other words, the application of general criteria to a specific situation requires professional judgement as to the goodness of fit. Beresford argues that knowledge uncertainty (which Fox identified many years earlier) is only one type, and by no means the most important type, of uncertainty faced by physicians in treatment decision-making. Uncertainty, he argues, is a fundamental and inherent characteristic of the decision-making process.

To date, the evidence-based movement has taken strongest hold in medicine and particularly among academic physicians (Evidence-Based Medicine Working Group 1992; Davidoff *et al.* 1995; Rosenberg & Donald 1995; Sackett & Haynes 1995; Sackett & Rosenberg 1995). But it is not confined to this particular health discipline. The journals *Evidence-Based Nursing* and *Evidence-Based Mental Health* have been developed to complement the original *Evidence-Based Medicine*. In addition, the British Cochrane Centre and its international satellites have taken on the task of synthesising, summarising and evaluating available research evidence on a wide range of clinical topics (although, interestingly, qualitative studies are not included in this database). They also develop recommendations based on the evidence (Kleijnen & Chalmers 1997; Department of Clinical Epidemiology & Biostatistics, 1998). Practice guidelines have been and continue to be developed in many clinical fields, primarily by professional organisations.

The phenomenal growth of interest in evidence-based practice in the last seven years (the term EBM was coined at McMaster University in Canada by the Evidence-Based Working Group in 1992) suggests that the medical profession, and to a lesser extent, other health care professions, are increasingly moving to portray their practice as a scientific endeavour grounded in the application of universalistic rules of scientific evidence to identify best practices from empirical research studies. In contrast, the so called 'art' of medicine, that is, the application of professional judgement, expertise and individual discretion in treatment decision-making has either been de-emphasised or, in some cases, downgraded to a kind of pre-scientific era of medical practice.

New knowledge and skills are required by physicians to practise EBM. They include knowledge of clinical epidemiology and biostatistics (so that physicians can understand the hierarchy of rules of scientific evidence used to evaluate the quality of intervention studies); computer search skills (to be able to conduct on-line searches for relevant studies and journal clubs in their clinical area); and critical appraisal skills (to be able to apply the rules of evidence to evaluate the scientific quality of different studies, i.e. to distinguish strong studies from weak.

Acquisition of these types of knowledge requires a different type of learning experience from that which students were exposed to in the past. Given the explosion of medical knowledge and the inability of physicians to keep up-to-date (Fox's first type of knowledge uncertainty), evidence-based physicians eschew clinical experience and judgment as essential tools for making optimum treatment decisions. Instead they argue that the physician's ability to retrieve, critically appraise and apply to his/her own practice relevant research results from rigorous studies around the world, indexed in large computerised databases, is the new essential ingredient needed to make optimum decisions.

There is no doubt that the EBM approach reduces physician uncertainty about what to do (which should not be confused with what the outcome will be), if one is willing to accept the premise that a particular type of research evidence should be regarded as the 'gold standard' by which treatment decisions made for an individual patient should be judged. Acceptance of this premise simplifies the decision-making process for physicians. If relevant high quality research evidence is available (a large assumption for some diseases), EBM offers an explicit statistical method for determining the 'best' treatment, meaning the most effective treatment, for a given clinical situation. Implementing clinical guidelines simplifies the decision-making process because someone else has already collected, evaluated and synthesised the research evidence and derived treatment recommendations from this review.

Clearly, research evidence is an extremely important input into the treatment decision-making process, but there are also limitations to this approach. First, as noted earlier, evidence from research studies typically comes in the form of probability statements about average outcomes for a particular group of patients treated with different interventions (e.g., A versus B, or A versus watchful waiting). The assumption is that if patients randomised in a clinical trial to receive treatment A do better on average than patients on treatment B, then A is the treatment of choice for an individual patient with a clinical profile similar to the study patients.

This assumption, however, ignores the fact that not all patients will do better with treatment A. Some will do better with treatment B, depending, among other things, on the patient's social circumstances, clinical history and degree of similarity to patients in the relevant studies. By focusing only on *average* outcomes for each group, the fact that some patients will do better with treatment B is completely masked. Moreover, since there is no way to predict which specific patients will do better with treatment A or B, using average group outcomes as the basis for determining individual level treatment decisions may not be appropriate unless one can be sure that the presenting patient is similar to those in the relevant study on a variety of personal, clinical and social characteristics.

Given the above, an important role for evidence-based physicians is to contextualise for each patient relevant research information on treatment outcomes. To do this, physicians need to rely on professional judgement to assess how closely a given patient fits the profile of patients benefiting from a specific intervention, and hence, how likely it is that a given treatment will be effective in this particular case. In short, even if treatment effectiveness has been established, professional judgement is needed to determine the appropriateness of a given intervention for each patient (Charles *et al.* 1997b).

Finally, patient preferences regarding the role, if any, that they want to play in treatment decision-making also create an irreducible element of uncertainty in clinical decision-making. The extent to which patients actually share the decision-making process will become clear only as the interaction evolves, as both physicians and patients reveal their treatment preferences and both work towards developing an agreement on the treatment to implement (Charles *et al.*, in press). When the patient's relatives, friends, and/or family doctor are also involved, uncertainty becomes even more pronounced because each person's views may need to be considered and weighed in the decision-making process (Charles *et al.* 1997a).

Conclusion

The EBM approach to treatment decision-making reflects a far different clinical mentality to that of the student physicians studied by Fox in the 1950s who, as an explicit part of their professional socialisation experience, were taught to accept clinical uncertainty as a normal part of everyday practice, to learn to live with uncertainty and to gain the confidence to use their clinical judgement to make treatment decisions in spite of it.

Ironically, acceptance of clinical uncertainty (with a more patient-centred than physician-centred focus) is now being advocated by a number of health professionals (e.g. Pozatek 1994; Binnie & Titchen 1999; Titchen 2000). These authors argue that in a postmodern era, health care providers should consciously adopt a therapeutic position of uncertainty ('sit with uncertainty') in their approach to patients. Adopting this position is seen as valuable to the therapeutic process because it recognises the complexity of each person's life, encourages providers to find out information about each patient's experiences, values and preferences through direct communication, promotes shared treatment decision-making, and reduces the likelihood of premature closure on the intervention to be implemented.

This argument can serve as a cautionary tale. The claim that research evidence should be given a privileged status over other types of information when making treatment decisions brings us full circle to a new form of paternalism. Other types of knowledge, including patient preferences and clinical judgement, need to be integrated into the treatment decision-making process if decisions are to be not only effective but also appropriate and consistent with patient values.

Acknowledgments

I would like to acknowledge the contributions of Sandra West, Colleen Mullavey-O'Byrne and Angie Titchen to earlier versions of this chapter. I am also very grateful to Joy Higgs for inviting me to be part of the fascinating group which met for a week in Leura in the Blue Mountains, Australia, to begin writing this book. I am extremely grateful to Stephanie Short for her support, intellectual stimulation, sense of fun and adventure as well as her spare bedroom which was my home base for much of the time I was in Sydney. My deepest thanks go to Rosemary Cant who invited me to the University of Sydney as a visiting scholar for three months in 1998 and who opened so many doors for me, including the week in Leura, during my stay. Final thanks go to Roy and H.G. for their hilarious contributions to my cultural education while in Australia.

Although they were not directly involved in this project, I also want to thank my research collaborators, Amiram Gafni and Tim Whelan at McMaster University, who have helped shape my thinking about both conceptual and empirical issues related to treatment decision-making. I assume sole responsibility for any errors appearing in this chapter.

References

Adelswärd, V & Sachs, L. (1996) The meaning of 6.8: numeracy and normality in health information talks, *Social Science & Medicine*, **43**, pp. 1179–87.

Anderson, T. F. & Mooney, G. (eds) (1990) *The Challenge of Medical Practice Variations*, MacMillan Press, Copenhagen.

Atkinson, P. (1984) Training for certainty, *Social Science & Medicine*, **19**(9), 949–56.

Beisecker, A.E. & Beisecker, T.D. (1990) Patient information-seeking behaviours when communicating with doctors, *Medical Care*, **28**, pp. 19–28.

Beresford, E. (1991) Uncertainty and the shaping of medical decisions, *The Hastings Center Report*, July–August, pp. 6–11.

Binnie, A. & Titchen, A. (1999) *Freedom to Practise: A Study of the Development of Patient-Centred Nursing* (ed. J. Lathlean), Butterworth-Heinemann, Oxford.

Chalmers, K. & Thomson, K. (1996) Coming to terms with the risk of breast cancer: Perceptions of women with primary relatives with breast cancer, *Qualitative Health Research*, **6**, pp. 256–82.

Charles, C.A. & DeMaio, S. (1993) Lay participation in health care decision-making: A conceptual framework, *Journal of Health Politics, Policy and Law*, **18**, pp. 881–904.

Charles, C.A., Gafni, A. & Whelan, T. (in press) Decision-making in the physician-patient encounter: Revisiting the shared treatment decisions-making model, *Social Science & Medicine* (in press).

Charles, C.A., Gafni, A. & Whelan, T. (1997a) Shared decision-making in the medical encounter: what does it mean? (Or, it takes at least two to tango), *Social Science & Medicine*, **44**(5), 681–92.

Charles, C.A., Lomas, J., Giacomini, M., Bhatia, V. & Victoria, V. (1996) Medical necessity in Canadian health policy: Four meanings and … a funeral? *Milbank Quarterly*, **75**(3), 365–94.

Charles, C.A., Redko, C., Gafni, A., Whelan, T. & Renyo, L. (1998) Doing nothing is no choice: Lay constructions of treatment decision-making among women with early-stage breast cancer, *Journal of Sociology and Health*, **20**(1), 71–95.

Curely, S.P., Eraker, S.A. & Yates, J.F. (1984) An investigation of patients' reactions to therapeutic uncertainty, *Medical Decision Making*, **8**(4), 501–11.

Davidoff, F., Haynes, B., Sackett, D. & Smith, R. (1995) Evidence-based medicine: A new journal to help doctors identify the information they need, *British Medical Journal*, **310**, pp. 1085–6.

Deber, R.B., Kraetschmer, N. & Irvine, J. (1996) What role do patients wish to play in treatment decision-making?, *Archives of Internal Medicine*, **156**, pp. 1414–20.

Degner, L.F. & Sloan, J.F. (1992) Decision-making during serious illness: What role do patients really want to play?, *Journal of Clinical Epidemiology*, **45**, pp. 941–50.

Department of Clinical Epidemiology & Biostatistics (1998) *Evidence-Based Health Care Newsletter*, An occasional publication from the Department of Clinical Epidemiology & Biostatistics, McMaster University, Hamilton, Canada.

Eddy, D.M. (1984) Variations in physician practice: The role of uncertainty, *Health Affairs*, **4**, pp. 74–88.

Evidence-Based Medicine Working Group (1992) Evidence-based medicine: A new approach to teaching the practice of medicine, *Journal of American Medical Association*, **268**, pp. 2420–5.

Fox, R.C. (1957) Training for uncertainty, in *The Student Physician: Introductory Studies in the Sociology of Medical Education* (eds R.K. Merton, G.C. Reader & P.L. Kendall), Harvard University Press, Cambridge, MA.

Fox, R.C. (1980) The evolution of medical uncertainty, *Millbank Memorial Fund Quarterly*, **58**, pp. 1–48.

Gabe, J. (1995) Health, medicine and risk: The need for a sociological approach, in *Medicine, Health and Risk: Sociological Approaches* (ed. J. Gabe), Sociology of Health and Illness Monograph Series No. 1. Blackwell Publishers, Oxford.

Iscoe, N.A., Goel, V., Wu, K., Fehringer, G., Holowaty, J.E. & Naylor, C.D. (1994) Variation in breast cancer surgery in Ontario, *Canadian Medical Association Journal*, **150**(3), 345–52.

Johnson, C.G., Levenkron, J.C., Suchman, A.L. & Manchester, R. (1988) Does physician uncertainty affect patient satisfaction? *Journal of General Internal Medicine*, **3**, pp. 144–9.

Katz, J. (1984) Why doctors don't disclose uncertainty, *The Hastings Center Report*, pp. 35–44.

Kleijnen, J. & Chalmers, I. (1997) How to practise and teach Evidence-based Medicine:

Role of the Cochrane Collaboration, *Acta Anaesthesiologica Scandinavica*, **111**(Suppl.), pp. 231–3.

Light, D. Jr. (1979) Uncertainty and control in professional training, *Journal of Health & Social Behaviour*, **20**, pp. 310–22.

Lomas, J. & Contandriopoulos, A.P. (1994) Regulating limits to medicine: Towards harmony in public and self-regulation, in *Why Are Some People Healthy and Others Not? The Determinants of Health of Populations* (eds R.G. Evans, M.L. Barere & T.R. Marmor), Aldine De Gruyter, New York, pp. 253–83.

Lupton, D. (1993) Risk as moral danger: The social and political functions of risk discourse in public health, *International Journal of Health Services*, **23**, pp. 425–35.

Parsons, E. & Atkinson, P. (1992) Lay constructions of genetic risk, *Sociology of Health & Illness*, **14**, pp. 437–55.

Pozatek, E. (1994) The problem of certainty: Clinical social work in the postmodern era, *Social Work*, **39**(4), 396–403.

Rizzo, J.A. (1993) Physician uncertainty and the art of persuasion, *Social Science & Medicine*, **37**(12), 1451–9.

Rosenberg, W. & Donald, A. (1995) Evidence based medicine: An approach to clinical problem-solving, *British Medical Journal*, **310**, pp. 1122–6.

Sackett, D.L. & Haynes, R.B. (1995) On the need for evidence-based medicine, *Evidence-Based Medicine*, **1**, pp. 5–6.

Sackett, D.L. & Rosenberg, W.C. (1995) On the need for evidence-based medicine, *Journal of Public Health Medicine*, **17**, pp. 330–4.

Seaton, A., Davidson, G., Schwarz, C. & Simpson, J. (eds) (1989) *Chambers Thesaurus*, W&R Chambers Ltd, Edinburgh.

Sutherland, H.J., Llewellyn-Thomas, H.A., Lockwood, G.A., Tritchler, D.L. & Till, J.E. (1989) Cancer patients: Their desire for information and for participation in treatment decision-making, *Journal of the Royal Society of Medicine*, **82**, pp. 260–3.

Titchen, A. (2000) *Professional craft knowledge in patient-centred nursing and the facilitation of its development*, University of Oxford DPhil Thesis, Ashdale Press, Oxford.

Tversky, A. & Kahneman, D. (1974) Judgment under uncertainty: Heuristics and biases, *Science*, **185**, no. 1124–31.

Wennberg, J.E. (1990) Sounding board. Outcome reach, cost containment, and the fear of health care rationing, *New England Journal of Medicine*, **323**, pp. 1202–4.

Chapter 6
Finding the Fifth Player:
Artistry in Professional Practice

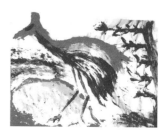

Lee Andresen and Ian Fredericks

'Teaching can be considered an art ... in the sense that teaching can be performed with such grace that, for the student as well as for the teacher, the experience can be justifiably characterised as aesthetic.'

(Eisner 1979, p. 153)

'Inherent in the practice of the professionals we recognise as unusually competent is a core of artistry.'

(Schön 1987, p. 13)

Programme notes

This chapter arose from a conversation. Although it is unconventional, we hope the form will be accessible to readers. Our goal is to add to that small body of work that studies the crossover where artistry and professional practices meet. Our field is artistry-in-practice within two 'caring professions', health care and education. Literature in this area typically addresses the appreciation of professional artistry *from the outside*. Written from the connoisseur's perspective, it either stresses connoisseurship and the language of appreciation, or urges a greater valuing of professional artistry. It tends to concentrate on description rather than analysis.

We ask whether it may be possible to step into the artist's world, hence to examine professional artistry *from the inside*. We ask what it is like to be an artist who practises as a professional; whether that might inform our understanding of what it means to be a professional who practises with artistry; and how artistry might then be cultivated among novices or apprentices in the professions. To explore this question Ian Fredericks operates as the musician/composer and Lee Andresen as the teacher and student of teaching. Reflective comment adds to the dialogue by reaching out to address the crossover of artistry in professional practice. Is artistry a metaphor illicitly stolen from the arts? Or does it comprise a deep *common ground* shared between the arts and other professional practices?

As in a piece of music, the separate 'movements' of this chapter may not at first appear to flow from one another. Be prepared for changes of tempo, sonority or rhythm. Each movement can be appreciated in isolation, but the integrity of the whole piece may not emerge until the end. This is not ordinary academic text. Its topic is crossover, so the text is a crossover between music and academic treatise. Like Schön (1987, p. 94), we 'willingly suspend disbelief' until, at our destination, we can look back and see where we have come.

The 'performance' is in five movements:

(1)   Prelude (autobiography)
(2)   Improvisatory piece (dialogue)
(3)   Variations on a theme (analysis)
(4)   Coda (terminological essay)
(5)   Epilogue (imaginary, reflective scenario).

Movements 2 and 3 are continuous, played/read without a break. All themes, whatever their presentation format, arise from the one series of conversations, and they uniformly strive to remain faithful to the spirit of that original dialogue.

Prelude

LEE ANDRESEN: My working life began as a schoolteacher. Ten years on, circum-stances and aspirations led me through curriculum development, teacher train-ing, and eventually academic staff development. That trajectory led me inexorably away from my own classroom, but it gave me three decades of privileged entry into the classrooms of literally hundreds, perhaps thousands, of other teachers. Through my observer and participant roles in those classrooms (appraisal, critique, feedback and guidance, support, problem solving, advising), I began to discern the qualities that distinguish outstanding from good, good from competent, and competent from incompetent, in the practice of teaching. It now pleases me immensely to have developed some feel for what I call the 'artistry of practice' among teachers. It has emerged out of innumerable notes, reports, observations and conversations. It comprises, at least in part, a grounded sense of appreciation of what good teaching looks like, and some facility with a language of appreciation for telling what I see and feel when in the presence of good (and sometimes great) teachers.

IAN FREDERICKS: I am a composer. The search for newness in art music has been the guiding light of many composers in the twentieth century and many new styles and genres have developed. However, this hundred years of exploration has left most art music lovers with a strong preference for the music of the eighteenth and nineteenth centuries. That is a fairly strong indictment of the twentieth century's compositional achievements. Nevertheless, the developing interest in electronic and computer music towards the middle of the century did bring the promise of something really new. With a mere 50 years of development this field is already beginning to blossom. That is quite remarkable, considering that the field encompasses new musical instruments, the performance practice required to play them and also the beginnings of a new music theory and composition practice. I find this to be the challenge in writing music for computers. Computer music is not merely a 'new style' or a 'new composition school'. It is a whole new musical aesthetic, perhaps a future universal world music.

Improvisation

Two-part dialogue with commentary

Question (Lee)
> Response (Ian)
>> *Commentary (Lee)*

1. How do you describe yourself nowadays, professionally?
> I specialise in writing music for computers. The allure here is the search for something really new in music.
>> *This tension between innovation and tradition: is it found in virtually every field of professional practice?*

2. Some say twentieth century music reached a dead-end. Has it really led nowhere?
> As far as audiences are concerned, that certainly seems to be the case. But I believe genuinely new music in the twenty-first century will take its lead from the use of computers as tools for composition, production and instrumentation. Here at last are the beginnings of truly new sounds and the promise of new musical constructs with which to compose them.
>> *Technology and innovative practice: do they go hand in hand, synergistically, in a similar way in music, in all the arts, and all the professions? Certainly technology is never separate from or necessarily antagonistic to human practices, since as Heidegger (1977) observed, it is itself a human practice.*

3. So what becomes of musical performance as we know it?
> For the first time in musical history, here is a musical field that is not restricted by corporeal gesture. No need here for physical virtuosity. A chance for a true music of the psyche! What then becomes of the art of musical performance is something yet to be documented.
>> *Do all practitioners experience the same sense of entrapment in corporeality? The sense that without our bodies we could do nothing, yet*

with them (and their limitations) we can achieve only so much of that to which we aspire. Does this promise of escaping from the bondage of corporeality help explain the excitement of computers in education? Or the inspiration of minds in tune with professional practice? Is the future of the interacting human being ('warmware') in education and the healing arts also something 'yet to be documented'?

4. And what becomes of all the great music of the past?

Computer music involves a whole new musical aesthetic but it will call upon sound structures from all previous musics as well as from nature herself.

> *Does each form of professional practice also have an aesthetic of its own? What does it comprise? Where do we find it? What is its relation to inherited standards and traditions (the previous musics) of our various practices?*

5. For you, how does the process of musical composition proceed?

It is characterised by continuous decision-making, decisions that are generally made entirely at the composer's discretion.

> *'Decision-making' appears in virtually all descriptions of expert practice in the professions; technical-rational decision making proceeds by following rules. But rules fail in the 'indeterminate zones of practice' (Schön 1987, p. 6). Is this our zone of interest, where practitioners exercise 'discretion' (or professional judgment) in the same way as any artist would?*

6. What criteria do you invoke in making these decisions?

There are none. More often than not I find I must adopt the egocentric position; I and I alone specify what will happen, simply because I say it will.

> *In art, the applicable criteria are almost entirely aesthetic. In the professions, however, surely other criteria must supervene? Surely they are instrumental criteria (practical outcomes) and moral/ethical criteria (honouring contracts with clients)? But do the professions acknowledge aesthetic criteria? Dare they?*

7. Egocentricity doesn't present a problem in your case?

Not necessarily; mostly I have my head entirely in the piece and the direction is clear, so ego is not actually a problem.

> *How, despite this 'egocentric' position of complete discretion, does ego remain nevertheless 'not a problem'? Well-deserved criticism of professional life is often directed at the unbridled egotism some practitioners display – like prima donnas in the arts. Iris Murdoch (1992, p. 86) speaks of the 'test of truth': '(In art) the temptation to the ego is enormous since it really does seem here to dispose of the god-like powers*

it secretly dreams of. Truth is always a proper touchstone in art.' Dare we wonder whether artistry's touchstone of truth might help other professions handle this dilemma?

8. How do you start, since there does not exist, at that point, any particular direction?

Using a computer you have a completely blank canvas: your greatest dilemma. No guideline, no procedure, no established theory, means you must simply stare into the abyss for a beginning.

Is an analogous 'abyss' faced in professional practice? When we face the client-to-be for the first time? The canvas is blank as we face the ultimately unfathomable question of a client's true needs. Will they ever say (in effect), 'This is what I want from you' (Frank 1995, p. 33)? And if they do, will we understand? Of all factors to influence our decisions, must we not unavoidably guess these needs through informed intuition?

9. But isn't facing the 'abyss' also the case in traditional music composition?

Sometimes, but the task is often set in terms of a commission, and it is often determined or implied by what instruments will be used. Often the genre will be 'given' by either the commission or personal preference. All this means that a procedure becomes evident, a theory of composition can be chosen and the work begun. Continuing decision-making is largely, if not entirely, directed by these existing paradigms.

*For other professionals the contract with the client likewise comprises the explicit 'commission'. But is there is also an **implicit** commission, which resides in our interpretation and framing of those needs? Either way, as in music, a 'procedure' must become evident before work can begin. 'You begin with a discipline, even if it is arbitrary ... you can always break it open later.' (Architect Quist in Schön 1987, p. 57)*

10. Do you deliberately try to abandon existing paradigms?

To adopt them would be at the very least restrictive, though one is often tempted to work from or at least simulate the traditional process if only to avoid the pain of searching the abyss for a beginning. But that would be to ignore (deny?) the freedom given by the computer.

The 'traditional process' in professional practice is of enormous importance. It defines what it is appropriate to do. It enshrines and invokes the 'know-how' criteria of competency. But are there not varying degrees of freedom even within it? Who knows where they begin and end?

11. But this pain of searching the abyss: isn't it a high price to pay for freedom?

This is a price the abyss demands of me if I truly aim to embrace the freedom the new instrument (the computer) gives. Now, there is no prejudice, no expectation, no rules, no constraints, no restrictions. But equally, there are no guidelines.

> *Art answers only to itself. Other professionals have **moral** obligations towards their clients – a duty of care.* For Mayeroff (1971, p. 4) the relationship between artist and art is one of care, analogous to care for another person. *Our 'caring professional' armoury of expectations, rules, constraints, restrictions, guidelines are all aimed at securing the moral contract. Nor can discretionary artistry exercised within the professions ever abdicate from that commitment. So what can be made of artistry's relationship to the 'rules of the game'?*

12. But somehow you must proceed with a theory – a set of beliefs or propositions – for *how to proceed with this particular composition*?

No, I can actually proceed without a theory and that's often viable, in the short term anyhow. But my preference is to develop at least an initial *'theory for the composition'* which tells me how to start the composition and then proceed. But it can take many different forms: a mathematical or abstract concept, a sociophilosophical position, anything whatever.

> *This is paradoxical. Perhaps in the professions we work with two such sets of propositions (what IF calls 'theories'). Theories of technique are well enough known; they come largely from tradition and are consistent with criteria of competence. But are there not also propositions or beliefs concerning appropriate style or form or enactment, with which we can be more open, experimental, discretionary? Where do they come from? How do we access them? How are they made available for critical reflection?*

13. Then the music begins?

Once this initial 'theory' is established, it can; the music begins to assume a life of its own; it begins to find its own way.

> *'A life of its own' ... in respect of technical competency this sounds like the 'autopilot' phenomenon; a function of routine, habit, sheer virtuosity. In regard to artistry in practice, however, it is rather more mysterious: perhaps the 'Fifth Player' of our title? 'Teaching', Eisner (1979, p. 154) noted, 'is an art in the sense that teachers, like painters, composers, actresses, and dancers, make judgements based on qualities that unfold during the course of action ... not dominated by prescriptions or routines but influenced by qualities and contingencies ... unpredicted.' That seems to be no less true of the healing arts.*

14. How does music find its own way? You seem to imply that you hear it giving you instructions. Are you in a trance?

The trick is to listen very carefully to the unfolding process. Eventually the work will start to talk back to me. It's a truly strange and wonderful experience because ego seems to cease to exist; one becomes almost transcended. But it's not being in a trance, because the rational mind remains very much a part of the process.

> *I'm reminded of a study by Bamberger and Schön (1991, pp. 188–9), where subjects who were engaged in hands-on problem-solving were seen to be 'improvising . . . on-the-spot experimenting in response to the new phenomena they were discovering. In short . . . "conversing" with their materials. Their conversations were more like the making and shaping of coherence in the arts than like the means-ends or instrumental logic usually associated with puzzles and problems.'*

15. It even sounds (dare I say it?) in some fashion 'spiritual' or mystical.

Certainly, because it is almost as though I have become the medium by which the music is able to realise itself (I'm not religious, mind you, nor in the least given to mysticism!). Nevertheless, something special happens, something difficult to describe in non-subjective terms. Yet the rational consciousness remains fully active. If it didn't I wouldn't be able to realise the music at all. Computers require considerable effort from the rational mind! And the rational mind is waiting in the background ready to swoop down and make notes and operate at a theoretical level.

> *Maybe this steps beyond even Schön; it now sounds closer to Bohm's theories of dialogue (Bohm & Peat 1987) or Gadamer's (1980) view of conversation. Each adopts a stance analogous to our 'Fifth Player' hypothesis to account for what seems to be the inexplicable happening, when that-which-we-do-not-yet-know emerges, seemingly of its own volition, declaring, 'this is what you were seeking but you did not yet know its name!'. The contemplation is not irrational; it is super-rational. Rationality is not suspended, it is heightened and transcended. The retention of (possibly enhanced) rational consciousness whilst being totally absorbed in action is a paradox of art and the professions alike, like the much-disputed 'reflection-in-action' notion (Schön 1983, p. 54). Can we reflect in action or only in the moments between action, when our minds turn from action to contemplation before returning to action before we have even become conscious of the interruption?*

16. But it's impossible to be in two states at once . . . isn't it?

I recently observed it when working with a dancer. He was performing the solo dance; at the same time calling technical directions to myself (music), to the lighting operator, and to the video cameraman. Whilst the body and parts of the mind were attentive to the artistic endeavour, part of the mind (and perceptions) was also busily overseeing the whole technical process. I can't think of a way of discussing this without sounding a bit weird!

Some descriptions of school teaching capture the same phenomenon, where it has been called 'pedagogic tact'. Presumably it is widespread throughout the professions. If it goes unnamed, this may indicate that it is largely unnoticed and its virtue unappreciated. But surely, here, the 'Fifth Player' (the 'muse' of the artist) was also present. So what, who, where, when and how is our own muse evident in education and health care?

17. You said the music 'talks back' to you. Can you expand on that?

Listening to what the music is telling you allows continuous modification (where necessary) of the initial theory. The spirit (ethos) of the music actually challenges that initial theory. Here is where I believe the real essence of creative work lies.

The artist is trying to follow a set of propositions that are themselves undergoing constant modification: this surely contradicts the basic tenets of technical rationality (TR)? Do we then conclude that there must exist some profound distinction between TR and the pursuit of 'professional artistry' (Schön 1983; Fish & Coles 1998, p. 41;)? If there is a distinction, need it be a conflict?

18. So the theory you start with is liable to be changing even as the composition proceeds?

One must be prepared to follow the initial theory up to the point where it allows the creative idea to gestate while at the same time being open enough to abandon it once the idea starts to live by itself. It's almost as if the theory is the mother of the musical gesture, and like any good mother it must know when to allow the progeny to leave the nest and grow by itself.

Different professional traditions grant their practitioners differing degrees of liberty to wilfully abandon established procedures and proven models directed at competent performance. Some, particularly in the health sciences, demand obedience at all costs; that is certainly the safe route. But does it lead to creative problem-solving? Or innovation? Or to comprehensively and authentically meeting client needs and honouring the client contract?

19. Are there times when the initial theory doesn't lead anywhere?

Yes, I must be prepared to abandon it and start all over again if it's not working. Otherwise the piece can turn out stilted and mechanistic, lacking musicality. It can be a frustrating time. It invariably leads to discord between the convergent being who has spent considerable effort developing a 'nice' consistent, logical theory and the divergent being who throws caution to the wind and 'rides the wild beast'. But this phase is crucial. It requires courage ... madness as well. Yet, there's a bridge between genius and madness. The trick seems to be to gaze into the abyss while (as Nietzsche might have put it) ignoring the abyss gazing back at you. It's a kind of schizoid state where part of one's being has surrendered to the primal intuitive (instinctive?) state.

> *Major (so far unanswered) questions surround the issue of the outcomes of professional practice. And we must remember that even artistry has its instrumental outcomes (Murdoch 1992; Scruton 1997). Courage and madness: an odd pair of virtues! It recalls what Iris Murdoch wrote about 'the courage which the good artist must possess' and how she related it to their need to invent their own tests of truth, otherwise their work is false, inauthentic, a forgery (Murdoch 1992, p. 86). How might these tests of truth inform the criteria for expert practice in the professions? Dare we recognise and reward them in the appraisal of professional excellence? There must be some interesting equivalent components of the 'schizoid state' in other forms of professional practice. Might it occur in trying to balance the client's needs with the profession's expectations? Or when balancing these with our own hopes, desires, values and aspirations?*

20. Are the steps in musical composition *sequential*?

No, and it's crucial to remember that. One phase does not necessarily follow from the other or lead to the next. It's not a series of steps. In the creative world, logic tends to exist in a three-dimensional space rather than along a one-dimensional line. It's crucial to maintain a cross-fertilisation of one phase into another; the phases are applied continuously and in a dynamic way.

> *Perhaps artistry and expertise are in this same dynamic, iterative (symbiotic?) relationship? If so, we would be wise to resist the idea that we become first competent and only then apply a veneer of artistry! But what are the options? If not sequential, perhaps artistry may be a possible (even highly desirable) quality to be cultivated in practice from the ground up, starting with the work of even the naïve beginner. This is certainly the case in all education in the arts. But could education programmes in our institutionalised caring professions accommodate such an idea? Perhaps artistry has its own inherent wisdom, able to inform (and profoundly enrich) practice at all stages of development, and in every situation, regardless of technical competency levels. How do we learn to recognise and value it and listen to it speaking, at all stages of our (and our students') development?*

21. What potential dangers must you be alert to?

Maintain constant vigilance for the 'theory trap': allowing adherence to the initial theory to obscure the desired end! If I devise a theory for the problem and then find a solution that merely fits the theory, I run the risk of falling into a tautology, infinitely regressive and ultimately fatal! The real universe is a complex one which cannot be reduced into component parts. If you attempt to do that you lose the essence; you lose everything.

> *The 'theory trap' has its parallels in professional practice: the 'following the rules' trap; the 'traditional' trap; the 'breaking the rules for the sake of breaking them' trap. The essence of professional practice needs locating. Where is it? What is it composed of? How shall we describe the heart of this human/practical purpose that intersects our lives with those of our clients, and brings our skills and sensibilities to bear upon their needs and their expectations, both of us and of the tradition in which we stand?*

22. Does this all constitute the 'Fredericks method' for the creative problem-solving process?

I think of it, in a sense, as something like a meta-paradigm for solving new problems in a creative way. It goes like this:

- Identify existing paradigms (in the Kuhn (1970) sense), and then abandon them;
- Examine the task from scratch, analyse it without prejudice, determine what part of the old paradigm is still applicable, then invent the initial theory for proceeding;
- Begin to apply this initial theory to the problem at hand, but beware of confusing the initial theory with the desired end-in-view, the composition you are searching for. The two are very different;
- Watch for the time the work begins to talk back to you;
- Dump the initial theory and proceed by letting the problem and the process of solution-searching lead you to your final solution.

> *Perhaps the 'reality' for professional practice comprises the human/practical situation of the client, and the needs deriving from that, which the professional must never confuse with anything else. Can we follow where our own sense of artistry leads, whilst never allowing it to usurp competence, care, and moral responsibility for clients? On the other hand, is the implied dichotomy a necessary one? Must it be one or the other? What are the alternatives?*

Postscript to the Dialogue

Already we are being tempted, lured, beckoned along the path of reductionism. We ask, 'What is the hidden essence?' and we intuitively (as good analytic scholars) wish to proceed to find it by analysing, fragmenting, breaking things apart in a frenzied search. Must it not also be a fruitless search? Will we admit that what we are trying to do is the impossible: to identify a whole amidst a heap of fragments? We *are* scholars, nevertheless. Our tools are those of scholarly representation, exploration and exposition. We are trained to analyse wholes into fragments and communicate about fragments in the hope that our readers will see the whole. What, then, do we do?

Having come this far, let us not lose heart. We can continue with our scholarly zeal, searching for the Gestalt amidst the pieces left over from analysis. Then, if the whole does ever become visible, our fears will have been in vain. If it never emerges, we shall have proved our point, that the whole is not, after all, the sum of the parts. We thus embark on the analytic pathway with trepidation and some foreboding. And, if our reader can sustain the effort, without even so much as a pause...

Theme with three variations on the idea of the 'Fifth Player'

Theme: Improvisation?

Let's look at the proposition that *improvisation* is a primary site for the creation (emergence, appearance) of original artistry. By that we mean a quality of practice whose precise form and substance could not have been known or planned in advance. Compared with the other use of 'improvised' (second-best or substitute) this *is* the real thing. But it is also transient, unable to be captured, something 'of the moment'.

Improvisation (the art of invention) is a foundational music tradition in many non-Western cultures. And it is right at the heart of jazz, as well as being ubiquitous in folk and rock. Jazz musicians and others '*feel* where the music is going and adjust their playing accordingly' (Schön 1987, p. 30). Indeed, all styles of Western music have their improvisatory forms (e.g. the 'cadenza' within the classical concerto). But let us consider jazz, for the present, as one instance where improvisation represents the very essence of performative artistry:

> '... jazz is set apart by its improvisatory nature. Jazz musicians participate in a shared culture ... carry common (but not identical) repertoires, and a common body of knowledge that allows them to make music together. The music is guided by a deep structure of chord progressions and themes. Using this unifying structure as a base, (they) create recurring and sometimes surprising variations on the underlying themes – weaving together varied qualities of tone, harmony, rhythm, volume, pace and voice.'
>
> (Oldfather & West 1994, p. 22)

Let us suppose that a jazz 'combo' comprises four players. Each plays for and responds to the other three. Each also plays to, and responds to, an invisible 'fifth player'. Without player five the playing may be competent, even clever or highly proficient, but it is not art because nothing creative or imaginative happens. Human conversation is likewise an improvisatory art, and conversation itself has been used as a metaphor for the *growth of human knowledge across the ages* (Oakeshott 1967).

For a practitioner, to be caught improvising (in this sense of the term) is to deserve the highest accolade: the mark of a true professional, displaying skill and sensibility that far surpass mere technical competence:

> 'Jazz exemplifies artistic activity that is at once individual and communal, performance that is both repetitive and innovative, each participant sometimes providing background support and sometimes flying free.'
>
> > (Bateson 1989, pp. 2–3)

Schön (1987, p. 30), in common with Bohm and Peat, Gadamer and others already cited, regarded spoken conversation as a pure improvisation. Following the argument to its limit, life itself is also an improvisatory art. Jazz becomes a metaphor for life and art.

Variation 1: *Who* is player five?

Every human event, Dewey argued, has an aesthetic dimension. Purely aesthetic events have only that dimension, whereas 'mundane' events have the aesthetic as *one of several* dimensions (see Dewey 1934, p. 11; also Coleman 1983, p. 12). Professional practice, in Dewey's sense, is thus a mundane event. That description in no way prevents us from celebrating its aesthetic qualities, however. The fifth player awaits the cue to enter the scene whenever we are ready for the entrance. But who is s/he?

Perhaps player five is part of each of us, but stands outside and beyond us, not any single player's 'property'. As a group consciousness perhaps? We each contribute something towards it, but it remains outside the control of any separate individual. Or it may be an independent entity entirely, summoned up by the power of the event, by the apt occasion, called forth by the collective consciousness and greater than it. 'The Muse' comes to mind: the benevolent entity for whom the poet or musician waits, whose truth will be dictated and revealed through the poet in its own time.

Variation 2: Artistry and/or competence?

The primary goal of professional practice is clearly not art as such. It is the fulfilment of expert practice, the outworking of a refined and cultivated professional discipline, the embodied demonstration of a way of being or a form of life (as physician, nurse, physiotherapist, teacher). It is performed not for its own sake but for the sake of others, for their health, education or well-being. That much is not in dispute. Moreover, the primary determinant of the success or value of a practice must remain the practitioner's competency or technical expertise. So, does this necessarily relegate player five to a secondary or ancillary role? In answer, we suggest two hypotheses:

(1)   It may be that the more we can discover, recognise, and then 'play for' and respond to the unseen player five, the more our competently expert practice becomes transformed (enhanced, augmented) from mere technical competence and becomes a form of professional artistry. Here artistry is a facilitative or enabling asset which unambiguously enriches or enhances the outcomes of competency.

(2)   A more challenging hypothesis might be that, *in the absence of player five* and the aesthetic sensibility that can accompany expert practice, what passes as 'mere competency' may even be demeaned and diminished in value. Mere competence may not, on this hypothesis, be enough in itself. Devoid of artistry's purifying virtue, it may emerge as a degenerate, self-limiting form of practice.

Variation 3: All in the mind?

The fifth player is as uncatchable as mercury, but can we learn where and when to recognise it? Perhaps the fifth player is being played for and responded to most critically at the *moment of decision*. That's when we make the choice: where to go, how to proceed, how to respond authentically to a never-before-encountered situation.

We could suppose the players to be, not separate identities, but *elements in conversation* in the psyche of the practitioner. We can even presume to name them, these four voices extemporising simultaneously within a practitioner's conscious or subconscious psyche:

(1)   The *perceived* (stated) *needs* of the client
(2)   The client's *interpreted needs*
(3)   The practitioner's *technical competency*
(4)   The practitioner's *ethical competency*.

These four, taken alone, can at best produce a Deweyan 'mundane' event. But let them be joined by the (as yet unnamed) player five. The object of our search now appears: artistry in practice. And is that where we must leave it, as a miracle/ mystery? Must we admit our scholarly aptitude's incapacity to make sense of something we intuitively know to be real?

Coda in the style of *The name of the rose*

Does the fifth player *have* a name? And who gives it the name – scientists, artists, or others? At Northwestern University, the Centre for the Study of Education and the Musical Experience (Reimer & Wright 1992) brought musicians and scientists together to research the nature of musical experience. Descriptors (names) emerging for the musical experience included:

- *Intrinsicality* (internal meaning)
- *Affect* (feeling, engagement)
- *Expectation* (unfolding, leads somewhere)
- *Meaning* (organised, connected with life)
- *Intelligence* (perceptual skill required)
- *Listening* (transforms the experience)
- *Sensuosity* (tangible effect on bodies)
- *Time* (movement forwards)
- *Reference* (as language, telling truths)
- *Greatness* (depth, profundity of meaning)
- *Inspiration and creativity* (imaginative decision-making)
- *Functionality* (social communion; the human condition).

This exemplary instance of a 'naming project' sets a standard to follow as we inquire into artistry in professional practice. Some valuable contributions have been made to that inquiry. The seven separate views presented in Table 6.1 all agree on the possibility of naming the player; they differ only in their choice of names. What's in a (particular) name anyhow? Maybe what matters is rendering the thing at least in principle nameable.

We rejoice to see how vocabularies for practice of health care are currently being enriched by the work of Fish, Titchen and others. We regret to note that in the world of teaching, certainly that of university teaching, we are still waiting for someone in this decade to 'name the rose' so that we can appreciate good teaching more fully through having a language with which to adequately render its praise.

Epilogue

When the show was over – foyer talk

The last sounds of music die away, there is that momentary pause when for a moment sweet silence reigns, broken immediately by the noise of seats squeaking, bodies standing and walking, the parade of an audience exiting home via the theatre's foyer.

In our case, home had to wait. After-show conversation, in a congenial local

Table 6.1 Naming the 'fifth player' (artistry).

Murdoch (1992)	Grace	Love	Loving attention/care
Fish (1998)	Composition	Symmetry	Movement
The object of the professional's love and respect	*Scale* Figure-ground Spatial relationships Viewpoint	*Volume* Gravity Mass Tonal shading Contours	*Light* Tone Texture Colour Space
Teaching: Eisner (1985) Axelrod (1973)	To develop taste or appreciation of artistic qualities in teaching we need to develop skills and languages of perception. The nature of artistry is largely hidden under the cloak of 'style'.		
Lee Andresen and Ian Fredericks The language of music	Nuance Interpretation Communication Evocation Noise	Uncertainty Vision Feeling Spirituality Integrity	Musicality/musical-ness ('Aptness') Phrase Phraseological structure Empathy/rapport
Titchen (2000) Professional artistry in health care	Being authentic as a person Using comportment to focus Creating a therapeutic environment Emotional and physical presence Engaged responses to patients' suffering	Balance between absence and excess of emotional engagement Dealing with negative or inappropriate emotions Using humour Comforting Being intimate, offering a form of moderated love	
Scruton (1997) Qualities of artistry in a work	Demonstrating aesthetic values: beautiful, sublime, elegant, ugly, unsightly Describing the effect of an object: moving, exciting, uplifting Describing aesthetic character: aesthetic perception, or taste	Everything that elicits our approval: good, great, a triumph Demonstrating virtues and vices: sentimental, cruel, noble, courageous, self-confident, truthful	

coffee house, soon turned to shop-talk. It emerged that we were all involved in preparing or upgrading professionals, working in professional 'schools' where craft knowledge is researched and taught. What should not have surprised us (but, as always, it did) was how, in due course, *our own* conversational 'fifth player' emerged of its own accord – the unmentioned issue suddenly demanding to be heard.

Skill, competence and expertise cannot easily be faked. Some were of the view that artistry, can, however. And the dependable technical 'virtues' can be 'turned on' more or less precisely as and when needed. But can artistry be invoked, summoned, commanded to appear? Faced by these qualitative differences between the worlds of art and of technique, we asked questions about reliability and confidence. And, as always, we asked about how you *educate for artistry*.

Should you take a particular theory of creativity and teach it as *the* way for students to be creative? Ian Frederick's theory works for him; must it work for everyone? Teachers of architecture argue over what is the best theory of design. Maybe we should look at competing theories, compare them, and let them talk to one another? In a true conversation, then, see what emerges for each individual student?

We talked in circles; the performance had raised more questions than answers. What do we do about them all? What difference should they make to us when we return to work on Monday and face our student class or supervise their clinical placement?

An inner circle stayed late, talking on into the small hours. It seemed to find a couple of things at least to hold onto (although we did not understand all the implications). They comprised a sort of challenge, with a sharp warning in its tail-sting. We certainly needed to learn how to construct the language of professional artistry *in our own discipline*. And to start talking it among ourselves, and with our students – to induct them into using it. Axelrod (1973, p. 8) had been spot-on with that point:

'... the art that Socrates created was improvisational. Neither he nor his intimates, neither his friends nor the strangers with whom he carried on an inquiry, could predict, when a conversation began, where it would lead ... and it is clear that the work of art was not created by Socrates alone ... it was created jointly by him and by every member of the group who entered into a relationship with him during the discussion. It is precisely that relationship which was crucial. More than any other factor, it determined the kind and the quality of the artwork that emerged.

... all members of the teaching–learning group – and not its leader alone – must become artists if a work of (educational) art is to come into existence ... They believe they are only talking ... but what they are doing is not simply talking, any more than a poem on a printed page is simply a sequence of words.

If the teacher has not been able to engage his students in the creative process, then he has failed as teacher–artist. Nor can he induce creativity in the learning group by calling attention to it, by exhortation, as art; the absence of self-conscious "creativity" is essential to the success of the teacher–artist's creation of art.'

That, we agreed, was the rub. Axelrod's unexpected point, that you cannot 'turn it on' or 'exhort' artistry into being, was surely true. We had often heard it elsewhere, not realising it was speaking about our teaching. Scruton (1997, p. 375) agrees:

'Friendship is undeniably useful ... one of the greatest benefits that life bestows ... But friendship comes only to the person who forgets its instrumental value. If I approach you with an eye to the benefit then I cease to see you as a friend.

... So it is with aesthetic values. We obtain much that is useful to us through the experience of art. But the experience is available only if we forget the use. We must consider the work of art as an end in itself; only then does it become a means for us.'

Night drew on, the comforts of home and sleep beckoned as we mulled over the most inscrutable notion of all. Somehow artistry and ethics had to be related. But how? For they each approached something like truth, though from different directions. Naturally, Keats came to mind: 'Beauty is truth; truth beauty'. And Eisner's plea: 'Should we ... regard the arts as irrelevant to matters of truth?' (Eisner 1993, p. 7). Perhaps it is no surprise that the language of artistry in the caring professions always picks up ethical qualities. Might it not therefore be that the ethical is perhaps one way of achieving the beautiful? Or should it be the other way round? We never did find out, on that occasion anyhow. But there's sure to be another.

Acknowledgments

Thanks to Della Fish (UK), Andrew Busuttil (UWS Hawkesbury), Robyn Holmes (Canberra School of Music) and the anonymous chapter reviewers, for corrections and enormously helpful suggestions for developing an earlier draft of this chapter. Without their loving, *care*-ful attention and generous help the final version would have emerged much less scrutable than this one is. All errors, confusions and annoyances that remain are the responsibility of the authors.

References

Axelrod, J. (1973) *The University Teacher as Artist*, Jossey-Bass, San Francisco.
Bamberger, J. & Schön, D.A. (1991) Learning as reflective conversation with materials, in *Research and Reflexivity* (ed. Frederick Steier), Sage, London, pp. 186–209.
Bateson, M.C. (1989) *Composing a Life*, Penguin, New York (cited in Oldfather & West, 1994).
Bohm, D. & Peat, F.D. (1987) *Science, Order and Creativity*, Routledge, London.
Coleman, E.J. (ed.) (1983) *Varieties of Aesthetic Experience*, University Press of America, Lantham, MD.
Dewey, J. (1934) (republished 1958) *Art as Experience*, Capricorn Books, New York.
Eisner, E. (1979) *The Educational Imagination: On the Design and Evaluation of School*

Programs, Macmillan Publishing, New York (especially Chapter 9 'On the art of teaching' and Chapter 11 'The forms and functions of educational connoisseurship and educational criticism').

Eisner, E. (1985) Aesthetic modes of knowing, in *Learning and Teaching the Ways of Knowing (Eighty-Fourth Yearbook of the National Society for the Study of Education, Part II)* (ed. E. Eisner), NSSE/University of Chicago Press, Chicago, IL, pp. 23–36.

Eisner, E. (1993) Forms of understanding and the future of educational research, *Educational Researcher*, **22**(7), 5–11.

Fish, D. (1998) *Appreciating Practice in the Caring Professions*, Butterworth-Heinemann, Oxford.

Fish, D. & Coles, C. (eds) (1998) *Developing Professional Judgement in Health Care: Learning Through the Critical Appreciation of Practice*, Butterworth-Heinemann, Oxford.

Frank, A.W. (1995) Lecturing and transference: The undercover work of pedagogy, in *Pedagogy – The Question of Impersonation* (ed. J. Gallop), Indiana University Press, Bloomington, pp. 28–35.

Gadamer, H. G. (1980) *Dialogue and Dialectic: Eight Hermeneutical Studies on Plato* (translated by P.C. Smith), Yale University Press, New Haven, CT.

Heidegger, M. (1977) *The Question Concerning Technology and Other Essays* (translated by W. Lovitt), Harper & Row, New York.

Kuhn, T.S. (1970) *The Structure of Scientific Revolutions* (2nd edn), University of Chicago Press, Chicago.

Mayeroff, M. (1971) *On Caring*, Harper & Row, New York.

Murdoch, I. (1992) *Metaphysics as a Guide to Morals*, Penguin, London.

Oakeshott, M. (1967) *Rationalism in Politics and Other Essays*, Methuen, London.

Oldfather, P. & West, J. (1994) Qualitative research as jazz, *Educational Researcher*, **23**(8), 22–6.

Reimer, B. & Wright, J.E. (eds) (1992) *On the Nature of Musical Experience*, University Press of Colorado, Niwot, CO.

Schön, D.A. (1983) *The Reflective Practitioner: How Professionals Think in Action*, Basic Books, New York.

Schön, D.A. (1987) *Educating the Reflective Practitioner*, Jossey-Bass, San Francisco.

Scruton, R. (1997) *The Aesthetics of Music*, Oxford University Press, Oxford.

Titchen, A. (2000) *Professional craft knowledge in patient-centred nursing and the facilitation of its development*, University of Oxford DPhil thesis, Ashdale Press, Oxford.

Chapter 7
Embodying Knowledges: Challenging the Theory/Practice Divide

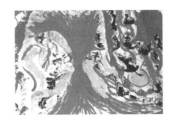

Debbie Horsfall, Hilary Byrne-Armstrong and Rod Rothwell

'...an altogether different approach to the politics of knowing and being known which ... advocates for the creation of a more hesitant and partial scholarship capable of helping us "to tell as better story"'

(Grossberg in Lather 1989, p. 28)

Professional practice needs to challenge the theory-practice divide. This chapter explores, through discussion and anecdotes, the mind/body, theory/practice split as a discourse that we take for granted in our professional lives. We propose that this taken-for-granted discourse:

- Is not just an idea, it has a material basis in our everyday language and social practices
- Remains invisible because we are born into it and it shapes every aspect of our lives
- Is based on the connection of power and knowledge
- Perpetrates practices that are not useful/ethical when working with people.

Our talk and everyday interactions shape our relationships and therefore our practices. Our communication is embedded in a set of assumptions about the world: a 'discourse', i.e. the systems of language and social practices that exist in the world. Discourses are not just assumptions in our heads, but are visible in our talk and in the social practices and conventions that make up society as we know it. In this chapter we unpack the discourse that separates 'theory' and 'practice'. Education designs programmes based on the notion that theory is a necessary foundation for practice, and that theory classes are separated from practice classes. However, most of us acknowledge in one way or another that the divide is artificial. So why do these practices persist? Our conversation, as people working in these fields, is strongly influenced by the power of social practices (we call separating theory and practice in education a 'social practice') in our disciplines to maintain the theory/practice divide. In other words, we are not going to argue the merits of theory or practice as such. We want to unpack the discourse that makes the priority of theory indisputable. In this discourse the priority of reason (on which theory is based) is closely associated with the separation of mind/body and the dominance of mind over body. The seductive quality of this notion is obvious in the statement by a lecturer in the following anecdote told to us by one of the co-writers of this book:

> *A mature student, after many years' experience working as a volunteer in her local community, enrolled at the local university to do a community work diploma. On the first day a teacher told the class that now they had entered university he wanted them to forget everything that they knew, because they were there to learn new things.*

> (Story 1)

We are saying that statements like this one belong to discourses which shape our professional arenas. Our belief is that we talk ourselves into existence (see also Davies 1994), that we are not in charge of language; rather, language and social practices are in charge of us. We want to make visible the way discourses are built into everyday social interactions in education and health settings and how these discourses remain largely undisputed because we take them for granted as the 'truth'.

It is this idea of truth that is central to our discussion. A discourse is formed by the connection between power and knowledge. Power and knowledge are connected by the idea of 'truth'. The mind/body, theory/practice split is supported by a discourse (in this context the rational, scientific discourse, or the 'sciences of man') which has at its centre the notion that there is a true knowledge which can be discovered through correct scientific investigations. Truth, power and knowledge are intricately woven together in a network of everyday talk and social practices. This talk produces our identities/roles (such as teacher, student, doctor, patient) and accords greater power/truth to the scientific way of knowing (spoken by the doctor or teacher) than other ways of knowing (the 'local' knowledge of the student or patient).

This chapter aims to make professionals aware of the way that discourses shape our everyday life, so that we can be more aware and act against these discourses when we think that what is happening is not ethical or helpful to the people involved (Horsfall 1998). We describe discourses as 'regimes of truth' (following Foucault 1980, p. 131) because they shape and are shaped by a set of rules and regulations that determine the truth and therefore what is said, how it is said, who says what, and where. We intend to investigate and unpack the particular 'regime of truth' that supports the theory/practice divide, making us believe that theory and practice are different.

The dominant regime of truth in health and education makes knowledge into a thing, separate from people, a commodity that can be possessed and given by one person to another. But all knowledge has historical origins in everyday human relationships. Knowledge is not separate from human beings and their relationships. When we fail to see these connections we end up with taken-for-granted pieces of knowledge that are useless, even ridiculous and often damaging. This is illustrated by the following story about a nursing practice still taught at one of our universities and still widely practised in hospitals:

> *Students need to learn to make a bed properly, according to traditional practices to be learned by students (i.e. the dominant discourse/practice). They go to the nursing lab at the university and are shown the 'correct' way to make a bed, with all the pillowslip openings facing away from the entrance of the ward.*
>
> *This practice has a concrete history. It arose during the Crimean war – to avoid the dust from passing horses' hooves blowing through the door into the pillows. This has now acquired the status of a standard practice serving some other purpose.*
>
> (Story 2)

This is an example of a taken-for-granted practice (knowledge) that has no relevance to the patient's comfort and well-being, yet it continues today. Why do conventions like this social practice persist? There are many examples like this around the arenas of health and education: classroom practices that inhibit learning, hospital practices that preclude compassion and healing. Examples are the way that human bodies are organised *by external agencies*, e.g. the physical constrictions of desk and chair, timetabling, forms of delivery. In hospitals the cleanliness discourse is an example (see Michaels 1990).

Before addressing this question we add two stories that are examples of other forms of social practice in people's everyday talk and actions:

> *Practitioners are not permitted to have contact with their clients outside the agency setting. Professional boundaries must be upheld to maintain the integrity of the professional relationship.*
>
> (From a manual for case workers in an unemployment agency) (Story 3)

> *Mike, a postgraduate student, has a wealth of life experience working with young people. In his first piece of written work, he draws heavily on his experience. While he shows that he has read some 'literature', he dismisses it all as elitist, inaccessible and too abstracted from his everyday life.*
>
> (Story 4)

The four stories above are examples of social practices in professional areas that objectify knowledge, separating it from human relationships. We are not judging them as right or wrong, we are making them visible:

- Story 1 illustrates a social practice found in universities which creates an environment that precludes people's experiences and knowledges, to promote discipline-based theoretical knowledge as the 'right' way of knowing.
- Story 2 is an example of a social practice that prescribes a routine and uses the power of the institution to promote it as a truth and therefore maintain it as a convention.
- Story 3 demonstrates a social practice that divides professionals/experts from the 'objects' they work with, the unemployed.
- Story 4 indicates a social practice which implies that knowledge is personal and owned by an individual and is therefore more relevant than other people and their knowledge.

Power and knowledge

What makes us think that conventional or accepted practices are right and 'true'? The answer lies in the connection between power and knowledge. Power is connected to knowledge because knowledge is produced in social relationships, and social relationships are formed by differences in position/power. When people are assigned a role within a discourse (e.g. teachers in universities, doctors in hospitals or social workers in unemployment agencies) they are granted positions/roles in a discourse from which to speak the truth according to the discourse.

Knowledge and power are interwoven in the positions/roles granted to people within any system. 'Who speaks' (e.g. lecturers, health professionals) (as in position/role) will give what they speak (knowledge) its validity. This is how regimes of truth are upheld and perpetuated. If, however, we adopt a sceptical position towards practices such as the pillowslip story, we might say making a bed is useful knowledge to have when working with people confined to beds. But is there a right way and a wrong way? Who determines this truth? What position do they have and what agendas are they upholding when they teach this? Whom does it most affect? Does the person in the bed have a voice?

In our position as academics in human science disciplines, we are aware of the power that these positions give us. We want to be aware of and not perpetrate social practices that reduce people's lives and relationships to object status (e.g. the human being becoming an object around which the practice of making a bed is accomplished). Students are not often taught to think about what/why something is taught (they have to acquire this knowledge through experience). For us, part of educating human science practitioners is to make them aware of the language systems and social practices shaping their environments so that they become critical thinkers who, although shaped by these discourses, can also practise, as appropriate, what Foucault (1980, p. 257) calls 'mobile and transitory points of resistance'. Our experience is that acquiring knowledge of the regimes of truth which inform any context produces people/practitioners with the ability to critically reflect and, when appropriate, to resist blind adherence to dominant regimes. This *critical practice* can challenge the unhelpful or often unethical practices that many regimes of truth perpetrate.

The next story, from Angie Titchen, is an example of critical practice:

A group of nurses wonder how they can intervene, resist the patronising and unhelpful attitude of the surgeon on his hospital rounds. Together they decide that instead of standing behind the surgeon, or at his side, as he talks at the patient, they will disrupt the way that the organisation of space is maintaining the surgeon's power. One nurse steps through the wall of doctors and crouches beside the patient facing the doctors. Another sits on the bed. This has an immediate effect on the surgeon and trainee doctors. The surgeon slowly moves into the crouched position as he speaks. The trainee doctors gradually move so that they are also sitting or crouching. When the doctor speaks, the nurse beside her asks the patient what she thinks; the relationship slowly changes – the patient is included in the discussion and the manner in which the surgeon speaks and listens to the patient changes.

These nurses analysed the social practices belonging to the dominant medical discourse and acted to challenge them. They realised that the social practices in force in this ward situation led to the isolation and objectification of people, making them objects to study and talk over rather than human beings whose knowledge of themselves might be just as or more relevant than medical theories. Medical discourse, with its particular ways of speaking and conduct (found in the positioning of the bodies around the bed), were shaping the relationships between people.

This example shows how discourses shape practices and vice versa. In other words, the knowledges produced in this scenario are constructed by the ways the people are relating to each other, which in turn are shaped by the medical discourse. Even though the nurses were part of the discourse, they critically reflected on it and intervened using other forms of knowledge. They used one of the social practices already in the arena (positioning of bodies) to reshape the power relationships. Their action created different relationships and therefore different forms of knowledge. They changed the relationship, not by direct challenge, blame or criticism, but by critically reflecting on the invisible, taken-for-granted practices supporting the medical discourse of which they were all a part. They did not tell/coach the patient to be more assertive. This would have implied that the patient was to blame (another common practice found in dominant discourses (and the psychology discourse is built upon it). For example, unemployment creates the unemployed, a category of person that is then worked on to be made better). They did not have a quiet word with the surgeon about changing his approach (which would imply that the surgeon was to blame). They simply positioned their bodies, shaped the space differently, and in so doing, changed the exercise of power and therefore the quality and number of voices contributing to the context.

Foucault (1984, p. 50) argues for:

> 'an attitude, an ethos, a philosophical life in which the critique of what we are is at one and the same time the historical analysis of the limits that are imposed on us and an experiment with the possibility of going beyond them.'

The health professionals in the above example recognised the practices shaping the space including its boundaries, and experimented with changing the relationships using the practices already in existence. To make such change it is necessary to make visible the everyday practices of dominant discourses (like those described in the ward round). But these practices are usually invisible to us, because they are once removed from our direct awareness or focus. For example, in the ward round the direct focus is on the patient's illness and as a result relationships and talk centre around this illness. If we commented about anything else in this context, the people involved would probably feel irritated with us.

But from a power/knowledge perspective, we would ask what discourse is shaping the space and how it is visible in the moment. In the above story, what was visible was the positioning of bodies in a hospital ward round and the way in which the positioning constructed certain forms of relationship. Changing the positioning of the bodies created different forms of relationships and therefore different knowledge production. Elements of the power/knowledge connection are found in many features, including the way that the ward is set up, the beds arranged and the pillowslips aligned, the positions of the patients, and the manner of the ward round (moving from bed to bed). They form a geography of power that maintains human beings as objects, maintains the sort of knowledge allowed (rational, scientific, objective knowledge) and maintains the relationships of power so that the knowledge of doctors and health professionals is considered more true/valid than patients' knowledge. Similar examples can be found in other professional contexts such as classrooms and university meetings.

The example of positioning of bodies in space is one category of social practice. The sorts of assumptions we have when we talk are another form of social practice. Other examples and their assumptions include the following.

Universalising practices

- In many contexts, the ways we talk about things we allude to a single truth 'out there' (Rothwell 1998) which we can discover. In this discourse truth is found through scientific method, and the institutions that uphold scientific method are the places where the truth can be discovered (forget all you know when you come to university because we will now tell you the truth).
- There is a single truth that can be applied across time and place. Theories and

practices, if scientifically proven, can be applied in all contexts (there is a right way to place pillowslips which can be applied all over the world for ever more).

Dividing practices

- The knower is separate from the known. It is possible to discover what is true through being objective, detached from any political or social agenda.
- Objective knowledge is the only valid form of knowledge (what one has experienced in life is not valid knowledge because it is subjective).

Individualising practices

- Differences in understanding are individual. For us to understand individuals we should separate and classify them according to the characteristics of standard human beings.
- Physical environments are organised to arrange bodies (or units) for the maximum efficiency of space and time (e.g. the classroom, the ward). They are not set up for learning or care.

Classifying practices

- People are classified according to norms. Personhood is redefined through this classification. For example a person becomes a 'student', rather than a person who is at university; we refer to a 'schizophrenic' rather than a person who has a mental illness, a 'Down's Syndrome' rather than a child born with a genetic syndrome and so on.

Normalising practices

- Objective knowledge is valid and true knowledge. Any other forms of knowledge are weird, abnormal, to be marginalised.
- Those certified as experts are responsible for decisions regarding how the truth should be practised.
- Truth is reinforced by a (scientific) method that generalises and universalises actions and behaviours. Professional practices are then arranged into standardised procedures. Diversity and difference of both the service provider and client, the student or the local context are silenced.

Surveillance practices

- People are observed in minute ways (i.e. placed in positions from which everything can be seen) in order to become a site for diagnosis (positioned in a bed at the centre of a ward round).

- This forces all of us to become the surveillors. We all learn to watch at a distance, and we see everything. But discourses determine what can be spoken about and what must be silenced. The bodies we watch, including our own, are arranged and identified according to certain knowledges. So knowledge becomes surveillance.

To illustrate these social practices further, the following is a story taken from our past practices as educators:

On the first day of the residential course, students were asked to complete a learning style inventory (see Kolb 1984) *and classify themselves as learners with particular learning styles called convergers, divergers, accommodators or assimilators.* (This process reflects the social practices of dividing people, assigning identities, classifying.) *A large cross was marked on the floor and students were asked to locate themselves in their quadrant* (reflecting the social practice of establishing boundaries, shaping the body, surveillance). *This would help them identify personal learning strengths and weaknesses and they could see where others in the group were positioned* (illustrating the social practice of normalising). *The next task was for them to work on themselves while at university to minimise their areas of weakness* (representing the social practice of individualising). *For their assessment, they were required to write reflective journals to articulate their process of personal growth through the learning styles* (demonstrating surveillance through a confessional procedure). *The role of the academic was to monitor the process of learning and to check the validity of the students' understanding of their learning style* (portraying surveillance and regulation).

We are of course describing a sort of educational practice that many people will be familiar with (even if it is more radical than some practices). Again, we want to emphasise that we do not think the practice wrong. (To do this would create another regime of truth.) But we want to maintain an open attitude, so we are questioning it.

Our disquiet is that activities such as this one are thought to be challenging of dominant educational discourses. Dominant educational discourses are built on several assumptions, such as the assumption that all human beings have the potential to become rational, coherent subjects through education. 'Potential' means that each person is born with inbuilt learning capabilities which are brought to the learning environment. Learning environments are therefore designed to facilitate the individual learner.

What are the limitations of this assumption? After all, it is an assumption on which education is founded. This assumption has a history that goes back to the seventeenth century and the birth of the human sciences, when people began to be regimented and organised into various forms of institutions to fit the growing requirements of capitalism. In order to shape people, the human body became individualised and made an object, so that it could be shaped and sculptured for political and economic gain, for dominance. (Individualising means that human beings are separated and isolated from each other, and treated like 'things'. This view belongs to modernism and is challenged by both structuralist and post-structuralist viewpoints that consider that there is no such thing as a self; the self can only exist as a relationship (structuralism) or as a process (poststructuralism). Lacan said, 'I am a poem not a poet' (in Truett Anderson 1995, p. 149).) In fact, before the seventeenth century there were few notions of individuality. The birth of the human sciences changed this. There emerged manuals with instructions for every minute gesture and moment of everyday life (see Foucault 1979) and out of these discourses the modern individual was/is produced (see Henriques *et al.* 1986).

Once individualised (seen as separate from relationship and context), both individual people and their knowledges can be dissected, classified, reduced, categorised and divided. Categories/identities such as convergers/divergers/dys-lexics/slow learners are assigned to people as well as to knowledge. (The limitation in this process is that this social practice reduces the complexity and beauty of people and their knowing to categories that are 'thin', abstract descriptions of life, rather than 'thick' descriptions with verisimilitude (Byrne-Armstrong 1999).) Knowledge categories include: visual, verbal, kinaesthetic or practical knowledge; propositional, personal or professional knowledge; intuitive or rational knowledge; explicit or tacit knowledge. Suddenly our language and social practices are filled with ever-increasing categories of things. Such individualisation produces knowledge as a commodity, as something that we individually possess or that is transmitted by experts. The social relationships and therefore the power relationships that produce knowledge are rendered invisible and go unchallenged.

Revealing the knowledge/power relationship

Instead of individualising and objectifying people, we can consider that discourses position us in relationship to others and this positioning of self and others will determine the sort of knowledge produced. This approach acknowledges that knowledge and power go hand in hand as they circulate through and around us, positioning us in relation to others. Our task as educators then becomes not one of focusing or diagnosing the sorts of knowledge and power that individuals possess or lack. We do not say that students cannot learn because they are easily distracted, or that the doctor on the ward round is responsible for treating the person in the bed as an object of science (although these things may also be true). Instead we ask, what is it in our culture, our institutions, and the classroom/hospital environment that invites us to label and position people? Is the label/position useful to the individual? Whose knowledge gets to count? Whose voice gets to be heard? What sort of questions can we ask?

An army of desks and chairs

Stationed on alert
Lecture tiers in numbered rows
Obediently waiting
Under lighting blinding with fluorescent zeal

Bodies arrive
Moving in slow motion
Mute, sleepwalking into position
As they comatose,
Fashioned by the space into slumped statues

An expert enters,
Proclaims the space
Hijacks the voices
Silences the bodies and flattens resistance
With proclamations of knowledge

The lesson has begun

Hilary Byrne-Armstrong 1999

This discussion, for us, is a political action. While practices and theories remain separated, while knowledge is considered ahistoric and apolitical, while the individual is seen as an object to be moulded in certain ways, the political, economic, institutional regimes of the production of truth (Foucault 1979) remain invisible and go unchallenged. The difference in approach is to transfer the focus away from individuals (and their psychosocial heritage) onto the social practices shaping the context. In doing this we are not accepting that the theories people espouse are separate from their practices. We are saying that the relationship between them constitutes (produces) the knowledge that is generated.

Until it is recognised that the theory/practice divide is propped up by a mechanism of power that maintains knowledge as a commodity and the human being as a recipient of the commodity, the domination of the sciences of man will remain. We work in institutions where, for example, there are lecture theatres where knowledge is passed on, certain books which must be read in order to 'know', assessment tasks which verify whether the person knows, codes of behaviour for each course, dress codes, and questions one is allowed to ask and questions one is not. Power, truth and knowledge are in collusion, supported by the institution, linked in discourses that regulate and legitimise knowledge as objective, abstract and rational, to be determined by independent observation/ evidence and empirical evidence, which can be generalised. Any knowledge that is not of this type (i.e. which is local, subjective, creative) is 'othered', seen as trivial, worthless, and too local to be considered seriously. Yet the power of the sciences of man to legitimise a certain form of knowledge also gives enormous energy and power to the 'othered' forms of knowledge. Hence the lure of experiential and problem-based learning.

As enthusiastic advocates of support for other knowledge, we turned our attention to uncovering subjective experience and natural learning processes (e.g. imagination, creativity, emotions), and to privileging life journeys (self-reflection and self-direction). Moving away from the headless automaton (the Borg) in a state production line of objective, rational subjects, a new regime of truth has emerged which privileges an organic, vital individual body following her/his personal dream (see, for example, Pinkola Estes 1992, or Bly 1996), which perpetuates the very individualism we were trying to challenge.

Why these things concerns us

The social practices that are part of any discourse form subjects (which Foucault in 1979 called 'docile bodies') who are silenced, their mouths shut, their vocal cords frozen, shaped by the circulating knowledge into a 'silent other' (Shor in 1996 termed this being 'in Siberia'). Most classrooms and hospitals provide illustrations. (We are not saying that people are consciously doing this to other people. We are saying that we are all shaped by social practices and sometimes we resist and sometimes we comply, knowingly or unknowingly.) For example, a patient not recovering in the predicted way does not like to bother the doctor with his/her complaints. A student, angry with a particular lecturer, talks about it to other students and not the lecturer. We could individualise the patient as cowardly, or the student as a troublemaker. We could, following our experientially-based practices, suggest communication workshops for the specialist or assertiveness training for the students (and therefore implicitly blame the student, specialist or the patient). Alternatively, we could join our voices and the voices of students/patients together to critically reflect on the regime of truth that is shaping the context and that may be silencing some knowledge(s).

Foucault (1977, p. 14) said that the aim is 'not to change people's consciousness ... or what's in their heads; but the political, economic, institutional regime of the production of truth'. The task for the budding professional becomes one of challenging the implicit social practices (and political agendas) that inform what is spoken, what is left unsaid, who and what is heard and who gets to speak. This is what we call education. Once students begin to think in this way, they can learn and think about what is relevant to their practices and to the people they work with. They can learn the importance of modifying and shaping their practices to fit the local situation. They can shape a practice that suits their style and local contexts. Professional practice shifts from a universal recipe and a prescriptive technology perpetrated on human bodies to a local, cooperative knowledge-finding investigation grounded in social, cultural and political issues.

So what?

What happens when theory and practice are not constructed as separate? We do not have a final answer; rather, our intent has been to ask questions and to share our knowledge about the topic in the hope that it will add to the existing questions on the issue. Grosz (in Lather 1991, p. 153) said that asking questions and musing creates 'a space in which it is possible to do otherwise'. This chapter is, therefore, a political intervention. Asking the question 'so what?' and challenging the theory/practice divide, can help us to move beyond received habits and taken-for-granted assumptions of what we know and do and to be sceptical of 'all that has been received, if only yesterday' (Lyotard 1993, p. 44). By making visible the regimes of truth, the space is opened up for other ways of being in the world.

Some of you may worry that deconstructing discourses and challenging everyday practices can lead to a blank empty space (Horsfall 1998). You may be asking, what does this mean to my practice? Do we not need to teach people knowledge or skills? We would say that of course people need skills/knowledge; without it they may be dangerous to themselves and others, as in the case of engineers, doctors, nurses, and people who drive cars. Critically reflecting on the connection between power and knowledge opens the space for more people and their knowledge(s) to have a voice. But the multiplicity of voices is only one aspect. The most important aspect is the connection between power and knowledge. If one has some (fluid) notion of social justice (see Gore 1993), then it is important to recognise that in any moment the knowledge being sung up is connected to the positions and the identities of those who are speaking and the discourses that grant them this position in the first place. Part of the ethical responsibility of any profession in which one has a consultant role in people's lives is to be aware of, and to sing up, this process.

We have referred to Foucault often, as we consider that he has opened the space for us to see alternatives to the previously unquestioned divisions and privileging of ways of seeing (see especially Foucault 1973). He has allowed us to see that the sciences of man are grounded not in foundations (a reality) outside of themselves but on a set of social practices that emerge from certain regimes of truth. We are thus not able to say that we have found a more truthful way of thinking about knowledge; we can only suggest that we have pointed to alternatives that open the way for other voices to be heard and other ways of doing to be revealed. Hopefully, this will help people to develop 'a politics of suspicion' (following Lyotard 1993) about the practices that privilege some discourses at the price of silencing others, privileging some people at the price of silencing many.

References

Byrne-Armstrong, H. (1999) *Dead certainties and local knowledge: Poststructuralism, conflict and narrative practices in radical/experiential education*, PhD thesis, University of Western Sydney.

Bly, R. (1996) *The Sibling Society*, William Heinemann, Melbourne.

Davies, B. (1994) *Poststructuralist Theory and Classroom Practice*, Deakin University Press, Australia.

Foucault, M. (1973) *The Order of Things: An Archaeology of the Human Sciences,* Vintage/Random House, New York.

Foucault, M. (1977) The political function of the intellectual, *Radical Philosophy*, **17**, pp. 12–14.

Foucault, M. (1979) *Discipline and Punish: The Birth of the Prison* (translated by Alan Sheridan), Vintage/Random House, New York.

Foucault, M. (1980) Truth and power, in *Power/Knowledge: Selected Interviews and Writings by Michel Foucault* (ed. C. Gordon), Harvester Press, UK, pp. 109–33.

Foucault, M. (1984) What is Enlightenment?, in *The Foucault Reader* (ed. P. Rabinow), Pantheon, New York, pp. 46–59.

Gore, J. (1993) *The Struggle for Pedagogies: Critical and Feminist Discourses as Regimes of Truth,* Routledge, London.

Henriques, J., Hollway, W., Urwin, C., Venn, C. & Walkerdine, W. (1986) (reissue) *Changing the Subject: Psychology, Social Regulation and Subjectivity*, Routledge, London.

Horsfall, D. (1998) *The subalterns speak: A collaborative inquiry into community participation in community health care*, PhD thesis, University of Western Sydney.

Kolb, D. (1984) *Experiential Learning*, Prentice Hall, New York.

Lather, P. (1989) *Deconstructing/deconstructive inquiry: The politics of knowing and being known*, paper presented at the American Education Research Association Annual Conference, San Francisco, March, pp. 25–35.

Lather, P. (1991) *Getting Smart: Feminist Research and Pedagogy With/In the Postmodern*, Routledge, London.

Lyotard, J. (1993) Note on the Meaning of 'Post-', in *Postmodernism: A Reader* (ed. T. Docherty), Harvester Wheatsheaf, Sydney, pp. 38–46.

Michaels, E. (1990) *Unbecoming: An AIDS Diary*, Empress Pub. Sydney.

Pinkola Estes, C. (1992) *Women Who Run With the Wolves*, Rider, Sydney.

Rothwell, R. (1998) Philosophical paradigms and qualitative research, in *Writing Qualitative Research* (ed. J. Higgs), Hampden Press, Sydney, pp. 21–8.

Shor, I. (1996) *When Students Have Power: Negotiating Authority in a Critical Pedagogy*, University of Chicago Press, Chicago.

Truett Anderson, W. (1995) *The Truth About Truth: Deconstructing and Reconstructing the Postmodern World*, Tarcher Putman, New York.

Chapter 8
Exploring Relationships in Health Care Practice

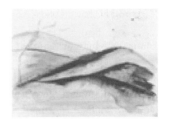

Dawn Best, Rosemary Cant and Susan Ryan

In health care the nature of the relationship we have with our patients is critical to the helping process (Davis 1998). Yet, as French (1997) reminds us, there is no such thing as one single ideal professional–patient relationship, since the type of relationship will depend on a number of factors. The most important of these relate to the individual client and professional, the client's condition and the specific situation.

In this chapter we explore professional relationships using frameworks from sociology to identify features of such relationships, and illustrate these with stories from professional practice. We also acknowledge that contemporary professional practice demands a much broader range of relationships than just that between practitioner and client. Relationships must also be established with government and nongovernment bodies, administrators and managers, colleagues, students, community workers, volunteers, carers and families. The practitioner must relate not just to the client but also to the community and other collectivities.

Professional practice is not static, but reflects the knowledge, attitudes and pressures of the time. It is constantly being modified to adjust to workplace issues. This chapter describes contemporary client practitioner health care relationships and concludes by identifying the current pressures on practice and the challenges for practitioners which will impact on interactions in the future.

A framework for professional client relationships

Talcott Parsons (1951) provides a useful framework for analysing professional client relationships. He identifies different characteristics or patterns of relationships which he calls pattern variables. These variables enable us to clearly distinguish the relationships between practitioners and their clients and to contrast them with, for example, relationships between two family members. His analysis serves to classify relationships as well as to pinpoint locations of contradiction, tension, stress and confusion in the roles people play. Parsons identifies the following pattern variables, naming them in terms of their different ends or poles:

- Affectivity/affective neutrality
- Universalism/particularism
- Ascription/achievement
- Self orientation/orientation to the collectivity
- Specificity/diffuseness.

If we consider the relationship between a mother, Beth, and her eldest son Jeff in terms of these pattern variables, Beth loves her son Jeff; that is, the relationship is suffused with emotion (affectivity). Beth loves Jeff because he is her child and not any other child and vice versa (particularism). Beth loves Jeff because he is her child (ascription) and not because of how clever he is (achievement). The family relationship between Beth and her son Jeff is functionally diffuse; that is, the relationship covers many different types of situation. The relationship is nurtured because it is fulfilling (self-orientation). On the other hand if we consider the relationship between Dr Brook and her client Jeff, Dr Brook's relationship with Jeff lacks emotional content (affective neutrality). Dr Brook relates to Jeff in the same way as she relates to Tom, Dick, and Harriette who are also her clients (universalism). Dr Brook manages the health problems which arise from Jeff's cystic fibrosis but is not concerned with Jeff's school problems or his sporting achievements (the relationship is functional specific). Dr Brook orders tests and treatment for Jeff not on the basis that this will increase her income but because she is concerned with what is best for Jeff and society (orientation to the collectivity).

For many children with chronic conditions, their therapy is carried out by therapists and other health practitioners as well as by their mothers. Mothers then are quasi-therapists, a position they often find tricky to negotiate precisely because their relationship with their child is different from that which the practitioners have with the child. We have just noted these differences in terms of Beth and her son Jeff, in contrast with those of Dr Brook and her client Jeff. Let us use pattern variables to push these differences a little further in order that the nuances of the relationship between the professional and the client become clearer.

Affectivity/affective neutrality

Affectivity/affective neutrality concerns the level of emotion or affect that is appropriate in an encounter. Affectivity is the motivational orientation of parent and child, while neutrality is usually accepted as a requirement of the health professional's encounter with each, although the emotional labour of professional caregiving is increasingly being recognised. Here we should distinguish between friendliness and friendship (Downie *et al.* 1974). Friendliness is usually considered an important part of the health professional's practice skills, while the special commitment of friendship, with its emotional overlay, has often been discouraged. Emotional detachment has been regarded as important if the practitioner is to engage in appropriate clinical reasoning, but recent literature repositions affectivity as an important part of the skilled practitioner's stance (May 1991; Titchen 2000). Titchen's (2000) work demonstrates how skilled companions bring their emotions therapeutically into their relationships with patients, at the same time protecting themselves against stressful or incapacitating over-involvement.

Special bonds between practitioner and client may exist, providing emotional support for the client, not as client but as adult person. Shared illness, accident or disability experiences between practitioners and clients may also facilitate easy rapport, even attachment, as well as deeper levels of understanding, as will be seen in the subsequent discussion. Schwartzberg (1992) reminds us that the sharing of similar stories with another can be a powerful influence on that person. By telling something about ourselves in a like situation we are giving the other person a message that we are trying to understand how they feel because we have experienced it as well.

Universalism/particularism

Parsons' view of the practitioner role was a traditional one. He saw it as proper that universalism characterises clinical encounters; that the practitioner's responsibility to the patient should be in terms of a set of professional principles rather than a particular loyalty to a particular client. He believed that the skills of the practitioner are applied regardless of client or status: that each case should receive the same attention. Although we might aspire to this, many of us reflecting honestly on our practice would probably concede that our practice does not reach the ideal. We are drawn to some clients, usually those whose problems resonate with us because we identify with them; we can imagine ourselves in their shoes; they are like us, or like people we know.

In comparison to the universalism approach, families may value particularism in clinicians. In a study of mothers of children with disabilities, Cant (1994) found that particularism, where it was perceived, was welcomed. Clients want to be perceived as special. Some of the mothers had chosen their GPs because of the opportunity for special treatment. 'Our GP is wonderful. He has been most helpful with Rochelle' (Cant 1991, p. 142).

Analysis of the teacher–student relationship has pertinence in the context of health care relationships. Downie *et al.* (1974) suggest that there are three ways of regarding clients as humans: first, clients as generic human selves; second, clients as idiosyncratic selves; and third, clients as general types or classes of person. Humanity in the first sense involves the notion that clients are persons rather than things. It implies that the practitioner should be reactive to them as persons as well as reacting to them just in terms of their medical condition. Relating to clients in the second sense, as idiosyncratic selves, involves a greater commitment than is usual in the client–practitioner relationship. This is the nature of the skilled companionship role that Titchen (2000) advocates. What many clients often want is that the practitioner takes an interest in them as individuals, an interest which would not be shown to others; that is, the relationship would take on the additional layer that is typical of friendship, an issue explored above. For some clients, however, this individual interest is unwanted, and functional specificity or a relationship similar to a trader relationship is preferred. This issue is discussed further below.

The third way of regarding clients as human, by recognising them as general types, recognises a client's special needs as a member of a particular class of people. Thus sensitive practice recognises that male practitioners may be unacceptable to middle eastern women, and that older men may prefer older male practitioners.

Relationship categories based on shared gender, shared experience, shared class or race and so on are often valuable but give rise to a mass of contradictions, complexities, and tensions in practitioner–client relationships. Health professionals' codes of ethics therefore are wary of encouraging such other relationships alongside the therapeutic one. However, it remains an anomaly that they countenance the existence of a financial relationship existing alongside and indeed argue that a financial relationship enhances the therapeutic one.

Finally, it is apparent that this kind of sensitive practice which incorporates aspects of both universality and particularity presents difficulties. Since one practitioner does not relate equally well with all clients, we need health professionals with a diversity of personal characteristics which enable them to relate to clients in the contemporary world. Moreover, as Binnie and Titchen's (1999) study shows, a conducive culture and effective personal and professional development support in the workplace facilitate close and even loving relationships with 'unpopular patients'.

Ascription/achievement

Parsons' pattern variable of ascription/achievement concerns whether qualities attracting different behaviours are attached to ascribed status or allocated on the basis of performance. This variable at one end of the scale focuses on who the person is and the expected behaviours arising from that, and at the other end of the scale on the actual performance. Parsons assumed that medical decisions would be based on objective diagnoses and scientific reasoning. The client's achievements should not render some individuals more worthy of treatment than others. Class (an achieved status), income or insurance status should be irrelevant to the decisions made. However, where health care resources are rationed, responses may take into account clients' ability to pay, their culpability for their illness or their compliance with exercises or lifestyle changes.

Self orientation/orientation to the collectivity

Therapists tend to be censorious where clients do not follow their directions. 'Mothers lie to me. They say they do the exercises and they don't,' a speech pathology student reported. The mother was self-oriented in that she was perhaps lying to preserve her child's access to a rationed service. The therapy student believed that her time would be better spent with a more compliant client. What may be missed by the therapist is the range of other factors which affect the client's behaviour. The child may react so badly to having to do the exercises that the mother may feel that persisting will endanger her relationship with the child. She may also have conflicting instructions from other members of the health care team. The paradox of a parent's position is that the orientation required as parent tends to be the opposite of that required as co-therapist. This may lead to role strain. It may be difficult for the parent to be emotionally neutral while giving treatment. This difficulty was recognised by the parents of children with cystic fibrosis, who through their voluntary association fought for and obtained home help to administer the daily prescribed physiotherapy treatment (Cant 1991).

Functional specificity/diffuseness and the professional agenda

In the earlier example, the speech pathologist was acting with functional specificity, unconcerned with anything outside the child's speech progress. The functional specificity that Parsons saw as appropriate for the practitioner–client relationship is often less applicable to some health care roles than others. The changing nature of illness is seen in an increase in chronic conditions for which there is no cure, but which are improved by the intervention of a number of health professionals. In addition, family care, support and therapy administered or supervised by family members are important to client well-being. High functional specificity, where orientations and obligations are narrow and specific rather than extensive and diffuse, is common in medical encounters with specialists and to a lesser extent with speech and physiotherapists. It is lower in encounters with GPs and occupational therapists, where the focus of practice may be less specific.

A lack of functional specificity in medical encounters was noted by Fisher and Todd (1986) in their study of the negotiations between doctors and clients of decisions to use oral contraception. They describe the way in which both medical and nonmedical matters of lifestyle choices were interleaved, and the irritation of many patients at this approach. In other situations, specificity may result in noncompliance because the practitioner fails to appreciate the complexity of the client's situation. Where there is a relationship between practitioner, mother and child, or practitioner, wife and husband the situation will usually be more complex than a clinician–client relationship. This complexity can be partly attributed to the family member's position as both co-worker and co-client. Practitioners often view mothers as clients, while the mother's perception of her role is that of co-health worker.

We propose that life experiences of practitioners may help them to appreciate the complexity of their clients' situations. Empathy can develop between people because they have had similar experiences, as discussed earlier. Practitioners may recognise certain features of the situation that others with less practical exposure fail to notice. For instance, a baby's cry may send particular messages to an experienced listener. A nursing study by Holden and Klingner (1988) found that paediatric specialists and students with their own children could identify the causes of the baby's cries, whereas students without children were not able to discern these differences. This practical experience creates an immediate bond of understanding. Others who have not shared such experience, nor had sufficient experience working in like situations, have to develop empathy in other ways.

Responding to change

The frameworks used in the discussion in this chapter are micro-approaches which focus on the characteristics of the interactions themselves. Macro-approaches focus on the importance of social structures in understanding the social world, and complement the previous approaches. The most significant macro tools of analysis are class, gender, age and ethnicity. Many changes in society challenge our past assumptions about relationships in practice. The next section identifies some of the current key issues facing practitioners.

Responding to social change in the recruitment and selection of health care practitioners

There has always been an apparent divide between the persons administering health care and those receiving it. In Europe in the early centuries this duty fell to the lay brothers in monasteries who administered hospitality to travellers and the poor in the hospitals. Through the centuries, health care became more specialised and doctors with particular knowledge became the professionals. From the beginning, society granted professionals positions of considerable trust. They had autonomy to do what they considered right, at the right time in the right way (Fish & Coles 1998). Being well-educated, they came from the upper-classes which were able to afford the lengthy education demanded. In the twentieth century, with further emancipation and wider educational possibilities, the middle classes entered medical education and the newly created therapies developed. This broadening of educational opportunities has continued at a varying pace in different countries throughout the world.

The issue of class is also relevant to ethnicity. French and Vernon (1997) highlight the difficulties in providing health care services for people from different racial backgrounds. In addition to the obvious barriers imposed by language, disabled people from ethnic minority groups may not know about available services or facilities, or the service may be inappropriate to the beliefs and attitudes of their culture. Whilst governments typically support main-streaming of health services as an efficient method of delivery, effective service delivery may require ethnospecific services. As communities grapple with implementation of equal opportunity legislation, it is clear this would be much easier if the multiracial mix of communities came to be reflected in graduates from health science programmes. A challenge is presented, to nurture secondary students from disadvantaged groups so that they too have access to tertiary training.

Utilising technological advances

The end of the twentieth century heralds a new age of communication that will affect relationships of all kinds, including those in health care. According to Neubauer (1998), there is an increasing unification and interconnectedness among nations and between those citizens fortunate enough to own and use technologies such as e-mail and the internet. However, there is competing inequality in respect of those who do not have such resources or who are not literate in their use.

In the USA and other western countries many elderly and disabled people who are confined to their homes have found new chat groups on e-mail list-servers. Different educational interactive courses on the internet provide learning and social opportunities undreamed of before the advent of this technology. Access to the most up-to-date medical knowledge is available to all who have this tech-nology. The easy access to knowledge and the opportunities for telemedicine and videoconferencing shift the parameters of the client–practitioner relationship. The art of developing rapport via satellite presents a new challenge.

Adapting to the changing economics of health care

The costs of health service delivery have escalated internationally. Although countries have addressed this funding crisis differently, many have adopted health service reforms which focus on strategies to increase efficiency and contain costs. International trends include the restructuring of facilities, contracting services out and the rationalisation of services. Many countries have adopted a system of prospective funding based on the USA casemix classification system. This system calculates health care cost according to diagnostically-related groups (DRGs). These homogeneous groupings assume that all people with the same diagnosis cost the same. When funding relates to the resources needed for managing a diagnosis rather than the specific health care requirements of an individual patient, practice is defined by the management protocols developed for that diagnosis, that is, the critical pathway, but not necessarily one related to individual needs.. One of the effects of casemix funding is an increased throughput. Patients are discharged from acute care facilities after shorter hos-pital stays. In terms of Parsons' pattern-variable framework, it is being demanded of practitioners that they consider the interests of the collectivity, as well as the interests of their patients. The collectivity provides the funds which underwrite the costs of health care. Managed care and funding, based on DRGs, attempts to balance self orientation with orientation to the collectivity, but caught in the middle are the practitioners.

Ferguson (1998) interviewed occupational and physiotherapists working in Melbourne in acute hospitals after radical restructuring and funding cuts. She reports that the changes created a workplace where there was little time: 'We barely have time to tell them our names'. The practitioners felt they could find out from the patient only what they needed to know, not what the patient needed them to know. With such limitations on time, these clinicians felt that the relationship critical to the recovery process was in jeopardy: 'No-one has enough time to care these days. Decision-making is made on the run with a focus on time and money.' The clinicians reported a change in priorities – the patients are not a priority: 'Well we'll have to start looking at the patients as not a priority, and I can't quite come to grips with that.' The focus on throughput inherent to this system becomes the bed: 'The bed has become the focus rather than who's in bed' (Ferguson 1998). Such depersonalisation takes Parsons' affective neutrality pattern variable to a new dimension.

Ferguson's study identified the emergence of new roles which were based on much more generic skills. The clinicians described a triage approach where patients were assessed with little attention to their needs. An increased predominance of assessment skills with less opportunity to follow up with management and discharge resulted in a decrease in job satisfaction: 'All I do is assessment only [not the] treatment part and I feel I am a bit disconnected from what happens to the client at the end of the process.' (Ferguson 1998.)

Adopting a corporate approach to health care

Compton and Robinson (1997) believe establishing a culture that is customer focused is the greatest challenge for allied health professionals. Their definition recognises that there are internal and external customers who affect and are affected by work processes. They recommend health professionals shift their focus on profession and service delivery to customer needs. This notion, adapted from large scale industry management, defines customer focus within a set of best practice principles which aim to improve productivity and quality with a focus on the customer. However, there is a fundamental difference in health care, since the practice of health professionals is also dominated by a duty of care, which presumes that their actions will be in the best interests of the patient.

A legal perspective is provided by Tucker (1998, p. 373). He views the doctor–patient relationship as highly complex, with unclear obligations to patients:

'Diverse legal and social influences have seen this relationship alter in a significant and sometimes conflicting manner due to the application of fundamentally different legal doctrines.'

Whatever the legal issues, it is obvious that practice today demands that the practitioner–patient relationship also involves many other relationships. Christianson and Baum (1997, p. 593) clarify some of these relationships in their definition of 'client centred' as:

> 'a collaborative relationship between individuals in the client's environment (family, teachers, independent living specialists, employers, neighbours, friends) to assist the client to obtain skills and make modifications to remove barriers that would create social disadvantage.'

Not only does this definition extend the range of external clients, it also provides for a diffuse scope of practice. Yet the shift of responsibility to the client may result in the instigation of short term contacts developed between practitioners and clients for specific health care management. Such a move would significantly move practice relationships on Parsons' specificity/diffuseness pattern variable towards more closely defined practice objectives.

In best practice language, 'internal customers' refers to the other members of the health care team as well as the administrative and general staff involved. The reality for those working in acute care environments after radical funding cuts indicates the difficulty of communicating internally:

> 'There is conflict between different disciplines because everyone is under pressure to discharge. The nursing staff are under pressure as well to get people out of hospital so they are pressuring the doctors who are pressuring us ... it is all part of a vicious circle and everyone, instead of working together and trying to get someone home as quickly as possible, everyone is blaming everyone else for reasons that they are not being discharged and it's a huge and real communication problem.'
>
> (Ferguson 1998, p. 116)

Davis (1998) outlines the effect that managed care has had on health care delivery in the USA. Although it has brought about cost containment and shifted the burden of responsibility to patients and their families, it has also produced ethical dilemmas for practitioners. When health care as a service is managed as a business, and access to treatment is controlled by prepaid health organisations, practitioners may be torn between ethical responsibilities to clients and contractual obligations to the funding organisations. In such a climate the relationship between the practitioners and those who fund the service becomes as important as the therapeutic relationship between client and practitioner.

Conclusion

Traditionally the primary focus of health care delivery has been on the important relationship between client and practitioner. We have explored some of the complexities and the attendant tensions of this relationship, and the value and dangers of a multilayered relationship between practitioner and client. The focus was broadened to analyse relationships of family members with clients, a different type of therapeutic relationship. Practitioners need to understand the interests not just of the family, but also of other stakeholders in the practitioner–client relationship. However, economic reform has had dramatic effects on practice. The primary patient–practitioner relationship is under threat and in some cases has already changed. On the one hand, there is a move to a more collaborative relationship in client-focused or even customer-focused care; on the other, this move is threatened by governments more tightly controlling resources. How this move is eventually reconciled with the concurrent funding reforms remains to be seen. It seems certain that if practitioners are to have any control in the new system, it is vital they develop closer relationships with policy makers and health funding bodies.

References

Binnie, A. & Titchen, A. (1999) *Freedom to Practise: The Development of Patient-Centred Nursing*, Butterworth Heinemann, Oxford.

Cant, R. (1991) *Tending work*, PhD thesis, University of Newcastle.

Cant, R. (1994) Just caregiving. Whose work? Whose control?, in *Just Health: Inequality in Illness, Care and Prevention* (eds C. Wardell & A. Petersen), Churchill Livingstone, South Melbourne, pp 257–70.

Christianson, C. & Baum, C. (eds) (1997) *Occupational Therapy: Enabling Function and Well-Being*, Slack, Thorofare, NJ.

Compton, J. & Robinson, M. (1997) *National Allied Health Best Practice Industry Report*, Commonwealth Department of Health and Family Services, Commonwealth Government Printer, Canberra.

Davis, C. (1998) *Patient Practitioner Interaction*, Slack, Thorofare, NJ.

Downie, R.S., Loudfoot, E.M. & Telfer, E. (1974) *Education and Personal Relationships*, Methuen, London.

Ferguson, K. (1998) *The nexus of health reform and health professional practice: narratives of health professionals in times of change*, DEd Dissertation, Graduate School of Education, La Trobe University, Bundoora.

Fish, D. & Coles, C. (1998) *Developing Professional Judgment in Health Care: Learning Through the Critical Appreciation of Practice*, Butterworth-Heinemann, Oxford.

Fisher, S. & Todd, A.D. (1986) *Discourse and Institutional Authority: Medicine, Education and Law*, Ablex Publishing, Norwood.

French, S. (1997) Why do people become patients?, in *Physiotherapy: A Psychosocial approach* (ed. S. French), Butterworth-Heinemann, Oxford, pp. 104–19.

French, S. & Vernon, A. (1997) Health care for people from minority groups, in *Physiotherapy: A Psychosocial Approach* (ed. S. French), Butterworth-Heinemann, Oxford, pp. 59–72

Holden, G. & Klingner, A. (1988) Learning from experience: Differences in how novice vs.

expert nurses diagnose why an infant is crying, *Journal of Nursing Education*, **27**(1), pp. 23–29.

May, C. (1991) Affective neutrality and involvement in nurse-patient relationships: Perceptions of appropriate behaviour among nurses in acute medical and surgical wards, *Journal of Advanced Nursing*, **17**, pp. 552–8.

Neubauer, D. (1998) *Impacts of Globalization on Health and Health Care Policy*, Occasional Paper No. 1, Centre for Professional Education Advancement, The University of Sydney.

Parsons, T. (1951) *The Social Science System*, Free Press, Glencoe.

Schwartzberg, S. (1992) *Self disclosure and empathy in occupational therapy*, paper presented to the Occupational Therapy Conference, Dublin, Ireland.

Titchen, A. (2000) *Professional Craft Knowledge in Patient-Centred Nursing and the Facilitation of its Development*, University of Oxford DPhil thesis, Ashdale Press, Oxford.

Tucker, P. (1998) Good faith: In search of a unifying principle for the doctor patient relationship, *Journal of Law and Medicine*, **5**, pp. 327–91.

Chapter 9
Technology and the Depersonalisation of Knowledge and Practice

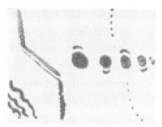

Charles Higgs

The context and processes of tertiary professional education world-wide are undergoing constant and major change. One factor which effects these changes is technology, particularly the technology associated with communication and learning. This chapter explores the effects of technology and current practices in the marketplace and education system on the creation and utilisation of knowledge. The principal arguments presented are firstly that technology can either serve or enslave its users; it is not neutral and has effects that can be depersonalising. Similarly the shift in focus away from the needs of the individual to the needs of the marketplace is potentially depersonalising of both knowledge and practice. Secondly, it is argued that professional practice and education need to be primarily about people, not economics, and technology needs to be used as a tool in these settings, not an end in itself.

Changing patterns in education

We are experiencing an era where information overload is becoming the norm and the rapid rate of change in our lives is reaching a crisis point for many people. Education systems are rushing headlong into 'on-line learning', 'location-independent learning' and 'flexible delivery'. At the same time we are seeing the emergence of the business model of education management with its penchant for 'economic rationalism', 'downsizing' and 'resizing'. Notwithstanding the potential merits (e.g. greater access and convenience for students) of flexible delivery, the combination of freer but more technology-dependent modes of education with economic constraints can result in technocentric learning systems which are depersonalised. Already, we are seeing in many places a shift away from academic control of education to managerial control, and a paradigmatic shift away from the pedagogical needs of the individual to the needs of the marketplace.

Universities are forming stronger links with industries and, with governmental support, industries are gaining greater control of vocational education curricula (see Fooks 1998). ('Vocational' in this chapter refers to career-oriented education across both the technical and higher education sectors.) With so many vested interests there is a potential conflict between what people should learn in order to meet specific industry needs and what world-wide society needs people to learn. Industrial sponsorship or underwriting of educational programmes can result in calls (or demands) for tailor-made graduates to enter directly into the sponsor's workplace without the need for specific on-the-job training or workplace socialisation by the employer. By comparison, society needs flexible, adaptable multitalented graduates capable of problem-solving and engaging in lifelong learning to meet the needs of a variety of workplaces over their working lives.

A principal goal of higher education is 'the education of appropriately qualified ... (persons) to enable them to take a leadership role in the intellectual, cultural, economic and social development of the nation and all its regions' (Higher Education Council 1992, p.12). Central to the achievement of this outcome is the expectation that students will acquire not only discipline-specific knowledge and skills, but also a range of generic skills relevant to these broader goals of higher education. Similarly, in the technical education sector graduates need to acquire skills in flexibility, workplace adaptation and self-directed learning to manage their career paths and continue to expand their work-related competencies. Increasingly, the community expects both types of graduate to be skilled in interacting with people as well as competent in technical work areas.

Technology and information

At the beginning of the new millennium there is increasing speculation as to how the world will look and what our lives will be like in the future. Will the global community bring us significant improvements or will the future be as bleak as some predict? What is the place (positive or otherwise) of technology and information processes in this new world?

Neil Postman (1985), in the introduction to *Amusing Ourselves to Death*, considers the information revolution in the light of two visionary books, George Orwell's *Nineteen Eighty-four* and Aldous Huxley's *Brave New World*. In *Nineteen Eighty-four* Orwell presented a world in which the masses were controlled by 'Big Brother', whose tyrannical suppression was built upon the action of hiding the truth from the people. When 1984 came and went we breathed a collective sigh of relief and continued to rush headlong into the technology revolution. Huxley's concern in *Brave New World* was that the truth would be made irrelevant through information overload within a societal framework dominated by entertainment and leisure. Postman (1985, p. vii) writes, 'Huxley feared those who would give us so much (information) that we would be reduced to passivity and egoism'.

Today we are experiencing an agglomeration of the Orwellian notion of Big Brother's information management/control and the Huxleyan notion of information overload. We have access to such a quantity of information that we are becoming increasingly reliant upon technology to help us manage, filter, process and make use of available information.

Such is the nature of the rapid rate of change in today's western society that the technology revolution is already being supplanted by the information revolution. Technology is becoming a ubiquitous tool and knowledge is no longer just 'power', knowledge is becoming the new currency. The management of information and knowledge is not merely a critical business tool, it is also potentially the means of mass manipulation and propaganda. Examples of this are the influence of global broadcasting empires such as CNN or, closer to home, the influence of the Fairfax and Murdoch presses. Waitley (1995, p. 8) describes these new empires and their relationship to knowledge as follows: 'We must understand that the empires of the future will not be built of concrete, with walls of stone, turrets, armies and gates. The empires of the future will be empires of the mind.'

Data and information form the building blocks of our knowledge creation and we have greater access to data and information in western society today than ever before. Technology has enhanced this access, and CD-ROM databases, on-line library access and the internet are only a few examples of how this 'brave new world' of technology can aid us. The volume of information is reaching such proportions that we not only need technology to access the data but are becoming increasingly reliant on technology and software to help filter, transmit and manage the information. Data General's *Managing Business and Technology Change for Success in the New Global Economy* demonstrates the impact of software on the information revolution: 'Business spent US$1 trillion on information technology in the last decade – but showed little gain in efficiency. Now, productivity is finally bursting out, thanks to better software and reorganization of work itself' (Data General 1996, p. 1).

People filter information based on their personal and social frame(s) of reference. This information is then utilised in testing hypotheses, challenging existing beliefs and creating new knowledge. In a postmodern epistemological (knowledge generation) perspective, our individual world views allow for the existence of multiple realities and inter-subjective frameworks for viewing the world. But what happens when our epistemologies become influenced by technology? Technologies (e.g. the internet) have an inherent *Weltanschauung* (world view) which impacts upon its users. For example, Becker and Dwyer (1998) found that groupware (computer software and hardware for group decision-making and communication) enhanced the learning of students who had a visual learning style while students 'who preferred learning more verbally found significantly less enhancement from the use of groupware and did not feel that the groupware helped the project process as much' (Becker & Dwyer 1998, p. 1). In this example the use of groupware technology favoured the learning style that was congruent with groupware's inherent world view. In addition, groupware enhanced the learning of visual learners who were also computer literate and had access to the technology. Talbott (1998) suggests technology will have a detrimental effect on modern education if we allow it to be used inappropriately. Although there are many benefits to be had from the use of technology in education, there are associated risks. By its nature the:

> 'central focus of information technology upon the reliable, precise, and quantifiable transmission of well-defined bits from one place to another, and the emphasis upon algorithmic procedures for manipulating this information, accord perfectly with
> - the 'shovelling facts' style of education;
> - the increasingly cosy relationship between education and businesses, whose primary concern has more to do with operational effectiveness than with depth of understanding; and
> - the rigid 'credentialization' and standardization of society, which, in turn, amounts to a denial of the life of the individual.'
>
> (Talbott 1998, pp. 6,7)

There are many proponents of the use of technology in education but for the purposes of this argument I have chosen to consider the associated risks and not the benefits. Technology is not neutral and unbiased, and it raises significant issues regarding standards, privileges and access. An excellent example is to consider technology from a gender perspective: 'Men have more computers, spend more time with them, and are more the dominating presence in cyberspace.' (Spender 1995, p. 166). At best only 30% of the internet population is female (Lowe 1996) and only 20% married women with children (Roy Morgan Research Centre Pty Ltd 1996). Similarly, the question of access is of concern as only a small percentage of the world's population has access to a computer, leaving a distinct imbalance between those with and without access to the information revolution.

The imposition of technology's inherent technocentric perspective, information volume and business' reductionist/objectivist perspective creates a volatile situation where people are being alienated from their work practices, and their ownership of knowledge is being depersonalised. 'Our advanced technological society is rapidly making objects of us and subtly programming us into conformity to the logic of its system. To the degree that this happens, we are also becoming submerged in a new "culture of silence"' (Shaull 1970, p. 15, in the foreword to Paulo Freire's *Pedagogy of the Oppressed*). The influence of lack of neutrality of technology is in part a question of how technology is used. Freire recognised that technology and the media could be used as tools of emancipation and enlightenment as well as oppression.

Managerialism in education

Historically, education has been accused of being insular and slow to adapt to the changing needs of society. This has been the catch-cry of those opposed to education being controlled by academe. As the managerial model replaces the academic model in our educational institutes we are seeing a growth in 'business-run' schools and privatised research departments and a decline in general and liberal education courses. Critics say Melbourne University's proposed plan to set up a private body will be its undoing. The Postgraduate Association, for instance, says the university has been 'overtaken by corporate-driven lust' (*The Bulletin* (Education Section) 25/08/98, p. 44). For some, such a move, in the face of substantial reductions in government funding, could be seen as economic necessity or survival, or indeed a far-sighted plan for prosperity. In the context of this discussion, the key issue is the impact of the management structure and ethos on the way *people* learn.

Modern managerial practices have supplanted people as the centre of our educational focus and have focused on the needs of the marketplace as opposed to the needs of the community. This focus is often based on reductionism and objectivism and is, to some extent, diametrically opposed to a holistic 'people' focus. In *Who's killing higher education? (or is it suicide?)* Talbott (1998, p. 7) suggests that the ultimate extension of modern educational management practices, coupled with information technology, is a model of education that leaves 'little room for schools or, ultimately, students'.

Green (1998, p. 38) reinforces the view that universities need to be cautious in their adoption of the managerial model of education. 'The purpose of universities is to foster learning and independent thought in that we may understand ourselves and our world as conscious human beings. This requires that we constantly work to maintain some spaces in our individual lives and in our society which are not dominated by the money-market-management mantra.'

An example of this humanistic objective is the current debate about training and education. Training meets the immediate needs of business whereas education has a long-term focus to meet the needs of people today and in the future. 'The primary direction of change for students ... is away from learning-to-learn skills, and towards techniques that will be obsolete in the short run. This trend is disastrous because the world is now changing so fast that people who do not develop learning-to-learn skills will inevitably be marginalised' (Theobald 1998).

Freire (1970) describes the 'culture of silence' that prevailed in Brazil earlier in the twentieth century as the direct result of educational oppression. Educational oppression can take many forms, one of which is censorship. The corporatisation of education is a form of inverted censorship. The needs of business and the marketplace are promoted in our education systems in preference to the needs of humanity. This is seen, for instance, in the emphasis placed on competencies and the 'hard' sciences in vocational and professional education and in the intro-duction of vocational training curricula in high school.

The humanities and the notions of liberal education and education for life are hit hard by this marketplace trend. Nussbaum (1997, p. 38), for instance, writes of American University courses, '...I have also found, and more frequently, a large number of creative proposals that promise a rich future for democracy – if only they could continue to receive the institutional and social support they require.' Nussbaum suggests that an increasing emphasis on vocational training and 'mean-spirited attacks on the humanities' threaten these proposals.

With so many vested interests in the funding and outcomes of vocational education the corporatisation of education must impact on academic freedom. 'By academic freedom I understand the right to search for truth and to publish and teach what one holds to be true. This right implies also a duty: one must not conceal any part of what one has recognised to be true. It is evident that any restriction on academic freedom acts in such a way as to hamper the dis-semination of knowledge among the people and thereby impedes national judgement and action' (Albert Einstein, attrib. in Lewis 1997). In this age of accountability, it is evident that academic freedom cannot (and should not) be an absolute freedom to teach in the absence of any control. Rather freedom must be mirrored by responsibility to the good of society. Thus the loss of academic freedom is not just the mourning of privileged individuals, but also a shifting of the responsibility for the fostering and management of learning and the gen-eration of knowledge from the academic 'knowledge-generators' to the business 'knowledge-controllers'.

The managerial tightrope: commercial interests versus educational integrity

The fostering of learning and academic freedom comes at a price and the goal for academic administrators is to achieve a balance between the needs of the uni-versities for revenue and patronage from the private sector on the one hand, and protecting academic integrity on the other. Considerable pressures are being placed on the universities to accommodate the requirements of the private sector in their curricula (Noble 1997, 1998; Talbott 1998). A recent survey by *Computerworld* magazine found that 'the latest trend (for companies) is to negotiate outsourcing contracts [using an external contractor to provide support services] in which a university provides courses and technical degrees customized for a particular business. In fact, 40% of large corporate training groups planned to create "corporate/university partnerships" in 1998, according to a survey of 100 business trainers' (Ouellette 1998, p. 1).

Many universities world-wide are commercialising their research. Research that was 'formerly pursued as an end in itself or as a contribution to human knowledge, now became a means to commercial ends and researchers become implicated, directly or indirectly and wittingly or not, in the business of making money for their university' (Noble 1998, p. 1). The commercialisation of research is a complex issue, as the need for a university to generate income in order to provide quality education has to be considered in these times of economic rationalism, yet how far should a university go? Many institutions are now commercialising their 'core instructional function, the very heart and soul of academia' (Noble 1998, p. 1). This certainly is a watershed in academia, with corporate interests now impacting upon the very core of higher education. John Ralston Saul (1995, p. 179) suggests that 'the sensible thing for the University community to do now would be to turn away from its self-interest in order to take on a leadership role ... They might discover that disinterested action of this sort would strengthen the role of the universities by pulling them away from colla-boration with the corporatist model. Back towards the wider obligation of humanism'.

The Taylorian approach to knowledge

Two distinct streams have emerged within organisation theory (Hatch 1997). One of these, typified by the works of Durkheim, Weber and Marx, is the sociological stream, focused on the social issues associated with society and the impact of industrialisation. The second stream is the classical management theory that was shaped by Taylor, Fayol and Barnar, among others. Frederick Winslow Taylor was the founder of scientific management, a system that used scientific methods to discover the most efficient working techniques for manual forms of labour. Using the scientific method, Taylor shifted the focus from the worker to the manager. Henry Ford's Model T car production line was an excellent example of Taylorism in practice, as each worker had a unique task in the production line. 'Taylor's system undermined the authority of the workers and their master craftsmen by introducing managerial control and supervision.' (Hatch 1997, p. 30). Taylorism 'failed to perceive the experiences and judgements of the workers as a source of new knowledge. Consequently, the creation of new work methods became the responsibility of managers only.' (Nonaka & Takeuchi 1995, p. 36).

The depersonalising aspect of the Taylor model has parallels in management practices today. While the working unit of an organisation may be the worker or small work team, technology is the new automation and knowledge is the new product. Once again the system has become the focal point and not the people within. As an example, Total Quality Management (TQM) has been criticised by postmodernists because of its Tayloristic practices that focus on objective measurement in preference to subjective measurement (Hatch 1997).

Many firms are now downsizing their workforces and outsourcing work, while at the same time there is a growth in the practice of flexible work practices such as working from home. While there are many benefits from being able to work flexibly there is a hidden cost. In Tayloristic fashion the worker can become just one 'node' within a greater system and these nodes have to combine to build new knowledge and practices. For instance, in some systems the task is assigned to a team, members having their input in shifts, and the final product belonging to the team or even being completed by another group. The individual loses a sense of pride and ownership in the finished product and any individual is more easily replaced.

While this approach has obvious managerial advantages it raises questions about ownership and control. Christiansson (1998, p. 1) writes of the knowledge node concept, 'this development will be even more accelerated as the globe shrinks to a global village with much higher utilization of available human resources.' Once again the focus is away from the person to the system and this approach raises the same questions of ownership, access and privilege. Some elements of the node concept are appearing in academia as teams of academics and technical support people are formed to produce flexible learning packages. Major concerns in this context are the danger of producing a technically excellent product without retaining intellectual oversight, and the potential for producing a learning programme that maximises consumer satisfaction rather than quality learning. A further concern for academics is the issue of intellectual property that is linked to individual professional responsibility as well as to individual ownership and opportunities for progression.

Taylorism is clearly being introduced into the education system in some areas. Noble (1998, p. 1) writes, 'the trend towards automation in higher education as implemented in North American Universities today is a battle between students and professors on the one side, and university administrations and companies with "educational products" to sell on the other. It is not a progressive trend towards a new era at all, but a regressive trend, towards the rather old era of mass-production, standardization and purely commercial interests'. Green (1998) argues in a similar vein that traditional teaching is being replaced by automation (e.g. internet learning and hypertext-based books), despite studies indicating that 'traditional' methods and books were preferred by students.

'Economic rationalism' appears to overtake humanitarian interests and we have to ask, 'why are we educating people?' Is it for their good, the good of the community or the good of the marketplace?

Professional response

This chapter is not meant as a 'call to arms' for cyberspace luddites, rather it is a challenge to us as professionals to consider what sort of pedagogical stance we are going to take. There are many benefits of utilising technology in our practices. As an example, the internet was a tool of academia before being commercialised, and the use of the internet and e-mail is commonplace in our universities today as tools for teaching and learning, research, administration and communication. Note though the emphasis on a *tool* of academia, not a replacement for the rich and varied range of teaching, learning and research methods available.

Noble (1997, p.3) reminds us that 'universities are not simply undergoing a technological transformation. Beneath that change, and camouflaged by it, lies another: the commercialization of higher education. For here as elsewhere technology is but a vehicle and a disarming disguise.' Thus we need to look beyond the face of technological change to the puppet masters and agendas behind the scenes. In doing so we identify that technology as a means of commercialisation, managerial models and educational Taylorism are all depersonalising our knowledge and practice. They move the emphasis away from the individual and towards the marketplace (as already shown). The paradox is that these moves benefit the privileged few (those with access to technology, knowledge and power) and disadvantage those without. The overall gain to humanity is certainly questionable and arguably negative.

Are we going to partake in this new 'culture of silence' or are we going to take a more holistic and people-centred approach? Freire's idea (in true Socratic style) was that no matter how submerged in a culture of silence, a person is capable of critically examining the world through dialogue with others. We need to openly question, debate and challenge change and strategies used in the creation of knowledge, in order to determine if they are serving the interests of humanity and not just the marketplace. Knowledge is not the property of the marketplace; it belongs to society. Also, knowledge is a dynamic phenomenon undergoing constant change and requiring personal and public validation, rather than a product or manufactured position statement to be purchased or promulgated unquestioned through education or mass media systems.

People first

Educational institutions need a supportive and flexible structure to survive in these times of change and economic constraints. Unfortunately, the dominant paradigm underpinning the management of educational institutions appears to be positivist; dominated by economic theory, objectivism and a pursuit of a 'solution' to the 'problem(s)'. These practices point towards the belief that structure and reason are of primary importance and humanist issues of secondary importance. Yet it is the people (both internal and external) and their needs that are central to education. We need to consider humanity before (but not exclusive of) economics, 'a world in which individuals have rescued control over their economic destiny' (National Board of Employment, Education and Training 1996).

We cannot operate in an ideological or environmental vacuum. We need education systems that consider equity and access issues as well as economic ones. We do not live in a perfectly objective and ordered world as the reductionist managerial model would suggest, and we have to consider education holistically as a means of growth and development, not compliance and commercial expediency.

The emphasis on tertiary education, in particular on the use of advanced technology in education, needs to shift from the reductionist cause-and-effect view to a complex, holistic, interactive system with a focus on people. Knowledge is about people. Note Denham Grey's interpretation of knowledge and its focus: 'Knowledge is the full utilization of information and data, coupled with the potential of people's skills, competencies, ideas, intuitions, commitment and motivation ... For knowledge to be of value it must be focused, current, tested and shared.' (Grey, quoted in The Knowledge Management Forum 1996, p. 1). Technology can be used successfully to promote the creation of knowledge or alternatively it can be used to depersonalise knowledge; the challenge is to use and not be used.

Conclusion

Technology has the potential to either serve us or to depersonalise our knowledge and practice. As education professionals we need to be able to function within an environment where technology is considered a tool, not an end in itself. Technology has much to offer, but it should not be seen as a replacement for sound teaching and learning practices. Technology should enhance education and not simply be used as a cheap alternative to traditional teaching practices.

Our work practices should also be seen in context. In the current climate of funding restrictions and potentially depersonalising work practices, the temptation is to focus on the economic issues and lose sight of the purpose of education. Education is about enabling people to develop the skills, knowledge and capabilities to enhance their lives and to make a contribution to society. As education professionals we need to maintain our focus on the humanistic objective where our practices, attitudes and commitments remain people-centred.

References

Becker, D. A. & Dwyer, M. (1998) *The impact of student verbal/visual learning style preference in implementing groupware in the classroom*, http://www.aln.org/alnweb/journal/vol2_issue2/becker.htm, 28/03/99.

Christiansson, P. (1998) *Knowledge communication in the building industry. The knowledge node concept*, http://www.delphi.kstr.lth.se/reports/ cibw78bled96.html, 08/07/98.

Data General (1996) *Managing business and technology change for success in the new global economy*, http://www.dg.com/technology/ white_paper/4528.html, 21/08/96.

Fooks, D. (1998) Industry partnership: Leaning on a broken reed, *Training Agenda,* **6**(3), August, pp. 15–16.

Freire, P. (1970) *Pedagogy of the Oppressed*, Continuum, New York.

Green, M. (1998) Machine minders of ACADEME, *The Australian (Higher Education Section)*, 11 March, p. 38.

Hatch, M.J. (1997) *Organization Theory: Modern Symbolic and Postmodern Perspectives*, Oxford University Press, New York.

Higher Education Council (1992) National Board of Employment, Education and Training, *Achieving Quality*, Australian Government Publishing Service, Canberra.

Lewis, M. (1997) *Eclectic Quotes from Albert Einstein*, http://www.geocities.com/Athens/Delphi/4360/q-eins.html, 23/03/99.

Lowe, S. (1996) Proof that it can be a woman's virtual world: Post-feminist guide to the Internet, *Sydney Morning Herald*, 20 August, p. 5c.

National Board of Employment, Education and Training (1996) *The development of knowledge and attitudes about career options and Australia's economic future: report of focus groups*, Commissioned Report No. 46, Australian Government Publishing Service, Canberra.

Noble, D.F. (1997) *Digital diploma mills: The automation of higher education*, http://www.firstmonday.dk/issues/issue3_1/noble/, 23/08/98.

Noble, D.F. (1998) *Digital diploma mills, Part II*, http://www.uwo.ca/uwofa/articles/di_dip_2.html, 30/03/99.

Nonaka, I. & Takeuchi, H. (1995) *The Knowledge-Creating Company*, Oxford University Press, New York.

Nussbaum, M. (1997) Democracy's wake up call, *The Australian (Higher Education Section)*, 5 November, p.38.

Ouellette, T. (1998) *Corporate training programs go to college*, http://www.computerworld.com/home/print.nsf/all/98041341FA, 31/03/99.

Postman, N. (1985) *Amusing Ourselves to Death*, Methuen, London.

Roy Morgan Research Centre Pty Ltd (1996) *Internet Usage July 1995–June 1996*.

Saul, J.R. (1995) *The Unconscious Civilization*, Penguin Books, Toronto.

Shaull, R. (1970) Foreword, in *Pedagogy of the Oppressed*, P. Freire, Continuum, New York, p. 15.

Spender, D. (1995), *Nattering on the Net: Woman, Power and Cyberspace*, Spinifex Press, Melbourne.

Talbott, S. (1998) *Who's killing higher education? (or is it suicide?)*, www.oreilly.com/people/staff/stevet/netfuture/1998/Oct1598_78.html, 23/03/99.

The Knowledge Management Forum (1996) *What is knowledge management*, http://www.3-cities.com/~bonewman/what_is.html, 08/08/96.

Theobald, R. (1998) Robert Theobald and the healing century. Program three. Learning to learn: The lifelong challenge, *Radio National Transcripts*, Radio National, Sydney.

Waitley, D. (1995) *Empires of the Mind*, William Morrow & Co., New York.

Chapter 10
The Research Sensitive Practitioner

Anne Cusick

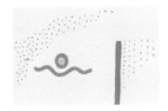

This chapter explores research as one important source of knowledge in practice. Most professionals are aware that research is a key foundation for practice. But how many practitioners actually use research to define their practice roles? How many use research findings on a daily basis or adopt research approaches to solve practice problems?

In this chapter I propose that doing practice research or using knowledge from research is an essential part of being a professional and that all practitioners should be 'research sensitive'. Research sensitive practitioners have a research orientation to practice: they have an awareness of research, and use systematic knowledge gained through research to guide their practice. Some individuals may become investigators themselves. Regardless of the research role adopted by practitioners, truly professional practice requires a sensitivity to research, as this is a defining feature of professional status. This chapter examines the rationale for and ways to achieve a research sensitive approach to practice.

Case study

Kim had been working on the clinical team for about three months. It was time for another team meeting. The team leader profiled the new clients, and the team began a discussion to allocate clients to case managers. The first client was allocated to someone notorious for hoarding his client list and refusing to refer clients on for specialist assessment and intervention. Everyone on the team knew it, but seemed to live with it to avoid unpleasant conflict such as had occurred in the past. Kim thought this was wrong as it meant that clients missed out on needed services. As the client was allocated, various team members rolled their eyes knowing they would never get to see the person. She decided today was the day she would take this issue on. 'I think I should see that client,' she said.

The team stopped their discussion and stared. This was very unusual, and she had only recently started with them. Perhaps she didn't understand how things were done. 'I beg your pardon,' said the team leader. Kim swallowed. 'I said I think I should see that client, he clearly has a need for specialist assessment, and from my experience, I can tell he will require my programme, so I want to get in and help him early by seeing him now.' The team was getting restless. 'Look,' said the leader, 'the case manager will assess and he will determine whether or not this guy needs to see you. OK?' Kim started to feel she was losing ground. 'But everyone here knows he doesn't refer. You all just sit there and complain but never do anything about it. And why did you hire me anyway – I am the expert in this field! I know when people need my services! What would he know – he is trained in a totally different area, he has almost no experience of these sort of clients, and you only have to look at the discharge profile he produces to know something funny is going on as most of them all come back!' She couldn't believe she had said what she was thinking. But it was too late to go back now.

The team was stunned. One of them looked at her sympathetically and said, 'Look, you're new, you're keen, but we have all been here a long time and we know what works. You need to use your energy to help us move forward, otherwise you'll just burn yourself out like the last two we had here.' Kim felt crushed, but more was to come. 'And look here,' said the team leader, 'you have made some pretty hard comments, and as team leader I can tell you a few home truths you should take on board before opening your mouth again. The only reason you're on the team is because management says the other centre has one and they are our main competitors. You might say you have success, but the two before you were a hopeless waste of space. What's so different about what you do? Why can you be so sure that you make a difference?' The team leader stared at the ceiling and sighed. 'Now look, we like your energy, you like your clients, and until now we have liked you. Just take a break for a few minutes, have a walk around, take a long hard look at yourself, and then perhaps you can come back in, apologise and we can get on with our business.' Kim walked out of the room. She walked around thinking. Then she was ready. She went back in.

The team seemed pretty relaxed. 'Clearly this has happened before,' she thought. 'Everyone, I'm sorry I got so heated. It wasn't the right way to go about things. And thanks for letting me know I've got potential here. But what we do, and my clients, our clients, are important to me. I think that what I said is true, and I'm going to prove it.' The team looked around at each other. 'What, another impassioned soapbox speech?' said one. 'No, I'm going to put my money where my mouth is and look at what evidence is around for what I do, what we do, and how we could be doing it better. And then I'm going to test whether it's working.' Silence. The team leader then said, 'Well good for you dear, we'll see how long that lasts. I started a research project years ago and it was just impossible with all the other things going on. You go and do that, but don't you expect I'll approve any work time for it. And you'll need to get our famous non-referring case manager on side. He's the only one here who knows anything about research. He has a PhD.'

Being in a profession

To be a member of a profession means having autonomy or independence in practice; mastery of a body of knowledge that is identified to be specialised in some way; a prerequisite educational programme; practice that can be seen as unique; a service orientation which means a focus on meeting socially important needs in the community regardless of personal reward; and special status which can be seen in the privilege or power of professionals compared to others. Professionals also work with a community of colleagues who might study in similar patterns, work in similar organisations or fields, share similar ideas and approaches and contribute to the overall development of the field through group activities and efforts, thus thinking of themselves as 'members' of a profession.

Of all these factors, the 'body of knowledge' has traditionally been considered the most important in defining, developing and directing professions (Pavalko 1971). It is critical to professional status, because without a special body of knowledge there can be no education programme to prepare professionals, no unique practice, no special privilege, no community of colleagues who share similar approaches. Without a body of knowledge there could also be no autonomy, as practitioners would have nothing on which to base day-to-day decisions about situations that confront them, other than their own common sense.

Research is only one way to generate knowledge, but it is an approach that is critical to the attainment of professional independence because it can validate professional practice (Fawcett & Downs 1986). It can thereby justify the autonomy, privilege and trust given by the community. In addition, knowledge generated through research has special status in a society which highly values science, technology and objectivity. For professions, two kinds of research have relevance (Patton 1990). Applied research investigates specific questions in the field and aims to generate knowledge which can inform practice and solve problems; basic research generates theory, discovers 'truth' and is important for developing the academic discipline that supports the profession.

In the case study, Kim considered herself to be a professional. She had undergone specialised training at university; she identified herself to be an expert in her area with specialised knowledge and skills; she considered herself autonomous enough to make decisions about whom she should be seeing and what she should be doing to help them; she had a commitment to her field; she identified herself as having an obligation to serve her clients and her employer, and she thought such service should be accountable. To address her professional responsibility Kim chose to tackle the problem which seemed to her to underpin the practice habits on the team. This meant confronting the issue of what knowledge was used in practice, and how it was used. The most strategic way to do this was through a commitment to research. In doing so she demonstrated a highly developed sense of professionalism through a commitment to using knowledge generated both within and outside her immediate sphere of practice.

Research has been found to improve service delivery because it identifies uniqueness of service, meets practitioner needs to solve practice problems, and provides information to demonstrate and enhance the efficiency and effectiveness of services (Selker 1994). Research is critical to quality service, since without a knowledge base generated through research, 'we have only the insistence of the individual that his or her practice is scientifically based' (Basmajian 1975, p. 607). Kim's choice to pursue a research strategy to defend and improve her practice came from her commitment to develop the profession's knowledge base and practice, as well as from a personal motivation to provide quality service to clients.

Within professions, individual members will vary in the extent to which they contribute to research efforts. However, each member should be responsible for contributing to knowledge generation in some way and for employing research to inform practice. Research is not an 'auxiliary professional activity' that only some practitioners consider (DePoy & Gallagher 1990, p. 59). All professionals should demonstrate involvement in research through a research orientation to practice. Smith and Hope (1992, pp. vi–vii) describe a research orientation to practice as follows: practitioners enquire 'into their own and others' practice . . . reflecting on their decisions and actions in the light of research so that their own practice can be continually improved'. If this approach is taken, research then becomes an objective for every practitioner, where 'every clinic [site] is a potential laboratory in which questions can and must be answered' (Baum *et al.* 1984, p. 267). Bernard and Gabelko (1987) characterised people with such an orientation as 'research sensitive practitioners', which is the theme of this chapter.

Research in practice

Doing practice research is a challenge for professionals. Practitioners by definition have a primary role of providing service, not doing research. A narrow view of research in practice which requires professionals to conduct studies as part of their daily work is unrealistic. This is why the notion of a 'research orientation to practice' is more inclusive and encouraging to practitioners who want to provide quality professional service. Here practitioners are clearly focused on service provision, but at the same time are sensitive to research as a useful foundation for practice decisions. A number of factors can contribute to the research sensitivity of practitioners: roles, research activity, collaboration, managing research, and relevance. These are now explored.

Research roles in practice

Research sensitivity can manifest itself in a range of practice activities and roles: consumer, advocate, evidenced-based practitioner, collaborator, and investigator. *Consuming* research can occur through reading, conference attendance, topical seminars, discussions and so on. *Advocating* for research happens through raising research funds, being positive about research efforts of others, making management decisions which support research activity, or encouraging learning about research. *Applying* research occurs through evidence-based practice, for example in research-based protocols, policy informed by research, or administrative decisions based on evidence. *Collaborating* in research happens when practitioners assist investigators in activities such as data collection, recruitment or trialing interventions. Finally, the role of *investigator* occurs through conducting research projects alone, or in teams as practitioner-researcher (Barlow *et al.* 1984; Cusick 2000, 2001). Each of these roles gives a practitioner a different yet important focus on research as an essential part of their knowledge for practice.

Research activity

Most practitioners will not be 'investigators'. In occupational therapy, for example, only a minority of practitioners self-select the role of investigator. To pursue this role they need to learn special knowledge and skills to conduct their enquiries (Cusick 2000, 2001). Common activities include: reviewing and critiquing the literature to see what has been done and discovered before; formulating a topic or problem, sometimes in the form of an hypothesis but not necessarily so; designing a research plan to investigate the problem; addressing ethical issues to ensure participants and others are not harmed or exploited; collecting data; analysing data; reaching conclusions and making recommendations; disseminating findings to others (Dumholdt 2000). Most practitioners have an understanding of research which includes these activities, even if they do not know how to do them all or have not done research themselves (Cusick *et al.* 1999). Kim, as a practitioner who has an interest and motivation to become an investigator, will need to engage in these activities to adequately address her practice problem.

Research as a collaborative activity

Collaboration in practice research means working jointly with others to develop, implement, analyse, and document a project addressing questions of concern to practitioners. Collaboration can occur among practitioners in similar or disparate disciplines who find they hold a common practice concern. It can also occur between practitioners and professional researchers such as academics (Cusick 1994). Collaborative research has the advantage of bringing together diverse skills, knowledge and attitudes to focus on the project. It also means more people carry the project workload, which can be important in practice positions where research is rarely the organisational priority. Collaborative research is, however, not always plain sailing. Collaboration usually occurs because a range of different abilities and resources is required. This very difference among participants can mean a variety of expectations, requirements, contributions and research performance skills in the team. Consequently it is common for collaborative research projects to have 'ups and downs' where interpersonal negotiation, conflicts and team building activities absorb participant time and energy.

One strategy to minimise negative consequences of collaborative research and maximise the benefits is the 'colleague model of collaborative investigation' (DePoy & Gallagher 1990), where a seven step process serves to guide practitioner and academic collaborators through the research task. These steps are: identifying a common research interest; role taking; planning and design; negotiation; implementation; completion; evaluation. In the case study, Kim could use this model to work productively with team colleagues or to recruit the participation of academic researchers.

Managing research in the practice setting

Those practitioners who choose to do research need to adopt strategies to ensure that their research projects or programmes are sustained and concluded in spite of the many organisational factors in practice settings that make service, not research, the daily priority (Cusick 2000). It is these organisational factors that can often lead some practitioners, such as the team leader in the case study, to give up research efforts or to consider research by others in the practice setting as a waste of time or drain on practice resources. Strategies to manage the practice environment to get the research done might include (Cusick 2000, 2001): knowing the system (resources, procedures, policies, players), actively managing key aspects of the environment (enlisting the support of key people and gaining access to necessary resources), and driving the research through the course of one's working life (through strategies such as time management, setting priorities, identifying and articulating values). If Kim is to be more successful in completing research than her team leader, she needs to think ahead and consider how best to manage the system in which she works to ensure the progress of her research. She needs to think carefully how she can 'manage her manager' to get even limited support for her research.

Relevance in practice research

Practitioners want research that is relevant, that is focused on practice. Research not relevant to practice will not be used by practitioners. Kim, as she searches through the literature, will want material that is relevant to her practice setting, her client base, her field, and in the first instance, her profession. It would be easy to envisage Kim becoming frustrated or even angry with researchers, if there is nothing in the literature to help her, or worse still, only opinion articles telling her what she should do but giving no evidence for why she should do it or whether it works.

Irrelevant research has been identified as a major problem in practice professions (Barlow *et al.* 1984). Hunt (1981) for example, suggested that nurses do not use research findings because they may not believe them, may not understand them, may not know about them, may not know how to apply them, or may not have the opportunity to use them. In the case study, Kim used her experience knowledge to justify her worth to the team, demonstrate her effectiveness and prove the need for clients to see her. While this knowledge is important, it requires validation to convince others of its worth. Such validation can come through research. Consequently, Kim needed and decided to generate information directly relevant to her practice problem, thus making interest and application more likely. But what of other researchers who may be interested in practice issues that go beyond their own team or centre? How is the problem of potential relevance dealt with?

Making research knowledge relevant and useful

Practitioners can enhance research relevance and 'use-ability' by considering the following: where research questions come from; research methods used; implications for clients, colleagues and sites where research occurs; the way in which work or community systems affect research and the way research might affect the system; the way in which findings might be applied in practice, and strategies which facilitate this application. In each of these considerations, explored further below, the role of the research sensitive practitioner is critical.

Generate questions from practice

The research sensitive practitioner plays an important role in generating research by identifying practice problems or research priorities (Tighe & Biersdorff 1993; Wade 1995). These can help guide research development in practice fields. Kim had particular problems of her own which she wanted to explore, but they touched on themes of practice efficacy, role definition, accountability mechanisms and teamwork, which are key issues that can apply to many practitioners. Consequently, she could search the literature for studies in these general areas to deepen her understanding of the situation.

Choose research methods which are 'practice friendly'

Practitioners are not generally trained to do independent research. Most practitioners who do research have either had special programmes of research study (such as honours degrees) or they have done postgraduate work which has given them additional knowledge and skill (like our case manager with a PhD). There is a tendency to think of research in practice as involving only those with this special training or skill. But in reality practitioners can take on a range of research roles (advocate, consumer, collaborator, investigator, evidence-based practitioner, investigator), each of which require different types of research knowledge and skill. Kim is clearly interested in taking on the roles of research consumer, evidence-based practitioner, and investigator. These roles will require her involvement in a range of research related activities such as searching and critique of the literature, and applying this information in her practice. The investigator role in particular, will mean that she needs to learn new research method skills and knowledge to conduct her project. For a practitioner new to research like Kim, her likelihood of starting and, more importantly, finishing her project will be enhanced if she selects 'practice friendly' approaches. These are characterised by: questions based on real problems, methods which practitioners find meaningful and easy to understand, strategies which can be applied in the practice setting with little change to service routines and priorities, and methods which will clearly provide the information to answer the question.

Consider practice values in research

Practitioners can find the thought of research daunting, not only because of the skills and specialised knowledge needed, but also because of the different values that underlie research and service. Traditional research, with its emphasis on analytical rigour, can be perceived to be at odds with a practitioner approach which commonly entails humanism, valuing clients as people, holism, and communication (Adamson *et al.* 1994). Indeed, some practitioners see any activity which is not direct service as separate to their professional role. Nurses, for example, 'are bound up in the care functions and feel that unless they personally deliver hands-on care, they have somehow abandoned the profession. They fail to see that influencing others to deliver quality care can have greater impact on the quality of care than any individual effort could' (Simms *et al.* 1985). It is therefore easy to understand why some practitioners experience a dilemma between doing research and providing service.

In addition to the apparent conflict of values, there is also a difference between the way in which researchers and practitioners value and use knowledge. Researchers are generally more interested in generating and expanding knowledge, practitioners are more interested in applying it and knowing whether it is adequate and plausible (Hardy 1988). Practitioners, therefore, have a tendency to value knowledge derived through subjective, unique experience, or handed down through tradition, rather than knowledge which comes from a research tradition. But are the two views of research mutually exclusive for the professional practitioner?

Kim, in our case study, had reached a point in which continuing practice under the same conditions and norms was becoming intolerable. She valued her patients, but had relied on knowledge that was subjective, based on her tradition of practice, and it was unique to her. To ensure her practice continued in the team and to improve service for clients, she needed to embrace other knowledge values. She recognised the need to reveal knowledge that was objective and empirical (so that other team members could readily understand it) and generalisable (so that the effectiveness of her profession and team interventions in the area could be considered). Practitioners like Kim, who value their clients as people, and use personally derived practice knowledge extensively, do not need to experience a conflict of values in relation to research. Practitioners who are aware of the values underlying research and practice knowledge can 'weigh up' the benefits and costs of doing and using research in the context of their central concern. They can keep practice and research values explicit, so that decisions about consuming, applying, and doing research are made in a manner that is ethically consistent with the practitioner's and profession's central concerns.

Use research findings in practice

Research sensitive practitioners play a pivotal role in the application of research findings to practice through a process known as research utilisation (Brown & Rodger 1999). They do this by applying research findings to situations they encounter in day-to-day practice, and reflecting on these situations in the context of research. They also do it by utilising theory generated through research and providing input to theory refinement through critiques, case studies, debate and so on. Research sensitive practitioners can see findings in terms of not only their statistical or theoretical significance, but also their clinical or practice significance. They are then able to incorporate them into their everyday practice by basing decisions on evidence. Kim's commitment to seeking evidence for her work is one example of a targeted approach to using research in practice.

Becoming a research sensitive practitioner

Doing or using research is fundamental to being a professional in practice. Research is recognised as essential for data-based decision-making, accountability, efficiency, credibility, and quality in practice. Through the research roles of consumer, advocate, collaborator and evidence-based practitioner applying research, and through conducting research as investigator, practitioners can develop their own identity and performance as research sensitive professionals.

Knowledge for practice is never complete, no matter how much research is available. An important part of being a professional is therefore 'being able to work within the uncertainty of an incomplete knowledge base' (Hardy & Hardy 1988, p. 201). For practitioners who are truly professional, such a situation is seen as normal, a daily challenge and a responsibility. Members of a practice profession should therefore have an expectation and an obligation to contribute to this incomplete knowledge base through their research orientation and chosen research roles. In this way research sensitive practitioners can further develop their expertise and complement knowledge derived from their practice experience.

References

Adamson, B., Sinclair-Legge, G., Cusick, A. & Nordholm, L. (1994) Characteristics of successful therapeutic outcome: A study of Australian occupational therapists, *British Journal of Occupational Therapy*, **57**, pp. 476–90.

Barlow, D.H., Hayes, S.C. & Nelson, R.O. (1984) *The Scientist–Practitioner: Research and Accountability in Clinical and Educational Settings*, Pergamon Press, New York.

Basmajian, J.V. (1975) Research or retrench: The rehabilitation professions challenged, *Physical Therapy*, **55**, pp. 607–10.

Baum, C.M., Boyle, M.A. & Edwards, D.F. (1984) The Foundation – Initiating occupational therapy clinical research, *American Journal of Occupational Therapy*, **33**, pp. 267–9.

Bernard, G.R. & Gabelko, N.H. (1987) Linking practice sensitive research-sensitive practitioners, *Education and Urban Society*, **19**, pp. 368–88.

Brown, G.T. & Rodger, S. (1999) Research utilization models: Frameworks for implementing evidence based occupational therapy practice, *Occupational Therapy International*, **6**, pp. 1–23.

Cusick, A. (1994) Collaborative research: Rhetoric or reality?, *Australian Occupational Therapy Journal*, **41**, pp. 49–54.

Cusick, A. (2000) Practitioner-researchers in occupational therapy, *Australian Occupational Therapy Journal*, **47**, pp. 11–27.

Cusick, A. (2001) The experience of clinician-researchers in occupational therapy, *American Journal of Occupational Therapy* (in press).

Cusick, A., Franklin, A. & Rotem, A. (1999) Meanings of research and researcher: The clinician perspective, *Occupational Therapy Journal of Research*, **19**, pp. 101–25.

DePoy, E. & Gallagher, C. (1990) Steps in collaborative research between clinicians and faculty, *American Journal of Occupational Therapy*, **44**, pp. 55–9.

Dumholdt, E. (2000) *Physical Therapy Research*, 2nd edn, W. B. Saunders, Philadelphia.

Fawcett, J. & Downs, F.S. (1986) *The Relationship of Theory and Research*, Appleton-Century-Crofts, Norwalk.

Hardy, M.E. (1988) Perspectives on science, in *Role Theory Perspectives for Health Professionals* (eds M.E. Hardy & M.E. Conway), Appleton-Lange, Norwalk, pp. 1–28.

Hardy, M.E. & Hardy, W.L. (1988) Development of scientific knowledge, in *Role Theory Perspectives for Health Professionals* (eds M.E. Hardy & M.E. Conway), Appleton-Lange, Norwalk, pp. 29–62.

Hunt, J. (1981) Indicators for nursing practice: The use of research findings, *Journal of Advanced Nursing*, **6**, pp. 189–94.

Patton, M.Q. (1990) *Qualitative Evaluation and Research Methods*, Sage, Newbury Park, CA.

Pavalko, R.M. (1971) The occupation-profession continuum: A conceptual model, in *Sociology of Occupations and Professions* (ed. R.M. Pavalko), F.E. Peacock Publishers, Florida, pp. 15–43.

Selker, L.G. (1994) Clinical research in allied health, *Journal of Allied Health*, **23**, pp. 201–28.

Simms, L.M., Price, S.A. & Ervine, N.E. (1985) *The Professional Practice of Nursing Administration*, John Wiley and Sons, New York.

Smith, D.L. & Hope, J. (1992) *The Health Professional as Researcher: Issues Problems and Strategies*, Social Science Press, Sydney.

Tighe, R., & Biersdorff, K. (1993) Setting agendas for relevant research: A participatory approach, *Canadian Journal of Rehabilitation*, **7**, pp. 127–32.

Wade, G.H. (1995) Is research in the practice setting feasible? *Journal of Continuing Education in Nursing*, **26**, pp. 253–6.

Chapter 11
The Practice Sensitive Researcher

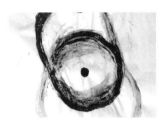

Dorothy Scott

Examples of practice research

Maternal and child health study

In the early 1980s I undertook a study which investigated the feasibility of broadening the role of community-based maternal and child health nurses from one of 'pediatric surveillance' (monitoring the growth and development of infants) to one encompassing 'maternal emotional and social well-being' (Scott 1987). Initially my plan was to develop and test an instrument which nurses could use to identify mothers who were depressed but I soon discovered that this was not how the nurses worked. 'We don't have a mandate to do mental state examinations', one nurse told me.

In similar research with maternal and child health nurses done elsewhere such instruments developed by researchers had been discarded as soon as the study was completed. Mindful of this, I didn't try to impose my research design on the nurses but invited them to tell me how they went about making a psychosocial assessment of the mother. One nurse, using far less dehumanising and clinical language, described the process as 'building up a picture' of the mother and her circumstances, and the picture metaphor better suited the creative and individualised ways in which the nurses went about doing this.

After hearing their rich case narratives and directly observing them in their interaction with mothers and babies, I was able to identify the factors to which they gave salience in their assessment and the unobtrusive and subtle ways in which they gathered and made sense of pertinent information. Complementing these qualitative methods of informant interviewing and observation with a quantitative approach, I administered a questionnaire to women using the service about their attitudes to the role of the nurse, and their post-partum emotional adjustment. The nurses found the study very affirming of their practice and the research has been used extensively in nursing education and professional development.

Child protection study

In a study of child protection practice undertaken in the early 1990s (Scott 1995), I sought to explore the ways in which different professionals working with the same family made their assessments, how they interacted with one another, and how the parents perceived their experiences with the service system. At the time of the study the issue of child abuse was the subject of intense media scrutiny, and there was much conflict between the different organisations involved.

All organisations gave their permission for the study and the major research method involved intensively 'shadowing' a small number of cases of alleged child abuse as they moved through the service system. The professionals involved in the cases were interviewed after each contact with the family, in unstructured interviews which sought to tap their 'think aloud' reasoning. Where possible their interactions with children and families were also observed. After the professionals' cessation of contact with the families, I interviewed the parents of the children in their own homes, in long, in-depth interviews in which they shared their view of their involvement with the services. Most of the parents saw the interviews as a valuable debriefing on what had been a very stressful experience. The published findings of the study were quite critical of a number of features of professional practice. This posed a dilemma for me in (seemingly) 'betraying' former colleagues who worked in a very difficult area of practice.

Practice research: what is it?

These case studies highlight a number of important issues about the nature of research undertaken in practice settings in the fields of health and social welfare, and it is likely that the issues are similar to those which would occur in other fields of professional practice such as education. This chapter discusses the nature of practice research and, using these case studies, explores the opportunities for and obstacles to undertaking such research.

What is practice research? In recent years the term 'practice research' has become more common in a number of professional fields. In the field of social work, the following definition of practice research was developed in the 1980s in collaboration with my colleagues Dr Len Tierney, Dr Lynda Campbell and Mr Stuart Evans (Campbell 1997, p. 29):

'Social Work Practice Research aims to improve social work practice. Undertaken by practitioners or through collaborative partnerships of practitioners, researchers and agencies, practice research seeks an understanding of the composition, operation and/or effects of a "slice" or episode of social work practice (be it a "case", a project, or a program). Typically the practitioners are active participants in the research design and execution, and a range of research methods may be used ("quantitative" and "qualitative"). Research activities include describing and classifying the population served, specifying and conceptualising the practice activities, and measuring outcomes for clients and agencies. Since the transferability of practice strategies across settings is a key issue in social work, practice research must include the broad context of practice (policies, ethical considerations, organisational and inter-organisational constraints and opportunities) in order to be "ecologically valid" or to produce generalisable findings. The process and outcomes must, in turn, be used to inform practitioners, administrators, policy makers and social work educators and students.'

The essential elements in this definition are also applicable to practice research in many other professions. These elements are that (a) the purpose of practice research is to improve professional practice, (b) the process is one in which practitioners are active participants, (c) the methodology is diverse and 'practice friendly', and (d) the findings and their implications are disseminated to the field. Some would argue that a missing element in the definition is any mention of the role of the consumer of services, with the implicit assumption that the consumer is not a partner in the research process but merely a research subject. In many examples of practice research the consumer's perspective is an important dimension, and it is an issue which has received increasing attention in recent times from researchers who are committed to involving consumers.

Opportunities for practice research

The practice setting, be it a residential setting, a neighbourhood-based service, a classroom or other professional context, is a unique ecological niche and a 'natural laboratory' of practice knowledge. To a significant degree, the knowledge of experienced practitioners consists of inductively derived tacit knowledge (Schön 1983). Among health professionals this type of knowledge has traditionally been known as clinical judgement, and in social work it has been known as 'practice wisdom' (Scott 1990).

Lawrence and Homel (1987, p. 3) describe expertise in the following way:

'What we can expect to find as the marks of experience and competence are: accumulated and formalised patterns of common details, rules for extracting cues and assigning weights, and some short-cut strategies that are tailored to fit recurring problems. These cognitive tricks of the trade assist the practitioner to build up mental pictures of what to expect in normal circumstances. They also trigger alarm bells that ring when discordant, unanticipated factors arise in what should be routine cases.'

Typically, such expertise is not expressed in explicit propositional form which can be tested in a hypothetico-deductive model of scientific inquiry or as general 'rules of thumb', but as something more akin to intuition (Scott 1990). It is thus recognised as the art rather than the science of professional expertise. The value of this clinical art was challenged in 1967 in relation to medicine:

'A clinician performs an experiment every time he treats a patient ... Yet we had never been taught before to give our "ordinary' clinical treatment the scientific "respect" accorded to a laboratory experiment ... We had been taught to call it "art" and to consign its intellectual aspects to some mystic realm of intuition that was "unworthy" of scientific attention because it was used for the practical everyday work of clinical care.'

(Feinstein 1967, p. 14)

A less mystical description of the process of tacit knowledge formation could be incipient induction, the implicit process of pattern recognition or the development of a cognitive schema which occurs from lengthy experience. In the words of Feinstein (1967, p. 12), 'in acquiring this experience, every clinician has to use some sort of intellectual mechanism for organising and remembering his observations.' While it may not be accorded scientific respect, such knowledge tends to be recognised and acknowledged by professional peers. Some empirical research demonstrates the soundness of practitioners' tacit knowledge.

In relation to the maternal and child health study, the research identified five main variables to which nurses gave salience as they assessed or 'built up a picture' of a mother's emotional and social well-being. These were:

(1) The characteristics of the baby (for example, infant temperament, feeding and sleeping problems)
(2) The mother's family background (for example, her own childhood experiences)
(3) The support available from key significant others (for example, her partner and her mother)
(4) Social support from others (for example, social networks in the neighbourhood)
(5) The presence of other concurrent situational stresses (for example, financial difficulties, illness in an elderly parent, adjustment to migration).

Quantitative studies using large samples have demonstrated significant correlations between maternal depression and all these variables (e.g. Brown & Harris 1978; Williams & Carmichael 1983; Tonge 1984), yet the nurses in this study were unaware of the research literature emerging at this time on maternal depression, nor had they had formal training in the recognition of depression or the factors associated with it. It is thus suggested that such practice wisdom deserves to be accorded respect, and recognised as a rich source of research hypotheses.

A practice sensitive researcher, whether a relative novice or an experienced practitioner, needs to conceptualise what may appear to be a concrete practice question in a form which enables the research to be enriched by studies which deal with quite different substantive questions which are similar conceptually. Thus, in the maternal and child health study, the research question was conceptualised as being fundamentally to do with changing the core and marginal roles of a profession. The study could therefore be informed by research from diverse fields such as investigations of the roles of Anglican parish priests and women police. Conceptualising the question in this way allows the researcher to search the literature using key words which are much broader than those relating to the substantive issue or profession. It also allows the findings of the research to be used by those in other substantive fields who face similar conceptual issues. To this end the researcher must have a strong and broad theoretical background in the behavioural and social sciences.

If the researcher wants to identify research questions which are important to practitioners and to generate some relevant hypotheses, practitioners may be asked to complete sentences such as 'I have a hunch that ...', 'I wonder if ...', 'What puzzles me is ...' and 'Something I have noticed is that ...'. Another method is to allow experienced practitioners, either individually or in a group, to give 'thick descriptions' of their practice which capture the concrete detail of their actions and the context. Observing experienced practitioners as they work and interviewing them immediately afterwards using 'clinical probe' style questions is another technique which is particularly useful to deal with what Schön (1983) describes as the fact that experts know more than they can say. In both the maternal and child health study and the child protection study, these techniques were used and the implicit principles which underpinned professionals' thinking and acting were extracted. To draw out this knowledge, the researcher needs the skills of listening carefully and respectfully and asking naive clarifying questions.

Tapping tacit knowledge is not an uncritical process, for it should not be assumed that all which passes for practice wisdom is wise. Cognitive and social psychologists working on how a cognitive schema is developed note that:

'sometimes people acquire schemas that are incorrect, either because they were exposed to non-representative instances, because they were taught an incorrect schema, or because a once correct schema no longer is consistent with reality.'
(Crocker *et al.* 1985, p. 199)

An illustration might be the practitioner who is exposed to a certain clinical population and on that basis draws incorrect conclusions about the factors associated with a particular condition. For example, a mental health professional, on the basis of a particular clinical population, could conclude that middle class women are more vulnerable to depression than working class women, although studies based on community samples show the reverse (Brown & Harris 1978).

Sometimes tacit knowledge contains implicit hypotheses which, if made explicit, can be operationalised and empirically tested, but not all tacit knowledge is capable of being expressed in propositional form. By its very nature practice wisdom is based on an ideographic rather than a nomothetic approach, a distinction made by Nagel (1961) in relation to different approaches to knowledge building. The nomothetic seeks to establish general laws for repeatable events and processes, while the ideographic aims to understand the unique and the nonrecurrent. In relation to complex human behaviour which occurs in particular social contexts defined by time and place, tacit knowledge may not be expressible in propositional form because of the number and complexity of interacting variables involved.

Moreover, some of the concepts which practitioners use are inherently low in falsifiability. They are seen as useful, however, because of their explanatory power. Concepts such as those of defence mechanisms are a good example. They cannot be operationalised and tested, yet are able to explain human behaviour not easily explained in other terms. Hence, it may be valid for professionals to use such concepts, albeit with a high level of caution. A professional knowledge base which lacked concepts related to hermeneutic understanding, the capacity to make interpretations about the possible meaning(s) which events and objects may have for individuals, would be a most deficient knowledge base in professions whose core task is that of working with people.

Obstacles in doing practice research

The practice sensitive researcher must grapple with many obstacles – practical, personal, political and ethical – in carrying out research in a practice setting. At a practical level, the very choice of a research design should be congruent with the realities of the setting. The constraints of the practice setting are numerous, particularly in pressured service systems where the primary purpose is service delivery, not research. Busy practitioners cannot be expected to carry the burden of collecting data unless it is easily integrated with their day-to-day practice. Research instruments used in practice research need to be designed and tested so that they are appropriate to the practice setting and the client population. Ideally, the research instruments used should also double as tools of practice which practitioners and clients would feel comfortable using and which do not assume a level of literacy beyond that of the particular client population. Some research instruments can be culturally insensitive and the demographic profile of the client population must be considered in deciding which tools to use.

At a personal level, the researcher may hold other roles, such as client or colleague, which interact with the role of researcher. In the maternal and child health study I was a consumer of the service at the same time as I was studying it, but I was not in a professional-client relationship with the particular nurses involved in the study. Nevertheless, being in the role of consumer was important at all phases of the research process. Traditionally it would have been seen as a source of 'contamination' of the research process. However, I have argued elsewhere (Scott 1997) that, rather than a source of bias, my being in the consumer role generated some of the most important hypotheses in the study.

In the child protection study I had previously been in the roles of colleague or teacher with many of the professionals in the study. This made it much harder to present findings which were critical of professional practice. The painful nature of the problems with which the child protection professionals dealt also aroused personal reactions, and as the study progressed I found myself identifying with some families which I saw as the victims of poor professional practice. It was important to work through these personal reactions to achieve one of the goals of the research, which was to identify the practitioner's perception of the case, a goal which required a respectful and empathic approach to professionals as well as clients. The significance of personal reactions and the nature of the relationships between the researcher and the researched have been described and analysed recently in relation to both the child protection study and an ethnographic study in the field of intellectual disability on deinstitutionalisation (Johnson & Scott 1997). In such circumstances the researcher may find it valuable to create opportunities with peers or with a consultant to explore personal reactions and consider their impact on the research.

The issue of subjectivity in research has been reformulated in the past decade or so, with qualitative researchers in particular being less likely now to present sanitised reconstructions of the research process. A feminist anthropologist has argued in relation to the research process that 'the experience involves so much of the self that it is impossible to reflect upon it by extracting the self' (Okely 1992, p. 8). Researchers have to struggle not only with the emotional responses aroused by the practice situation but also with the pressures to intervene to alleviate suffering:

'Naturalistic researchers ... must often struggle with the personally painful question of whether to throw in the towel on doing research, and give themselves over entirely to "helping" or to remain in the field as a chronicler of the difficulties' (Lofland & Lofland 1984, p. 34).

In the maternal and child health study this conflict became most apparent on one rainy afternoon during an immunisation session at a centre in a very poor locality. The nurse was overwhelmed with the number of parents and children, many with quite pressing problems. To remain in the role of the 'chronicler of difficulties' was impossible and I became the de facto nurse assistant, giving practical help as required. In this way I joined with the nurse. I believe I was able to chronicle the difficulties better as a result. In the child protection study there were occasions when the imperative to intervene became very strong, particularly when families seemed to suffer at the hands of the services. Yet I resisted the temptation to intervene directly in ways which would have resulted in being denied the opportunity to continue as the 'chronicler of difficulties'. Practice research can be fraught with personal dilemmas.

At a political level there are also obstacles involved in conducting practice research, which require enlisting the support of key stakeholders and fostering a sense of collective ownership of the project. These can be long and painstaking processes, but without a sense of collective ownership there will be less chance of gaining cooperation in executing the research and less commitment to implementing the findings of the research. Sometimes the tensions in the relationship between the researcher and the organisation arise at the end of the research process, when findings may reflect poorly on some aspect of the service. In the child protection study, the differences between some professionals and the researcher were presented in the research report in a way which attempted to be fair to both interpretations.

Issues about the differences in interpretation also arise when feedback occurs before the report is completed. While the participants' point of view about a social process is important, it is also self-interested and embedded in the power relations of the community. The final interpretation has to rest with the researcher, except in action research in which discussion and negotiation are a part of the research design (Commonwealth Department of Human Services and Health 1995, p.12).

The situation is further complicated when the research is commissioned by the host organisation and where issues relating to accountability, the prospect of future funding, political censorship and intellectual property pose threats to the integrity of the research and the researcher. For example, the organisation commissioning the research may, as a condition of the contract, impose restrictions on the researcher's freedom to publish the research or to speak to the media about the research. As universities are increasingly pressured to undertake contract research, real dilemmas arise, especially for those carrying out research in areas which are politically sensitive. These issues need to be addressed at the negotiation phase. At the same time, contract research can sometimes give the researcher greater awareness of organisational factors and greater capacity to assist in implementation of the findings.

At an ethical level there are also major challenges associated with practice research. Among these is the difficult issue of informed consent. The close collaboration which the researcher may wish to develop with the professionals in practice research may itself increase the vulnerability of clients, who may fear that what they say will be conveyed to the professionals upon whom they are dependent for a service or who may exercise power over them. The capacity to give free and informed consent may be compromised by the vulnerability of certain groups of consumers:

'Special problems are posed for researchers who wish to conduct research involving people, who, for whatever reasons are less able to consent than other members of the community. Among the categories of people who are thought less able freely or autonomously to agree to participate in research are: children; people with certain developmental disabilities; people with certain psychiatric or medical conditions; and people experiencing early or late stages of dementia.'

(Commonwealth Department of Human Services and Health 1995, p. 62)

While the parents of the children in the child protection study did not fall into any of these categories, they were vulnerable in relation to their capacity to make an informed decision at a time of crisis. While a decision was made not to involve children directly in any of the interviews in the child protection study, the issue of observing professionals' interviews with children through a one-way screen was problematic. While such observation was a routine event in the specialised clinic in a teaching hospital, it raised questions as to whether the informed consent of the child was required. Parental consent was given for such observations, but to what extent should parents be able to give consent on behalf of their child and at what age should the child's consent also be necessary?

When the researcher is also delivering a professional service, the ethical problems relating to informed consent can be compounded by those dual roles which may compromise the rights of clients in a dependent professional–client relationship if asked to be research participants. On the other hand, some clients may experience it as less intrusive to be asked certain questions by a professional they know and trust than to be asked such questions by a stranger. The boundaries between practice research and a clinical audit may also be blurred, leading to ambiguity as to whether informed consent is required. An issue which is not always considered by ethics review boards is that of the informed consent of the professionals involved. Just because the researcher has obtained the permission of those in senior management in the organisation, does it follow that staff are expected to participate in research? And what happens when new personnel join a team which consented to the study initially? Are they expected to participate as part of their employment or should they be given a choice, and could their choice jeopardise the completion of the research? Such problems are not always anticipated and yet can be major obstacles in practice research.

Conclusion

Practice research provides rich opportunities to develop the knowledge base of professions in a way which draws upon the expertise of experienced practitioners and which increases the probability that research findings will be utilised in practice. There are many challenges in developing research designs which tap the pre-existing knowledge of practitioners and which are practice-friendly and able to be implemented in the complex organisational world of professional practice.

There are many dilemmas facing practice sensitive researchers and we need to develop strategies to deal with them. In the words of one team of researchers referring to the twin ethical and political complexities in research in the human services:

> 'The best one can do is to consider the ethical and political issues in asking a particular research question, determine the areas of concern prior to the research, take into account professional standards that have been established and then consider the ethics of the entire research process as an individual case with its own social and political ramifications.'
>
> (Minichiello *et al.* 1990, p. 245–6)

While the ethical and practical obstacles to practice research can seem like a minefield, there is no alternative for a profession which seeks to be accountable than to undertake practice research. After all, in many areas of professional practice in the human services, practice is itself something of a social experiment, with the potential to harm as well as help. Practice research is therefore an essential tool for making services and professionals more accountable and for increasing the knowledge upon which practice is based. It can also be a source of immense satisfaction and intellectual stimulation for those who undertake it.

References

Brown, G. & Harris, T. (1978) *The Social Origins of Depression*, Tavistock Publications, London.

Campbell, L. (1997) Good and proper: Considering ethics in practice research, *Australian Social Work*, **50**, pp. 29–36.

Commonwealth Department of Human Services and Health (1995) *Ethical Research and Ethics Committee Review of Social and Behavioural Research Proposals*, Australian Government Publishing Service, Canberra.

Crocker, J., Fiske, S. & Taylor, S. (1985) Schematic bases of belief change, in *Semantic Anthropology* (ed. D. Parkin), Academic Press, London.

Feinstein, A. (1967) *Clinical Judgment*, Krueger and Co., New York.

Johnson, K. & Scott, D. (1997) Confessional tales: An exploration of the self and other in two ethnographies, *The Australian Journal of Social Research*, **4**, pp. 7–48.

Lawrence, J. & Homel, R. (1987) Sentencing in magistrates' courts: The magistrate as professional decision maker, in *Sentencing in Australia: Policies, Issues and Reform* (ed. I. Potas), Australian Institute of Criminology, Canberra, pp. 151–89.

Lofland, J. & Lofland, L. (1984) *Analyzing Social Settings*, Wadsworth Publishing Co., Belmont.

Minichiello, V., Aroni, R., Timewell, E. & Alexander, L. (1990) *In-Depth Interviewing: Researching People*, Longman Cheshire, Melbourne.

Nagel, E. (1961) *The Structure of Scientific Inquiry*, Routledge and Kegan Paul, London.

Okely, J. (1992) Anthropology and autobiography: Participatory experience and embodied knowledge, in *Anthropology and Autobiography* (eds J. Okely & H. Callaway), Routledge, London, pp. 1–28.

Schön, D. (1983) *The Reflective Practitioner: How Professionals Think in Action*, Temple Smith, London.

Scott, D. (1987) *Primary intervention in maternal depression*, MSW thesis, University of Melbourne.

Scott, D. (1990) Practice wisdom, the neglected source of practice research, *Social Work*, **35**, pp. 564–8.

Scott, D. (1995) Child protection assessment, PhD thesis, University of Melbourne.

Scott, D. (1997) The researcher's personal response as a source of insight in the research process, *Nursing Inquiry*, **4**, pp. 130–34.

Tonge, B. (1984) *Postnatal mood states, mother-child interaction and child development*, MD thesis, University of Melbourne.

Williams, H. & Carmichael, A. (1983) Depression in mothers in a multi-ethnic urban industrial municipality in Melbourne, *Journal of Child Psychology and Psychiatry*, **26**, pp. 277–88.

Part Three
Journeying in Professional Practice

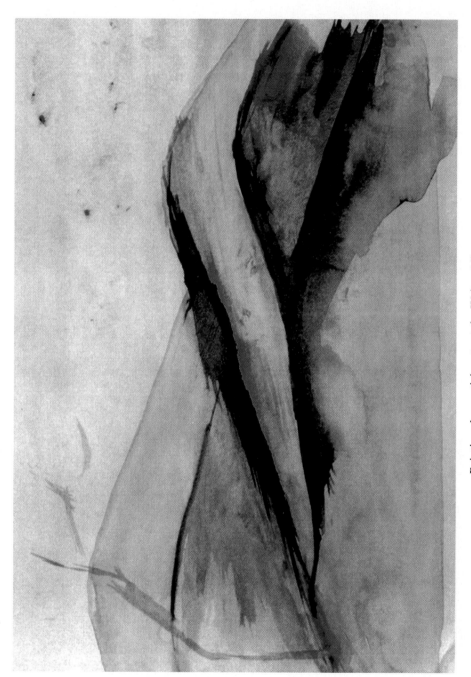

Paintings by participants at the Writers' Retreat.

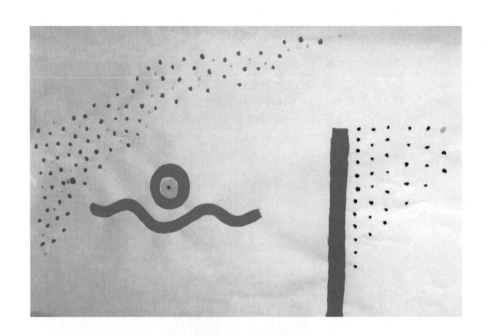

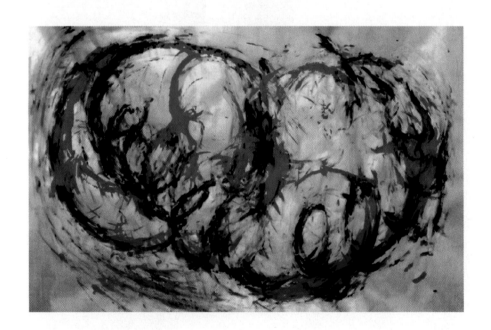

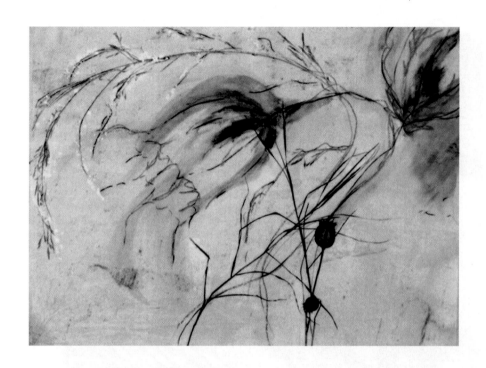

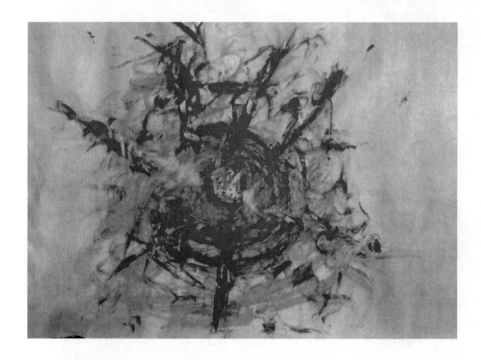

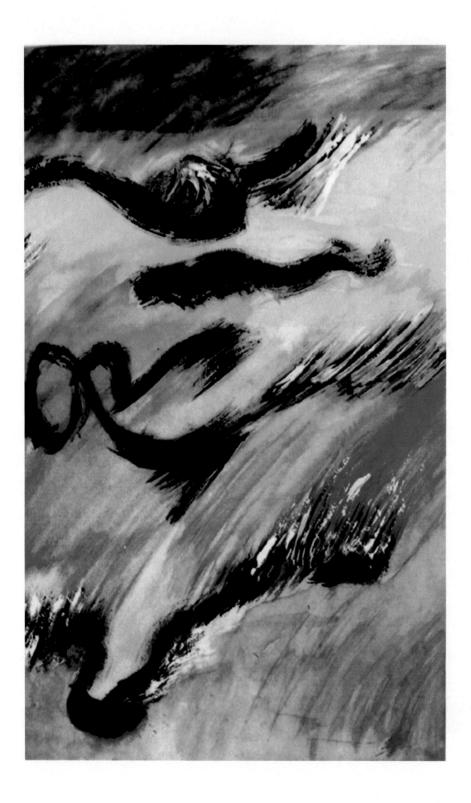

Chapter 12
Using Autobiographical Narrative and Reflection to Link Personal and Professional Domains

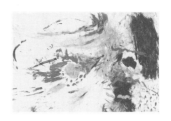

Sally Denshire and Susan Ryan

'There is no theory that is not a fragment, carefully prepared, of some auto-biography.'

(Paul Valery)

This chapter is a collaborative account of the telling of and reflecting on Sally Denshire's autobiographical narrative. Later, Susan Ryan discusses with Sally her life experiences. We talk about the usefulness of being aware of the links between life experiences and the way one practises in occupational therapy (OT). We reflect on how uncommon it is to do this and we show one way that it can be done. To begin, we introduce ourselves.

SALLY DENSHIRE: I have been an occupational therapist for 21 years and a mother for 12 years. I founded the Youth Arts Programme at the Royal Alexandra Hospital for Children in Sydney in 1984. I have published several articles about my approach to youth-specific occupational therapy and I have written about work, family and organisational development. My teaching is in the areas of occupation and communication in the OT programme at Charles Sturt University in Albury, Australia, where I have been a lecturer since 1995. My post-graduate research in the School of Occupation and Leisure Sciences at the University of Sydney is concerned with making linkages between personal history and professional practice by using metaphor analysis and lexicographic methods.

SUSAN RYAN: I am a reader in educational development in the health sciences and course leader for postgraduate OT programmes at the University of East London. My master's study examined the clinical reasoning processes of expert and novice therapists in the USA in the 1980s. This research led to a fascination with curricula and with module designs that would facilitate the integration of reasoning and reflection within professional knowledge. I am interested to see how undergraduates are helped to 'put it all together'. My qualitative PhD study uses narrative reflection. I have listened to the voices of newly graduated occupational therapists from two schools, one traditional and the other using problem-based learning. I have tried to understand how they view their present practice and how they make sense of their educational courses.

Today, both of us believe that it is impossible to separate our personal lives from our professional lives. From our working experiences, we can say that our personal and professional practice has become richer and more meaningful because of our awareness and acknowledgement of this blend of the personal-in-the-professional and the professional-in-the-personal. It was not always like that. We were both educated as occupational therapists in the 1970s and, at that time, the personal world and the professional world were kept separate. At that time, health care followed the natural science paradigm, the impact of which we will discuss later.

This chapter will show how we explored Sally's early life experiences so that she could reach a new understanding of the impact those experiences had had on her professional and personal life today. We hope that her new insights about these links will influence her future work. We describe the journey we took and outline the methods we selected. We both acknowledge that there are many other ways that could be equally effective.

Early work

Developing a focus

The focus of this chapter came from our participation in a larger, multi-disciplinary group at the writers' retreat at Leura, Blue Mountains, Australia, where this book was planned. The group spent a great deal of time brainstorming, sorting through and discussing ideas about personal and professional links and boundaries. We began by considering how medical practitioners in the eighteenth century had classified pathological symptoms and, as described by Foucault (1973), had envisaged mankind as distinct from its disease. We discussed the literature on self-development and the transformative awareness of personal growth which happens during the initial tertiary educational experience as student practitioners gradually assume professional behaviours. We examined papers that described interactive practice where themes such as empathy and self-disclosure between a therapist and a client were outlined.

While all this material centred around aspects of the personal and the professional, somehow these perspectives were not exactly what we were seeking. The group felt that this topic should be treated more deeply and holistically. We decided that looking at people's life experiences and then helping them make links to their present way of being would be more in keeping with the spirit of this book about new knowledges for practice. Sally offered to tell her story and Susan to help her.

Agreeing on a process

Susan had been working with narratives in other research studies to good effect, so we decided to use an autobiographical narrative account (Clandinin & Connelly 1994) of Sally's past. We agreed that Sally would talk about aspects of her past life which she felt had had an impact on her present work. She would edit the end result, so that she did not feel inhibited as she talked. Susan tape-recorded the story. We realised that this would simply be one version of Sally's memories and that other perspectives might surface if her experiences were recounted on another day.

Finding a method for analysis and interpretation

We chose to examine Sally's story by using a retrospective, four strand framework called 'Strands of Reflection' (Fish *et al.* 1991) which aims to delve deeper into a person's awareness with each successive strand. The main purpose of the framework is to develop insight over time into the way you are and the way you work. We preferred this reflective framework to reflective questioning alone because we wanted realisations and links to occur. The model facilitates in-depth exploration of the details of the initial story, any patterns that emerge, their relevance to a person's values and beliefs and how this knowledge could be used in the future. The group agreed that this framework would yield a holistic picture that would inform Sally's present and future work.

The 'four strand' approach

This approach is adapted from Fish (1995, pp. 139–44).

The factual strand

- Briefly describe the context where the story takes place.
- Tell the story about what happened, how did you think, feel and act, and why.
- Pinpoint any critical incidents or key moments in this story. Identify and describe any incidents which caused surprise or offered scope for learning. Describe the resulting feelings.

The retrospective strand

Look back at the entire events and processes as a whole and search for any patterns and new meanings. This helps you to draw theory from practice and develops sensitivity and imagination by asking how others might have viewed this event. Doing this helps you to consider a range of perspectives.

The substratum strand

This strand helps the discovery and exploration of assumptions, beliefs and value judgements that underlie events and the ideas which emerge from the factual and retrospective strands. It seeks careful consideration beyond the technicalities of practice. It should be assisted by consideration of a range of perspectives from formal theory which can be invoked. It helps professionals to tolerate a range of views.

The connective strand

This strand relates to the wider world of practical situations. It helps to see how both practice and theory can be modified for future work by examining the experiences, views, reflections, theorising and actions of other professionals: other personal theories and formal theory. A clear action plan can result from this new understanding.

Historical background

Before we tell Sally's story, we look at some of the broader influences on our lives. We believe these influences set up boundaries that stop the recognition that the personal and professional spheres are linked. This dichotomous way of viewing the world has shaped our professional behaviour; much of it comes from our educational knowledges and experiences.

Looking back on the history of the allied health professions such as OT and social work, we find that the majority of practitioners in the early days were female. This trend continues today. At the end of the nineteenth century and beginning of the twentieth century, when these groups were forming, their work was seen by others as a 'natural' extension to a paid workforce of the unpaid, caring, domestic work done by women (Fisher & Tronto 1990). In the middle decades of the twentieth century most allied health groups came under the direction of medicine and immersed themselves in the scientific world in order to become 'professional'.

In 1954, the sociologist Parsons wrote that only medicine and law were true professions. The main characteristics of these professions were autonomy, commitment to the community, an in-depth body of knowledge acquired over several years of study, and an ethical and moral stance towards work. Then, nurses, occupational therapists, physiotherapists, social workers and teachers were classed as semi-professionals. As a consequence, many of these groups prolonged their initial education and started to research their practice in order to be seen as true professionals. In countries such as the USA and Canada, further degrees and higher salaries flourished.

When we examined the literature of this period, we saw that the predominant practice and research approaches followed the laws of the natural sciences. Thus it was assumed, according to Fish and Coles (1998), that work was 'value-free' and 'context-free'. This was referred to as the positivistic, deterministic approach. Researchers aimed to be objective so that their data were not contaminated by personal bias. This was the way most medical and health related research was conducted and written about until quite recently. Sally talked about this ethos in part of her narrative:

SALLY: *During the early 1980s I began to publish papers about my work with young people in hospital. The journals preferred me to write in the third person and to present my work objectively. Curiously though, while I was writing these papers, I was aware that much of that work drew on my personal beliefs and experiences yet they were never alluded to. During the 1980s, if you wanted to be 'professional' this was what was expected, even in the non-traditional practice area of adolescent health. In effect my personal way of being was eliminated from my work. It remained unsaid.*

Propositional and nonpropositional knowledges

In those days, most of what was written was about the procedural and technical aspects of work, often referred to in the literature as propositional knowledge (Benner 1984). Later, as we will outline below, it was realised that much of the success, in the therapies at least, was also to do with interpersonal relationship and innovative practice. The personal part of practice started to be acknowledged from the late 1980s (Mattingly & Fleming 1994).

SUSAN: *Story telling, as in case stories, replaced the drier version of case studies. Suddenly many aspects of practice felt more dynamic. I noticed how enthusiastically the clinicians who came to my clinical reasoning workshops responded to these new approaches. My undergraduate students said they could visualise people's lives more easily although they needed help picking out the important points to look for. These subjective views of practice are becoming more prevalent.*

Sally's story

Preambles

Returning now to this study of Sally's life story, we emphasise that it is a narrative account, not narrative inquiry in which processes are used to analyse and synthesise a narrative account (Polkinghorne 1995). The use of narrative, in whatever form, is still relatively new in the health sciences and there are no generally accepted rules. Joy Goodfellow has written about the methodological messiness in this area (Goodfellow 1997). We both find this exciting because in our view it gives us a chance to be innovative and we hope that more organic work (such as this) can help to transcend some of the previous artificial divides and stimulate greater insights into practice.

Before we started recording Sally's story about parts of her life, we found a quiet place where we would not be interrupted. It is important not to be in a hurry, not to be in noisy surroundings, and to feel easy with each other and clear about what is expected. In this relaxed way, a story will flow more easily. It is not necessary for the person telling the story to have thought about it a great deal or rehearsed it in any way, although they do need some chance to decide on what to include or, at least, where to start. In this situation, Sally is a co-researcher with Susan, as well as the participant in the research. In earlier drafts, tensions were inevitable between the telling of Sally's story, her reflections on the story and Susan's interpretations. This was why it was essential to go back and discuss her interpretation with Sally.

The following section is the final self-edited, but not rewritten, version of her story. It is told in her own conversational style and in the order in which she told it. Often the mind does not work in a logical order and one recollection may trigger others. Her description corresponds to the first factual strand of reflection (Fish *et al.* 1991). Often it helps to read a passage such as this aloud, to feel the intonations and grasp the meaning better.

Factual strand data

Sally is talking about her childhood holiday experiences in Australia:

When we were at Currawong we would do all these tribal wonderful things, we'd collect shells, we'd go up into the bush and visit Aunt Maggie who had all these tribal statues in the garage (where) she lived on the top of the hill between Currawong and Mackerel Beach. We'd creep around in the bush and our parents would come and get us because we were out too late. We'd make ghost trains in the bush, we'd put on concerts and we'd play Cockie Laura. My dear friend Sarah was there as well and we used to do – ah, eleven year old things together – she'd have nail polish and jump-suits and we used to dress up in those and, ah, it was just a very free time.

I used to dig these sort of, um, underground houses and put a hole in the ceiling and then the sun would shine down through the hole and illuminate this little sand cave. I was probably about eight or nine . . .

We used to do lots of stuff with clay. There was a rock called Doctor's Rock that had these sort of sandstone benches on it. It was an enormous rock as big as this room and we would climb up on top of it and spend all the day doing this stuff using clay from the bush. So Currawong was very much a very free sort of space. It was about running around with this big throng of other kids and having all these adventures, playing all these imaginary games, and then collecting the shells as sort of memories of Cur-rawong. They would come back in a cardboard box, um, back to my house (in Sydney). I remember I had this collection of crabs' nippers in a steel wool box, an old blue Steelo box. I was quite imaginative as a child and I used to do these dances on the beach with these crabs' nippers and it was quite a sort of witchy type of a thing.

I suppose as I went to Currawong when I was a bit older, sort of about 13 or 14, when I started to meet boys there and do adolescent things. There was this guy called Malcolm who had Mao's Little Red Book *and, um, I thought this was very radical at the age of 15 and he had a copy of it. My friend Sarah, whose Dad was a university professor, had a volume of Yevtushenko poetry. It was seen as very bohemian to have this.*

So I suppose Currawong was a setting for my development as a kid and then growing into adolescence. It was like the other world of my childhood – you know – it was the sort of respite – the special place away from living in the suburbs.

And then it was in my twenties that I was in New Zealand and that was where I trained as an OT and that's really how I accomplished my adolescent separation – by moving to another country.

Travelling was very pivotal for me as a new graduate – and I travelled in the Middle East and Eastern Europe and was in a lot of very exhilarating and dangerous situations. In New Zealand I was mountain climbing somehow and I was doing [laughs] all these things that were really stretching me to the edge of my limits and that was both exciting and terrifying.

[Back in Sydney] I was drawn to working in a Rudolf Steiner Home for children in need of special soul care. I did that for 18 months and for me that was like a transition from the wild places overseas to coming back. So I worked in this alternative system for a while and that was very good for me but intellectually it didn't really extend me. I remember at that time I did some corporeal mime and a lot of dance and things, for expressive reasons not for performative reasons. Then I saw the job at the Children's Hospital and I applied for that.

My practice there was with young people – teenagers who came to hospital repeatedly. I seemed to have this strong drive to make this hospital, as a territory, better for them. So I did a lot of group work with young people. I got to know them really well. My practice then was very relational, um, I was very much with them as a youth worker would be. I worked very informally, was very anti the clinical view – yes – and did a lot of creative work about them finding their own voice and, in parallel, I was finding mine.

Then, once I had my first child I worked part-time and also became a childbirth educator and the heartwork that I had done at the hospital I began to do at home with my own children and so my work role became a lot more rational. I became much more interested in the conceptual and the philosophical rather than working so much with me as a person . . .

I have always liked writing – I have always written. I grew up with a lot of speech around me, a lot of words, and a lot of poetry. I would write poetry as a child. I've always been interested in etymology, in dictionaries, in language, in terminology. I studied Greek and Latin and so I have that language bias and I bring that to my occupational therapy practice, not only to understand the medical terms but also to deconstruct the language that we use as therapists because often I think we unwittingly use language that does not do our practice justice. I am very interested to evolve a language with my colleagues that is representative of our true work rather than sort of hybridise from medicine and social work.

[On her present role as an academic] ... Creativity and healing is really the heart of my practice. I founded the Youth Arts Programme and now that work transfers to creativity and learning and that's what I recognise and bring out in my students. I find peer learning and working with groups in a relational way is a very satisfying way to create a learning environment where students continue their learning in a number of modes not only using text. Where the students' voices are very much uppermost and I just create a place where the learning rises up ...

I use some of my personal experience in my teaching because I've been an OT for twenty years and that seems to mean something to the students. So I find great transferability working with people as a practising OT and then teaching students to work as a practising OT. I value that career progression ...

[About being a parent] My daughter drew this picture of Mummy that had all these clouds coming out of my head and I said, 'what's that?' And she said, 'Oh – that's your thesis'. They've just grown up and their parents each have these interests that they are part of – not excluded from. The whole household has things they do that are really important to them. So when I was younger I was more conscious of – of trying to keep my heart at home and my head at work but now everything is everywhere – Yes!

Retrospective strand data

On rereading the transcript after returning from the writers' retreat, Sally found there were eight key topics within her story. They were: the other place of my childhood; working in a Rudolph Steiner home; working with young people in hospital; becoming a parent; writing; creativity and learning; the family's interests; the blending of domains. Then, when we looked back on her story as a whole together, some clear patterns emerged. They were: creative occupations, dedicated space as a respite, giving a collective voice to those who do not have one, finding alternative ways, putting your heart into practice, finding language for practice, pushing personal and professional limits, and the power of transforming experiences as you move through life. When she read this, Sally began to realise that much of her occupational therapy practice, her teaching approach and the way she is bringing up her children was based on these patterns.

Substratum strand data

New realisations are interesting, but they must not be left at this level if deeper understanding is to emerge. Fish (1995) warns that one of the dangers of using these strands is to finish on the second strand. So, in order to reflect further on her story, Sally agreed to be tape-recorded again and interviewed more formally. By asking a series of probing questions about her assumptions, beliefs and value judgments, we tried to uncover and critically explore her underlying personal theories and get her to consider how these could be helped by formal theory. Through iterative and reiterative discussions, some clear themes emerged. Below we have described in Sally's words the six personal themes which surfaced after she considered her story further.

A broad spirituality

I've always been interested in myths and legends and as a child I read a lot of folk tales from different cultures. When I was working in the Steiner setting, the fairy tale was always a very instructive presence in the school or in the anthroposophical centre. I studied ancient history because I was interested in how people lived. My sort of relationship with religion has always been a bit problematic and I suppose I'm interested in a broad spirituality, rather than an organised religion.

Humanising institutions

The reason that I stayed at the Children's Hospital for so long was that I felt very strongly about making it a human place. It was very Dickensian architecturally, a very cold sort of place and I created change, that was quite a drive in me.

Underground practice

I have always been interested in informal work even when I worked in a medical setting and the medical people had all these structures, forms and terminology. I felt those of us who worked in allied health were pretty light on these and we were just called 'nonmedical'. I've always been interested to unpack our work and give it language and meaning. This work was often done in corridors and it was this that Mattingly and Fleming (1994) called the 'underground practice'. Although it sounds contradictory, I would like to systematise the informal.

Creativity, innovation and making the invisible visible

I value the creative world and anything to do with creativity and humans is important to me. It has certainly played a large part in my practice. Innovation is a sort of motif in my work and in my life. I like working with the new and the untried. It's like working 'on the edge'. Like other contributors in this book I would like to make what is often called nonpropositional knowledge visible. We need to articulate things that are outside the mainstream. So innovation is a key component of what I do.

Discovery

From my story you can see I've always been interested to go to new lands and discover new ways of doing things. Not doing the same thing day after day. I'm talking about something small, much more everyday moments of discovery.

Synthesis

I feel my work is like a synthesis of the free spirit within the limits of a sort of scaffold which may be some of the formal theories. Some of the work from occu-

pational science and theories from the creative process form the infrastructure. Institutional structures also play a part.

When we had finished going through the first three strands, Sally realised how closely her personal life experiences had formed the foundation for her professional work and her child rearing. By telling her story and articulating her feelings, making these realisations and linking them to her present life, she was bringing into sharper focus things of which she had previously been only vaguely aware. In addition, the substratum strand of reflection enabled Sally to engage in Mezirow's (1981) stage of theoretical reflectivity.

Connective strand data

Finally, to see how Sally's practice and theory can be modified we engaged in the connective strand of reflection, in which Sally concluded:

Now I hope to use these aspects of my work with students to counter the present technical rational way of viewing practice. I realise the value of discussing my ideas more openly and more often in the future. I also see that, for many therapists and students, working in an economically rational way fragments their therapy. To voice their personal theories and situate them within the existing formal theories I believe will enrich both themselves and their practice. In fact I think that this is pivotal for a new understanding of professional work. And finally, I am presently immersed in my thesis which is examining the development of my practice and the links between the different parts. The personal insights gained from collaborating on this chapter with Susan will assist me to make further connections between my personal values and attitudes and my professional practice by using metaphor analysis.

Where to from here?

If you are considering using this four strand approach to explore your own autobiographical narrative, here are some pointers for proceeding that we have drawn from our own experience combined with Fish's original theorising. We leave you with our invitation to try some of these ideas:

- What life experiences are being used in your practice at present? Include your client's experiences as well as your own.
- Think about your choice of practice area(s) and then reflect on any personal experiences that have informed your choices.
- How could you enhance or change your practice by including more of the personal in it?

In this chapter we have presented one person's autobiographic narrative and shown how aspects of life experience and professional practice can be linked by using successive levels of reflection to find new meanings. We have found doing this worthwhile and hope that, whatever your career stage, you will be able to make use of the strands of reflection to come to a new understanding of your practice.

Acknowledgements

We would like to thank Dawn Best and Rosemary Cant for their early input to this chapter. Thank you to the reviewers of the chapter, Lee Andresen, Joy Goodfellow, Debbie Horsfall and Angie Titchen. Your perceptive comments made reworking worth doing. Finally, a special thank you to Della Fish who has inspired many.

Website

You can visit Charles Sturt University's Creative Links website at http://www.csu.edu.au/faculty/health/cmhealth/creative.

References

Benner, P. (1984) *From Novice to Expert: Excellence and Power in Clinical Nursing Practice*, Addison-Wesley, London.

Clandinin, D.J. & Connelly, M.F. (1994) Personal experience methods, in *Handbook of Qualitative Research* (eds N. Denzin & S. Lincoln), Sage, California, pp. 413–27.

Fish, D. (1995) *Quality Mentoring for Student Teachers: A Principled Approach to Practice*, David Fulton Publishers, London.

Fish, D. & Coles, C. (1998) *Developing Professional Judgement in Health Care*, Butterworth-Heinemann, Oxford.

Fish, D., Twinn, S. & Purr, B. (1991) *Promoting Reflection: Improving the Supervision of Practice in Health Visiting and Initial Teacher Training*, West London Institute, London.

Fisher, B. & Tronto, J. (1990) Towards a feminist theory of caring, in *Circles of Care: Work and Identity in Women's Lives* (eds E. Abel & M. Nelson), State University of New York Press, Albany, New York, pp. 35–62.

Foucault, M. (1973) *The Birth of the Clinic: An Archaeology of Medical Perception*, Tavistock Publications, New York.

Goodfellow, J. (1997) Narrative inquiry: Musings, methodology and merits, in *Qualitative Research: Discourse on Methodologies* (ed. J. Higgs), Hampden Press, Sydney, pp. 61–74.

Mattingly, C. & Fleming, M.H. (1994) *Clinical Reasoning: Forms of Inquiry in a Therapeutic Practice*, F.A. Davis, Philadelphia.

Mezirow J. (1981) A critical theory of adult learning and education, *Adult Education*, **32**(1), pp. 3–24.

Parsons, T. (1954) *Essays in Sociological Theory*, Free Press, New York.

Polkinghorne, D. (1995) Narrative configuration in qualitative analysis, *International Journal of Qualitative Studies in Education*, **8**, pp. 5–23.

Valery, P. quoted in J. Olney (ed.) (1980) *Autobiography: Essays Theoretical and Critical*, Princeton University Press, Princeton.

Chapter 13
Students and Educators
Learning Within Relationships

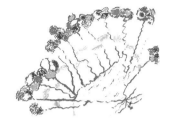

Joy Goodfellow, Lindy McAllister, Dawn Best,
Gillian Webb and Dawn Fredericks

Crucial moments in becoming a professional are often couched in terms of successful or unsuccessful relationships with others. The human potential to learn is founded within experience and the context of being in a relationship. Students and educators in the human professions often engage in quite demanding professional relationships during experiential learning programmes. The relationships between students and field-based educators in university health science and early child educator degree courses provide the context for this chapter.

This chapter has two sections. In the first section we present a story as told by Colin, a young physiotherapist. He recounts his experiences during fieldwork placements in his undergraduate education and early professional practice. In the second section of the chapter we explore our understandings about the nature of relationships and the critical role of relationships in learning through experience. Colin's story provides much of the material for these explorations. However, we also introduce the voices of other students and educators in order to illustrate important points. During our explorations, we reflect on the narrative accounts and reconsider the importance of relationships both in the development of professional competence and in socialisation.

Colin's story and the other quotes/voices used in this chapter come from true stories (the names of the participants have been changed to protect their privacy). These stories were collected in field-based settings. They capture the pressures and tensions under which both students and educators now operate in climates of fiscal constraint, reduced staffing and increased demands for productivity. Readers will note that the majority of stories and quotes come from females. This gender imbalance is typical of the health science and education professions, where the majority of practitioners are female. While acknowledging that gender issues can affect the development of relationships in the learning context, a detailed analysis of these issues is beyond the scope of this chapter.

Storying and relationships

Stories explore the nature of learning through experience and the importance of relationships within that experience. They provide a means through which there is an opportunity to look at the 'I' or the person within the story both as an object for scrutiny and as a reflective agent (Popkewitz 1997). Stories may be viewed as constructions in which knowledge is generated as we search for new meanings and new understandings of beliefs and values within our relationships with people. Human beings make multidimensional connections encompassing cognitive, social, moral, aesthetic, personal and interpersonal qualities. These connections, made within the context of relationships, contribute to our identity as individuals. The making sense of relationships is often revealed through the stories we tell.

Elicker (1997) speaks of relationships as:

'dyadic in nature; they develop over time, they are based on a history of interactions, they include emotional content and expectations produced by history, and they provide an experiential context that both supports and constrains the behaviour of individuals who are in them.'

(Elicker 1997, p. 6)

Developing professionals who are engaged in field experiences are active participants in a complex set of relationships (Zeichner 1985). These relationships are with people, with the chosen programme of study, and with the characteristics of the setting in which the field placement is undertaken. Experiences form the landscape within which personal meaning is painted through engagement in and reflection on that experience.

Experience is not finite but part of a pattern of dynamic human relationships within which practical knowledge is constructed (Beattie 1997). While both the social and physical environments provide important contexts for learning, the personal context (relating to our views of ourselves) is also particularly important. Clandinin (1985, p. 362) describes this as personal practical knowledge that is 'experiential, embodied and based on the nature of experience'. Personal practical knowledge requires reflective thought in and about practice rather than a process of direct transmission of information as we engage in life's learning journey. Such reflection and meaning-making is illustrated in Colin's story that follows.

Colin is a new graduate who has just gained his first appointment as a physiotherapist in a rural community. In his story, he recalls his journey as a developing professional and how relationships within his fieldwork influenced his learning. It is through understanding the relationship between elements of his story, the plot, the characters and the events and nature of the experience, that we can begin to gain insights into his ways of knowing and, at a broader level, into the importance of relationships within the context of knowledge and learning.

Colin's story (from an interview with Dawn Best)

The first year at university was really good. Being in a placement gives you the best idea of what it's all about. I remember watching a physio with an outpatient. She asked me if I had any ideas about what the problem could be. I didn't know ... In first year, before you have much knowledge, it's hard to know exactly what is going on. I think that really comes later on.

When I got to second year I went to a Community Health Centre for my two week placement. I really felt intimidated the whole time. My supervisor seemed very aggressive. She grilled me about the difference between rheumatoid and osteo-arthritis. When I told her that we hadn't covered it yet, she accused me of lying. She said, 'I've had that many students, I know. It's in my book' [the subject manual sent by Colin's university]. *She got out the book and flicked through it and said, 'Oh, you haven't done it, but anyway you should know it.'*

I really disliked that placement. I'd go there and I'd try my hardest and I'd read up on everything. No matter how hard I tried I could never please her and I hated that placement. It just got me down in the dumps. Every morning I'd wake up and I'd think 'Oh no!'.

I wanted to do well in clinics. I was really enjoying the course and I wanted to show I could do it, but the relationship with this supervisor was very negative – probably the worst I had ever experienced. I usually get along well with people.

I was glad when third year came along. I was bursting with theory. I felt that I really wanted to 'get my hands on'. I remember that I was very nervous and always conscious of doing something wrong. I really didn't function clearly the whole time. I tended to ask questions because they were on a list rather than finding out things about a particular patient. [The word 'patient' is most often used in medical settings. While the authors recognise that Colin has used the words 'patient' and 'client' interchangeably, they have chosen to use the word 'client' within their text.]

In third year, I had excellent supervisors. I had a really good year in three different placements. My first placement was at a big metropolitan hospital for my cardiothoracic clinic. Probably cardio was my weakest point. I struggled a lot and did not have the same enthusiasm. My supervisors were good. They were very knowledgeable. You read your notes and considered your options, but I don't think you have a full grasp of the situation. You speak to these professionals and they seem to be able to incorporate everything. They are so knowledgeable and so spot on.

The second placement in third year was a rehab setting for my neurology clinic. The supervisors not only knew so much, but they presented the knowledge they taught. I listened and it was up to me to absorb it all. I think this was a distant relationship. It wasn't negative, but it wasn't on an equal footing. It was very much based on 'knowing your place'. That rates as one of my best placements. I really loved it and I learnt a lot. I felt I could ask anything. They made me feel right at home from the outset. They gave me the chance to think things out for myself. They supported me, corrected me and gave me hints. When I was in this placement I wanted to go home in the evenings and think about my patients and discover the best way for me to manage their problems. I felt it was up to me and I felt I was in control. They really empowered me. [Colin was referring here to the empowerment that comes from knowing what to expect and being given responsibility for his own learning. He found this 'place' of ownership and self directedness empowering.]

My third placement was in a country hospital. I had two supervisors and they were close in age to me. We socialised and I felt relaxed in their company. We played netball together after work and I addressed them informally within social situations. Little did I realise that the informality of my greetings was considered to be unprofessional and, therefore, a subsequent cause of tension between us. When I got my feedback at the end of the placement I was told off for being unprofessional. I suppose in a way I had let my guard down a bit. But I liked the placement and I was keen to go back there to work.

I was lucky in my first fourth year clinic; they basically let me go. I was in a rehab setting in a big gym area where my supervisors could always keep an eye on me. They basically said, 'Well here's your patient, go for it and ask questions if you need to.' They gave me the chance to think things through. They gave me this freedom and, through this, the opportunity to make links between theory and the needs of this person. This was the first time I'd done that. Now I had to do it for the client, not for my assessment. I began to evaluate according to whether physiotherapy had met the client's needs. This was great.

Although at times I missed out on things, I thought a lot more thoroughly because I had more time and didn't have to keep looking over my shoulder to see who was watching me because someone was assessing what I was doing, or worrying about whether I was hurting the client. I think as long as you keep judging yourself you continue to learn. In fourth year it's good to have a placement where you are let go and you discover more about yourself.

I had had a couple of weeks with my own patients. They were getting better and that was when I started to feel like a physiotherapist. I was now involved in going to team meetings and selecting clients for the weekend lists . . . I felt part of the place. I was able to take initiative rather than being told what to do.

My last placement before graduation was difficult. My mum was sick and I had a hard time with my supervisor. She told me two weeks before I graduated that I should think about another profession because I was never going to make a physio. That doesn't do a lot for your confidence. She'd say, 'I know I'm pushing you hard and your confidence is rock bottom, but I'm going to get more out of you.'

I know I learnt a lot about physiotherapy practice. I also learnt a lot about myself and about life. This was a tough relationship, even worse than my second year experience; however, I did have confidence in myself. Even if you don't get along, it's important to show respect. Otherwise you feel like you can't do anything.

Now I'm back in the country. When I started here, it felt just like another fieldwork placement. For the first month, I felt I had to run what I was doing past someone. After a month I've realised that I don't have to justify what I do to anyone. Now I know that I am answerable to myself. I'm getting really good broad experience and I have a lot of support from the hospital and the private practitioners in the town.

Colin's story tells of his relationships with his supervisors during his fieldwork placements. These relationships and understandings had emotional undertones that impacted on his development as a professional. Colin's expectations and his responses were also guided by the subtleties of his beliefs and values, and his images of what a professional physiotherapist should be like. Positive relationships existed in situations where there was a sense of cooperation, a feeling of confidence in self and a recognition of self by the other. As these relationships developed and changed, Colin experienced new understandings of himself, both as a person and as a developing professional.

There are a number of elements within this story that are worthy of consideration in relation to learning through experience. Given the limited scope of this chapter, we focus on only a few of these elements throughout the rest of this chapter.

We recognise that learning seldom occurs in isolation. We take an interpretative view that gives a holistic, relational perspective and we reflect on the emotionality of relational knowing (Hollingsworth 1994; Elicker 1997). We consider these perspectives in conjunction with Colin's story as we explore his understandings gained through experience. His story highlights the importance of the context and the people involved.

The nature of relationships

Professional experience enables knowledge to be gained through encounters with others and through practising skills during engagement in professional activities, as well as through associated reading and reflection (Reason & Heron 1986). The encounters may be direct, as in being given direction, or contained within conversation, or they may be less direct such as through observation. Encounters most often contain an affective element indicative of being in relationship.

Making the connections

Bateson (1979) argues that learning is a holistic process which has affective, cognitive and conative features. Colin's story reveals differing affective states, from feelings of uncertainty, frustration and being 'down in the dumps' to emerging confidence in self as a professional and a feeling of self-worth. It is interesting to read how the challenges made by those in authority resulted in extra effort on Colin's part. Other situations dampened his enthusiasm, and yet there was no indication that he would withdraw from the programme. Always there was a regard for the 'knowledgeable' professional with whom he worked and a growing appreciation of what it meant to be a professional. The experience of working with professionals in a clinical placement enabled Colin to gain 'the best idea of what . . . [being a physiotherapist] is all about'.

Learning occurs through thoughtful action. Enactment or practical experience may provide the context for the development of understanding (e.g. different perspectives on the management of a client's condition) and the clarification of meaning (such as the appropriateness of differing strategies which are responsive to individual client needs). Understanding and meaning-making are contributing factors in developing relationships.

We next focus on aspects of entering and maintaining a learning relationship.

Trust, respect, authenticity, responsiveness

The importance of interpersonal relationships between students and educators has been discussed by Pickering (1987; 1989–90). Ann, a health science educator wants to 'know her students as people'. She realises that this takes time and commitment and 'imparting a bit of yourself'. Ann feels it is important to be open with the student, to be seen to be fallible, in order to build trust:

> 'I share a lot of my experiences and I also let them see that I'm fallible, because it's really important that they see that being a good professional is not about doing all the right things all the time. I think it makes me human; it makes them see me as someone who understands; it builds trust. [I seek to] work towards a relationship that is mutual where relationships can come up from both sides and be discussed.'
>
> (from interviews with Ann by Lindy McAllister)

Authenticity exists where there is openness about the 'personal'. To be open requires respect and trust. Respect and trust are also associated with developing confidence in self and in others. Where there is confidence, a feeling of security and a sense of openness, then learning is more likely to occur. To be respectful is to have a regard for the other and that regard means that the other person is accepted for who and what they are (Goodfellow 1998).

Entering a learning relationship

For both educators and students, the beginning of the learning journey can be a time of new environments, roles and expectations. Challenges to the maintenance and development of the learning relationship during the newness stage have a heightened emotionality. A mismatch of expectations, or negative emotions which are not acknowledged and managed, can interfere with the establishment of rapport. Rapport provides the medium through which trust, respect and authenticity can be developed.

According to Pickering (1987), educators have expectations that their students will be involved in the learning process as active rather than passive learners who are able to share their perceptions about the learning experience with their educators and are open to change. The expectations that educators have of students' knowledge, skills and attributes are often framed within their own 'pedagogical repertoire' of professional and personal knowledge and experience (Millies 1992, p. 28). While these expectations may be tacit, they guide educators' images and the expectations they hold of students. However, communication and relationship building at this stage are more readily facilitated in situations where these tacit expectations are made explicit. Such disclosure is more likely to occur in situations where both the educator and the student have confidence in themselves.

Learning in an experiential setting is about acquiring practical knowledge and building on propositional knowledge acquired in more formal settings (Higgs & Titchen 1995). Failure to understand the nature of the reorganisation and transformation of knowledge can create anxiety in students and educators. Field-based educators may be angry at the educational institution and resent having to teach the student. They may question what is taught at university and its relevance to the real world of practice. Colin's story shows failure of an educator to appreciate and understand the nature of the learning experience and how to help him. She expected Colin to come with pre-packaged knowledge pertinent to the type of work setting. She did not understand the role that experience in the learning setting would play in the growth of Colin's knowledge and skill.

At the start of any new relationship with students, educators will have their expectations of their educative roles; these expectations will most often be framed within their images of self as educator and practitioner, of students and of the profession. Successful educators have a strong 'sense of self' (McAllister *et al.* 1997). In the words of Ann, 'the most important thing you bring into any job is yourself and your skills and who you are'. This sense of self influences how educators perceive students, and their willingness to act in ways which support students' growth. For example, Annette, a health service educator also interviewed by Lindy McAllister, commented, 'I am always optimistic for [growth in] people and students. I always like to give them the benefit of the doubt. I'm happy to give them extra time'. Similarly, Ann aimed to help students 'grow as people'.

In order to fulfil their role effectively, educators need to 'know the philosophical arguments of their practice and to have a grasp of the traditions in which they are working' (Fish & Twinn 1997, p. 59). Educators may also have concerns about their knowledge, about being watched, and about the challenge of explaining their practice to students. While educators have expectations of themselves, students also have expectations of their educators and of themselves as they enter new learning relationships. Pickering (1987) identified that students expect their educators to share perceptions about the learning situation, to instruct when appropriate and to collaborate in learning as students become more independent, and they expect support for growth towards independence.

Colin's story illustrates some of the expectations displayed in the images he held of himself in relationships within the fieldwork context. Colin expected that he would be working within a supportive and therefore trusting relationship. He was not expecting his educator to be aggressive. And again, his image of himself as an effective communicator within a relationship was shattered when he was disciplined for informality with his educators. As his story of third year placements shows, he expected his educators to be knowledgeable and competent practitioners. As a final year student, he expected and received more independence from his educators, which in turn helped him on his way on his learning journey.

Students hope that they will be liked and will get on well with people in the learning situation. This does not always happen. Erica, a health science student, was shocked at her field-based educator's lack of interest, in a placement where she was not oriented by the educator and was left alone in an office for much of the day. She described how she felt: 'I was not welcome'. Sometimes this sense of being unwelcome stems from the time pressures under which many field-based educators operate (Ferguson & Edwards 1999). Students may be seen as another responsibility to fit into an already over-full day. In addition, students hope to perform well and pass assessments. They would like to successfully put into practice what they already know and to learn new things. Again the learning context within which they gain practical experience becomes an important contributing factor.

Affective aspects of relationships

Field placement responsibilities have varying emotional undertones for both educators and students. Educators may feel ambivalence about taking on the role of educator at all; they may have been coerced by the educational institution as was the case with Jenny, a relatively new graduate therapist, who would 'rather have had more time to consolidate skills before taking a student'. Others may be willing to be involved, but be anxious about how well they will fulfil the role. Given that few tertiary educators outside the school education system are prepared for their roles as educators, this is a not unrealistic concern. For the new fieldwork educator, feelings of inadequacy and discomfort are common. Jenny expressed this as 'self-doubt about whether I was doing the right thing and if another fieldwork educator would do the same thing'. (Quotes from Jenny and from Emma, below, are from interviews with Lindy McAllister.)

Many field-based educators are concerned about balancing their various roles. This need for juggling was apparent to Emma, who, new to her educator role, described it as 'juggling everything around time, everything being the clients, parents, students, people just popping in to ask a question'. Similar tensions were described by Lianne, an early childhood educator:

'My responsibility is for the children ... But I feel that my attention has been drawn away by the student ... in the last four weeks I have developed the student, but I haven't developed the children at all.'

(from interviews with Lianne by Joy Goodfellow)

Multiple responsibilities and accountabilities to different stakeholders may provoke considerable anxiety for educators. This becomes exacerbated with students who are at risk of failure. In these cases, educators may fear having their own professional and personal competence judged. After two failing students in a row Annette became self critical:

'I would have to turn around and have a good look at myself and what I was doing in my role as a fieldwork educator and ask myself had I completely lost the plot that I couldn't cope with two weak students in a row.'

(from interview with Annette by Lindy McAllister)

Students face a vast array of human problems and they may fear the responsibility that they will be given for the welfare of children or clients. In medical settings, students can be shocked by the reality of life-threatening illness and they may fear making mistakes (Best 1990) or harming their clients. Students worry that they do not know what they need to know or that their skills may not be adequate. They may also fear being on show, having to articulate their practice and being judged: 'Having to make explicit my knowledge in this way was really threatening initially' (third year physiotherapy student in interviews by Gillian Webb). Students hope for a learning environment where it is acceptable to ask questions, take risks, make mistakes, reflect and explore options.

Students report that they 'find it very difficult to give answers straight away. I always like to think about things before giving an answer ... [and] I feel if I ask too many questions they will give me a bad mark' (third year physiotherapy student). The fear of being judged is unsettling for some students, like Erica who said of her health science fieldwork placement: 'I really think the supervision wasn't a learning supervision; it was an assessment supervision'. Erica always felt that she was being critiqued and assessed, never supported to learn or being given the freedom to learn. Higgs (1993) has discussed the need for educators to create a liberating learning environment for students, not one which engenders concerns. The inevitable challenges to and tensions within relationships can be more readily addressed where such supportive learning environments exist.

Diversity within relationships

Building and maintaining a learning relationship is based on the rapport between learner and educator. Additional complexity and challenges arise in the relationship when there are differences in values, culture and communication or where expectations of teaching and learning vary.

Differences in culture and communication

Educators and students come from diverse backgrounds with their own social and cultural frameworks. Those frameworks may reflect many values which are unspoken, unchallenged and taken for granted. How we walk, talk, think and feel are culturally determined. Nonverbal cues are often misinterpreted. Since each of us works within our own framework of cultural values, it is necessary to develop an appreciation of shared understanding and open, effective communication. For effective communication to take place, values have to be made explicit if the implications of verbal and nonverbal communication are to be understood (Hofstede 1987).

In the learning setting, minority culture students face many difficulties. These students report that they find 'listening is the hardest'. They may have problems with active listening and simultaneously translating. Other comments reflect uneasiness with 'not knowing when to interrupt; difficulty understanding accents or slurred speech; an awareness that patients seemed less confident with non-Anglo Australian students; problems with having to speak out aloud about their reasoning processes; need an understanding of the local culture e.g. geriatrics; developing empathy when language by itself is difficult' (third and fourth year physiotherapy students).

Educators' judgements of student learning are often based on the ability of students to engage in social conversation and thereby develop a rapport with their patients. Within the health professions, students have reported communication difficulties and concerns about building relationships with their patients. Many students comment that they are unable to make the informal conversation needed in their interactions both with their clients ('I don't know anything about footy and I feel excluded') and with their educators ('I don't know if it is right in Australia to talk about someone's family'). Further, cultures view illness and wellness differently. These differences have important implications for the goals which students in health care settings develop with their clients, and how they approach their clients and communicate with them (Landrine & Klonoff 1992). Different cultures view the goals of education differently (Farver *et al*. 1995). Similarly, students from minority groups or disadvantaged backgrounds may present with particular cultural and communication assumptions and styles. Attention to cultural contexts and approaches to learning appears to be critical, if positive cross-cultural relationships are to be established. Educators need to demonstrate respect for cultural differences. Lack of cultural awareness, unwillingness to learn and poor cross-cultural communication competence in educators can be interpreted by students as racist behaviour, and can pose a major challenge to the maintenance of a learning relationship (Stewart *et al*. 1996).

Differences in expectations of teaching and learning

Lincoln *et al*. (1996) recommend that educators be aware of differences that exist in learning styles, and adapt their teaching styles accordingly. When educators impose their approaches to learning on students, disempowerment and anxiety can result. Learning styles differ noticeably across cultures. For example, the western acceptance of student participation in discussion and debate is different from that of the traditional Chinese classroom where the educator imparts knowledge and students are the recipients of that knowledge (Gallois & Callan 1997). This makes it difficult where students are required to express opinions, make decisions and justify them to their educator, with little time for reflection, perhaps in front of others, where to give the wrong answer has implications of loss of face and feelings of inadequacy. Time for reflection is important to allow for language translation and the complexities of reasoning and expression of that reasoning verbally (McLachlan 1997).

Students sometimes feel that 'clinicians are judging fluency of language rather than the efficacy of the interaction' (third year physiotherapy student). Chinese students often feel uncomfortable about confronting or disagreeing with their supervisors. The Anglo-Australian preference for informality and discussion is very different from the respect for their elders shown by Chinese students. 'In many cultures the educator's opinion is always right. Therefore [it is] hard to express [my] own opinion or even to form [my] own opinion' (physiotherapy student).

Colin's story highlights the importance of educators adapting their role and supervisory style to students' needs, stage of knowledge and skill. In third year he would have liked someone to be 'over his shoulder', but in fourth year he felt he could manage more independently. When educators do not or cannot adapt their style and their level of support to what has been referred to by Higgs (1993) as the learner's task maturity level, then maintenance of the learning relationship may be compromised. Some educators find it easy to offer high levels of support to their students, but are unwilling to challenge the students' thinking through the provision of critique, confrontation, negative feedback or an assessment of poor performance. Emma, a new health science educator raised her fear of 'not being liked' by the student with Lindy McAllister. This perception subsequently led to a prolonged unproductive learning experience, for, as Emma concluded:

> [the student's] 'apparent fragility was a bit of a façade that prevents people going further with her. I decided that a few more direct comments may do more good than harm. She's just not getting indirect messages. I became more assertive with her. If she was going to get anywhere, I couldn't be nice.'

Students commonly express that they want their educators to have positive interpersonal and communication skills, and good professional knowledge and skills. Poor interpersonal skills exhibited by the educator who 'intimidated' Colin did not provide a good role model or create a conducive learning environment. When referring to his second fieldwork experience, Colin highlighted the respect he had for the knowledge of his clinicians and how he regarded them as good role models. Subsequently, his growing professional knowledge and his ability to apply that knowledge in his placements allowed him to feel more confident.

Conclusion

Throughout this chapter we have given consideration to the qualities required of educators, to the assumptions, values and beliefs which influence educators' attitudes, and to the images, experiences and strategies which guide their practices. The educator does not act alone within the teaching/learning process. The responsiveness and individual characteristics of the learners also have a major role to play in the learning relationship dance. It is here, where the tune is one of accord and where students and educators have established and maintained successful learning relationships, that lifelong learning is most likely to take place. Titchen (2000) uses the metaphor of critical companionship to highlight the importance of the relationship between experienced practitioner and learner in the development of professional craft knowledge (practical know-how). When the relationship is based on mutuality, reciprocity and respect for the person, and where individual differences are taken into consideration, then the challenges of learning are balanced within a supporting environment. Educators engage in artistry as they choreograph the relationship dance and act in creative and responsive ways to support student learning.

The stories included in this text reveal experiences of learning which demonstrate a concept of knowledge as being embodied within us. Knowledge is also relational and practical. Knowledge develops over time. We construct new meanings as others respond to our interpretations of experience. However, as lifelong learners, our learning journey is most often a shared one within the domain of human relationships.

References

Bateson, G. (1979) *Mind and Nature*, Ballantine, New York.

Beattie, M. (1997) Fostering reflective practice in teacher education: Inquiry as a framework for the construction of a professional knowledge in teaching, *Asia-Pacific Journal of Teacher Education*, **25**, pp.11–128.

Best, D. (1990) Supervising creative clinicians or competent clones, *Proceedings of the 3rd International Congress of Physical Therapists*. Hong Kong, p. 470.

Clandinin, J. (1985) Personal practical knowledge: A study of teachers' classroom images, *Curriculum Inquiry*, **15**, pp. 361–85.

Elicker, J. (1997) Introduction to the special issue: Developing a relational perspective in early childhood research, *Early Education and Development*, **8**, pp. 5–10.

Farver, J.A.M., Kim, Y.K. & Lee, Y. (1995) Anglo-American preschoolers' interaction and play behavior, *Child Development*, **66**, pp. 1088–99.

Ferguson, K. & Edwards, H. (1999) Providing clinical education: The relationship between health and education, in *Educating Beginning Practitioners: Challenges for Health Professional Educators* (eds J. Higgs & H. Edwards), Butterworth Heinemann, Oxford, pp. 52–8.

Fish, D. & Twinn, S. (eds) (1997) *Quality Clinical Supervision in the Health Care Professions: Principled Approaches to Practice*, Butterworth Heinemann, Oxford.

Gallois, C. & Callan, V. (1997) *Communication and Culture: A Guide for Practice*, Wiley, New York.

Goodfellow, J. (1998) There's a student teacher in my centre: Cooperating teachers' perspectives, *Australian Journal of Early Education*, **23**, pp. 36–45.

Higgs, J. (1993) The teacher in self-directed learning: Manager or co-manager, in *Learner Managed Learning: Practice, Theory and Policy* (ed. N. Graves), World Education Fellowship, London, pp. 122–31.

Higgs, J. & Titchen, A. (1995) The nature, generation and verification of knowledge, *Physiotherapy*, **81**, pp. 521–30.

Hofstede, G. (1997) *Cultures and Organisations: Software of the Mind*, (revised edn), McGraw Hill, New York.

Hollingsworth, S. (Ed.) (1994) *Teacher Research and Urban Literacy Education: Lessons and Conversations in a Feminist Key*, Teachers College Press, New York.

Landrine, H. & Klonoff, E.A. (1992) Culture and health related schemas: A review and proposal for interdisciplinary integration, *Health Psychology*, **11**, pp. 267–76.

Lincoln, M., McLeod, S., McAllister, L., Maloney, D. & Purcell, A. (1996) A longitudinal investigation of reported learning styles in speech pathology students, *Australian Journal of Human Communication Disorders*, **23**, pp. 13–25.

McAllister, L., Higgs, J. & Smith, D. (1997) *A sense of self: A core concept in describing and interpreting the experience of being a clinical educator*, paper presented to national conference of Speech Pathology Australia, Canberra, March.

McLachlan M. (1997) *Culture and Health*, Harper-Collins Publications, New York.

Millies, P.S.G. (1992) The relationship between a teacher's life and teaching, in *Teacher Lore: Learning From Our Own Experience* (eds W.H. Schubert & W.C. Ayres), Longman, New York, pp. 25–43.

Pickering, M. (1987) Expectations and intent in the supervisory process, *The Clinical Supervisor*, **5**, pp. 43–57.

Pickering, M. (1989–90) The supervisory process: An experience of interpersonal relationships and personal growth, *National Student Speech Language Hearing Association Journal*, **17**, pp. 17–28.

Popkewitz, T.S. (1997) A changing terrain of knowledge and power: A social epistemology of educational research, *Educational Researcher*, **26**, pp. 18–29.

Reason, P. & Heron, J. (1986) *Research with people: the paradigm of cooperative inquiry*, Working paper, Centre for the Study of Organisational Change and Development, University of Bath.

Stewart, M., McAllister, L., Rosenthal, J. & Chan, J. (1996) International students in the clinical practicum: Problems with English language proficiency, cross-cultural communication and racism, paper presented to the ISANA 7th Annual Conference: *Waves of change*, Adelaide.

Titchen, A. (2000) *Professional Craft Knowledge in Patient-Centred Nursing and the Facilitation of its Development*, University of Oxford DPhil thesis, Ashdale Press, Oxford.

Zeichner, K. (1985) The ecology of field experience: Towards an understanding of the role of field experiences in teacher development, *Journal of Research and Development in Education*, **18**, pp. 44–52.

Chapter 14
Becoming in Professional Practice: an Exemplar

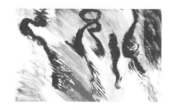

Robyn Ewing and David Smith

This chapter explores the notion of 'becoming' in professional practice, through a description of a teacher development programme which has evolved in a sub-urban Sydney primary school. It aims to bring together challenges for teachers, beginning teachers and teacher-educators. These challenges include the need for teachers to continually develop their skills professionally with ever-decreasing financial support; for beginning teachers to experience school-based opportunities over extended time frames; and for teacher-educators to make their courses meaningful, bridging the gap between university courses and classroom practice. As such, it not only provides an account of professionals at work in their action context, it also provides one model for bringing about changes in practice through professional learning at the site of the practice.

The main body of the chapter is written by the mentor who entered the primary school to advise on professional development and the development of the school programme. The school principal and project coordinator made comments which have been used in revising the chapter. A second voice is provided by an external researcher who has recently evaluated the project for the National Innovative and Best Practice Project. This second voice is indicated in italics and provides a reflective commentary on issues related to the knowing, being and becoming aspects of professional practice as revealed in the project.

A brief description of the background to the project is provided initially. It should be noted that the project was centrally concerned with increasing the learning outcomes of students. Thus a major part of the data gathered is derived from interviews with students. Since this chapter is principally about issues of professional practice, the main data reported here concern teachers' professional learning, knowing and becoming. Further details of the complete project are available elsewhere (Cusworth 1997; Ewing *et al.* 1998).

Background: North Curl Curl Primary School

North Curl Curl Primary School is located on Sydney's northern beaches and has about 450 students, 20% of whom are from language backgrounds other than

English. Student backgrounds are diverse, with a large number of students from a lower socioeconomic background.

So professional practice occurs in 'real' and authentic contexts with people whose lives and needs are diverse. Such contexts demand complex and sophisticated knowledge bases that force professionals outside their own values and life experience. Such demands are an important source for both knowing and becoming.

From the outset the project has been concerned with improving student literacy outcomes and developing strategies to implement the K-6 (primary school years of kindergarten to year 6) English syllabus (NSW Board of Studies 1994). The project has evolved over the last four years. It can best be described in three phases, as detailed below.

Thus professional practice is purposeful and moral and should act to further the interests of the clients, in this case, the students. Professional learning is continuing and developmental, often best structured as a spiral, building new learnings on previous ones.

Phase 1 (1994): Identification of priority needs: literacy with years 3 and 4 and initial planning and implementation

Possible involvement in the Innovative Links Project (a nationally funded initiative in Australia from 1994–96 to link schools and universities in a mutually beneficial partnership) led to staff discussion and consensus that, initially, the project at Curl Curl North would centre around the literacy needs of year 3 and 4 students. There were several reasons for this.

First, the English syllabus had been published in its initial form in 1994, providing the catalyst to focus on improved literacy outcomes in the K-6 years. Previously, there had been some resourcing of early childhood (stage one) literacy needs with the appointment of a K-1 literacy teacher to Curl Curl. The school had also been an exemplar in the development of the reading recovery programme, particularly for stage one students. Early literacy had also been well supported with the introduction of the state-developed early learning profiles in 1994, with initial units written in the school to support them. Thus there had also been a concentration of professional development at stage one. It seemed, therefore, that the continuum of student and teacher learning needed support at the junior primary level.

Second, the emphasis on an outcomes-based approach to assessment and programming in the syllabus necessitated a shift in pedagogy to a focus on student learning outcomes in talking and listening, reading and writing, rather than teacher purposes at each stage. The syllabus document itself did not contain explicit guidance about how this was to be achieved and then communicated to parents. It was decided that it would be better for the school to focus on one stage of development than to try to achieve this simultaneously across all stages.

In addition, an externally determined short time frame for implementation of the syllabus caused teachers concern. The professional development opportunities offered by the NSW Board of Studies and employing bodies to help teachers implement the syllabus were limited, with short workshops or seminars following a 'train the trainer' model, despite evidence that mandated change from central bodies does not produce lasting or significant change and that teachers need ongoing professional support over time (Fullan 1994). It was clear that the professional development opportunities provided by the NSW Department of School Education needed supplementation if real curriculum reform was to occur at the school.

> *Being a professional means being a lifelong learner, continually becoming and 'rebecoming', keeping pace with changing knowledge and practice in the professional field, and responding to changing political and social policy contexts and mandates, which themselves often demand new professional knowledge and skills.*

Using some of the initial funding, year 3 and 4 teachers were released once a week to examine the intended outcomes for junior primary in the document. They explored ways of using the syllabus outcomes and developed more explicit pointers or indicators to demonstrate when outcomes had been achieved. The teachers trialled different 'user-friendly' assessment proformas and concentrated on targeted children in year 3. Taking very successful and less successful year 3 students, they attempted to assess the students' stage and levels of achievement using the syllabus outcomes. It became obvious that this approach was both excessively time consuming and totally assessment driven. It seemed that teachers needed more support in the use of the methodology of the functional model of language (NSW Board of Studies 1994) before strategies for assessment could be examined effectively.

> *Because of the intense and demanding nature of professional practice, often the only way in which ongoing professional learning can occur is through external resourcing and support (Fullan 1994) facilitating release from professional duties. This was a very important feature of the project described here.*

While the first six months of the project had been useful for the year 3–4 teachers directly involved, the end of the year saw staff changes and recognition of the need to find a way of involving all staff in the project. The funding had provided:

- Time release for professional dialogue to identify priorities
- Opportunities for staff to discuss documents and trial various assessment strategies

- Opportunities to examine the individual needs of the students at the school in context.

Phase II (1995): The involvement of a mentor

In 1995, classes were organised to maximise the opportunities to meet the needs of individual students through:

- Establishment of a year 3/4 class of more able students
- Establishment of a year 4/5 class of boys and a year 4 class of girls as a direct strategy to improve educational opportunities
- The recruitment of a mentor to work alongside classroom teachers to support change in pedagogy which staff saw as vital in order to implement changes implicit in the new English syllabus.

From term 2 of 1995, a mentor, Robyn (Cusworth) Ewing, from the University of Sydney's Education Faculty, was recommended on the basis of her work at a nearby school (Cusworth & Dickinson 1994). The executive staff met with Robyn several times to establish her brief which is summarised as: to support teachers in improving the literacy outcomes of years 3 and 4 students at Curl Curl North Primary School. This was to be achieved through focusing on changes in teaching and learning strategies necessitated by a functional approach to English. Changes in teaching and learning programmes would lead to improved assessment using the syllabus outcomes and profiles to identify students' achievements and needs. The usefulness of the outcomes-based approach in profiling year 4 students would also be monitored.

Robyn met with the whole staff on several occasions and had input to the staff professional day on literacy. She also presented her research on newstime (Cusworth 1995, 1996) to the staff and to the early childhood group which met at the school.

The mentor's work in each class varied according to the individual teacher's needs. It initially included working on report writing with the extension 3/4 class, using drama to develop narrative writing with the year 4 girls' class, and developing critical literacy skills with the year 4/5 boys' class. The year 3 class teacher chose to meet with Robyn regularly in order to participate in a professional dialogue based on his own identified training and development needs. From this came the concept of an optional collegial group in which individual teachers could share their expertise with others. This group met throughout term 4.

Data about outcomes from this mentoring phase were collected at the end of 1995 through two questionnaires, one administered to all staff and one to participating teachers. Positive features identified included:

- Staff not directly teaching in years 3 or 4 expressed a desire to be more involved in the project
- Classroom teachers involved were happy with the team-teaching approach used by the mentor
- Staff as a whole felt that professional development had been ongoing and successful and met individual needs; that is, it followed a concerns-based professional development model (Hall & Hord 1987)
- The units of work generated by the joint programming had been effectively implemented and were available for other staff.

Difficulties identified included time constraints and the delayed arrival of some resources. Possible ways forward suggested in the evaluation were:

- Further exploration of integration possibilities: programming across all the KLAs (key learning areas in primary school curriculum)
- Further development of the articulation between a functional approach and grammar, especially in facilitating children's understanding of how language works
- Continued use of drama strategies to enhance literacy development, perhaps monitoring children's responses more formally for assessment purposes
- A conscious effort to ensure involvement of all staff in the programme whilst not detracting from the outcomes of the programme.

Mentoring is a powerful strategy for professional learning in the context in which the practice occurs. It involves a more experienced colleague who, in a relationship of equals, has a strong commitment to assisting a professional colleague(s) who is a neophyte in the area of the mentoring (Hatton & Harman 1997). Effective mentoring entails being with the neophyte and working with the developing concerns and needs of the neophyte, as further illustrated in the next section. Because it is more a relationship of equals, successful mentoring results in mutual learning and becoming for the mentor and the mentee(s).

Phase III (1996–8): Ongoing professional development K-6 and school-based drama programme

Phase III of the project supported links across K-6 rather than only years 3–4. This met the desire for more teachers to be directly involved. The mentor worked individually with a key teacher in each grade, so that specific needs and concerns could be discussed and programmes developed which were focused on the issues identified by the teacher. In this way the teachers' self-identified needs drove the mentoring, rather than the reverse. Examples of teachers' concerns addressed in 1996 are:

Year 6:   To extend understanding of the English document, e.g. to refine teaching of grammar using a literature-based and functional approach.

Year 5:   To use a range of strategies to help develop the children's writing, specifically in the area of argument (Olympics in Sydney – term 3) and narrative (in the *Rowan of Rin* activity – term 4), while providing support for a beginning teacher in terms of planning and programming specifically in English.

Year 4:   To use a range of drama strategies to facilitate a cooperative classroom climate. Focus strategies included encouraging readers to use a 'theatre mantle' and to use collage (see Cusworth and Simons (1997)).

Year 2:   To use drama strategies to enhance literacy development, specifically the development of research skills in report writing.

Year 1:   To use 'hot seating', 'frozen moments' and oral discussion to enhance children's writing and understanding of multiple meaning in a range of literary texts.

Kindergarten: To develop students' oral storying as a precursor to written narrative.

Each teacher involved in the mentoring in turn mentored other teachers. The mentoring allowed teachers to take greater ownership of English across the school, sharing their expertise and ideas rather than working as individuals in isolation in their classrooms. The development of a collegial climate was thus facilitated.

In addition, teachers on the school's English Committee were released to work with Robyn on the development of a new English policy and the organisation of the school's English resources. The acquisition and organisation of English resources across the school had been a major concern for members of the English Committee. 'Links' funding allowed careful consideration of the direction in which the staff needed to go, in resourcing the English key learning area. For example, it enabled multiple copies of quality literary texts to be purchased, as well as some appropriate factual material to support the literacy needs of students at each stage and level in the outcomes framework outlined by the syllabus document. In addition, units were organised around these texts to support teachers in their implementation of the new English syllabus. 'Links' allowed time for planning and professional dialogue in a considered way, so that decision-making could be coherent across the school. The mentor was made a member of the English Committee and offered her expertise alongside that of other committee members.

Professional practice is intensely people-centred and interactive. In the daily work of the professional there is little opportunity for private time for deliberate reflection on decisions being made instantaneously in the action context. Deliberate reflection, however, is central to professional learning, development and becoming. The resources of the 'Links' programme provided release and opportunity for this essential reflection, and thus enabled professional learning to take place. Just as important, this reflection possibility was presented to teachers in their workplace, optimising both time and opportunity for participation.

School-based drama programme

There was a growing awareness of the importance of drama strategies to enhance the development of critical literacy. The syllabus contained a listing of many drama ideas but there was little professional development available in that aspect. A school-based university drama programme was developed by the mentor and staff at the school. In this programme, final year university students in a primary teacher education degree who were completing a drama major were allocated to each class. Each week for ten weeks in both semester 1 and 2 the students used drama strategies in English or other key learning areas during a 40 minute lesson, modelling the use of drama as a powerful teaching methodology across the primary curriculum. After school, both drama students and teachers attended a professional development seminar to continue to refine their expertise.

Teachers in surrounding schools were invited to the after-school seminars at minimal cost. The programme aimed to:

- Enable student teachers to work alongside experienced teachers, sharing expertise in an ongoing relationship over the year
- Enable cooperating teachers to directly experience the use of drama as a powerful teaching methodology across the KLAs and to experience ideas suggested in the English syllabus
- Share the professional development in drama and literacy with surrounding schools and teachers.

The school-based preservice component also demonstrated that resources can be used in a flexible way to effectively reach teachers at all stages of their professional journey. Developing a collegial partnership across the education continuum can be empowering for all concerned. In their course evaluations the student teachers commented frequently that the seminars alongside 'real live teachers' had been very beneficial. Hearing the teachers comment about ideas and strategies as they related to their classroom contexts provided a valuable dimension to the course.

Over 1997 and 1998 the mentoring continued. The mentor worked with all but three teachers in the school. The non-participating teachers were initially unsure about the concept of having another person in their classroom. Another component of the mentoring support in 1997 was the development of a reporting framework incorporating the writing outcomes from the K-6 English syllabus, so that they could be communicated more effectively to parents.

The successful inclusion of the school in the innovative and best practice national evaluation in term 4, 1998 and term 1, 1999 led to the writing of a number of English and Arts units for implementation at each level, as well as a comprehensive evaluation of the whole initiative by a researcher external to the innovation. The researcher, David Smith, facilitated seven focus discussions with students from each grade across the school who had worked with the mentor. He also interviewed both the principal, the 'Links' coordinator and six teachers who had been involved in the mentoring programme and the school-based drama professional development programme. The interview information was combined with the earlier questionnaire data and with student teacher evaluations of the drama unit at the school.

Teachers were unanimous in positive, unequivocal support for the mentoring process. They were also unanimous that it should continue. Major gains in both their own professional development and students' learning outcomes in literature and drama were perceived. Factors identified by teachers in the success of the innovation included:

- The *voluntary* nature of the programme, in that no teachers were pressured to be involved
- The *release* time provided by the funding to *plan, discuss and assess* teaching and learning strategies and issues
- The *longevity* of the project, enabling less confident teachers to see the process work successfully and to become involved over time
- The *sharing* of experiences at meetings and through student performances at assemblies (e.g. 'I have learnt a lot and been able to pass on ideas and strategies to other staff members')
- The *modelling* process and the credibility of the mentor (e.g. 'seeing Robyn work in *my* classroom with *my* kids'; 'the mentor provided me with a window into what my students didn't understand'; 'Robyn is prepared to roll up her sleeves . . .')
- The *essentially practical nature* of the school-based drama and literature course (e.g. 'I believe that this kind of mentoring programme is an effective facilitator of real growth and change')
- The *personal and professional relationships* that grew between staff, students and mentor.

In thinking about ways in which the programme could be improved, teachers suggested that larger blocks of time with the mentor might be useful. For example, instead of the mentor coming for 40 minutes once a week over a term, it might be fortnightly for a whole (morning or afternoon) session and over a longer time frame. In addition, more sharing opportunities at staff meetings might also be productive. Teachers also felt that opportunities for grade meetings with the mentor would also be valuable.

> *There are some important aspects reflected in the teachers' comments. First, without exception, they all describe powerful personal professional learning that has given them new confidence and efficacy in professional knowledge and practice: learning that has resulted in new becoming. Second, this has occurred because the learning has been in response to their professional needs derived from their own work, and the learning opportunity has been voluntary and provided in their own classrooms and school. Third, the learning opportunity has been delivered by a mentor perceived to have strong credibility in classroom practice because of her success in working with the teachers' students in the teachers' classrooms. The mentoring relationship has been based on equality in which both mentor and mentees have learned through mutually investigating their professional practice through being together. As a result both parties have used their being and learning together as a platform for their continuing professional knowing and for their becoming, both as persons and as professional practitioners.*

Conclusions

A major outcome of the 'Links' programme at the school was the opportunity for teachers to grapple with the changes in pedagogy necessary for true reform. The leaders of the school community saw the need for coherent, ongoing professional development for teachers if real change of major significance was to occur. The process was thus ongoing and continually evolving to meet the needs of the individual teacher as well as those of the school community. The teacher-driven nature of the professional development was a crucial feature of its success.

Students at the school experienced a range of broad teaching and learning activities which enhanced their literacy development. Student teachers were provided with more opportunities to trial strategies and ideas learned in theory alongside experienced classroom practitioners.

For the mentor, it was important to be welcomed and made part of a school community. She learned much from being in K-6 classrooms each week alongside teachers interested in changing their practices. Her understanding of the pressures facing classroom teachers was maintained. She was able to stay authentic.

> *Professional work is a holistic activity. It demands the effective integration of the personal self and the professional self. Professional practice is based on decisions deriving from perceptions and beliefs that arise both from professional education and personal life experience and biography. Thus any authentic and lasting*

change in professional practice demands a reassessment of the professional's beliefs, perceptions and actions. Authentic change can occur only within the individual. It cannot be mandated or imposed by others. Arguably, it is only change based on self-directed learning that can be the catalyst for the continual becoming of the professional. Such learning and change require support and release from the busy action context of practice. Professionals need to feel that such professional learning and the time to undertake it are valued by the leaders of the organisations in which they work. In short, the continual learning that is essential to being an effective professional and person occurs most successfully in an organisational culture that explicitly values and is committed to fostering and supporting such learning. The school and programme described in this chapter provide some important insights into how such learning can occur and how such a professional culture can be established.

Acknowledgements

The authors acknowledge with thanks the input from Patricia Cavenagh, Principal at Curl Curl North Primary School and Kerry Scott, Links Coordinator.

References

Cusworth, R. (1995) The framing of educational knowledge through newstime in junior primary classrooms, PhD thesis, The University of Sydney.

Cusworth, R. (1996) Newstime and oral narrative, in *Talking to Learn* (ed. P. Collins), Primary English Teaching Association, Sydney, pp. 25–36.

Cusworth, R. (1997) *School based teacher education alongside professional development: Changes, challenges, chances.* Paper presented at Practicum Experiences in Professional Education Conference, Adelaide, February.

Cusworth, R. & Dickinson, A. (1994) *Changing the curriculum: A case study.* Paper presented at AARE Conference, Newcastle, November.

Cusworth, R. & Simons, J. (1997) *Beyond the Script*, Primary Teachers Association, Sydney.

Ewing, R., Cavenagh, P. & Scott, K. (1998) *Celebrating best practice: Developing links across the primary-secondary-tertiary continuum.* Paper presented at the International Practitioner Conference, University of Sydney, July.

Fullan, M. (1994) *Change Forces. Probing the Depth of Educational Reform*, Falmer, London.

Hall, G. & Hord, S. (1987) *Change in Schools: Facilitating the Process*, State University of New York, Albany.

Hatton, N. & Harman, K. (1997) *Internships Within Teacher Education Programs in NSW*, NSW Department of Education and Training and University of Sydney Faculty of Education, Sydney.

NSW Board of Studies (1994) *English Syllabus and Support Documents*, NSW Board of Studies, Sydney.

Chapter 15
Transforming Practice

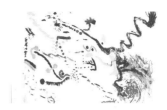

Angie Titchen, Jim Butler and Robert Kay

In our dynamic times professional practitioners face many external pressures which create and demand changes to our work environments and practices. The active (chosen) transformation of practice by practitioners is part of a professional responsibility to continue to provide quality and relevant services, and part of the drive of professions or organisations to retain or enhance their viability in a competitive and accountability-seeking context.

This chapter focuses on practice development which involves external facilitation. It addresses the general question of how outside facilitators (academics working in institutions that focus either on practice development or theory development) can relate with practice organisations, so that the people in the practice organisation are encouraged and skilled to pursue their own growth patterns and transform their professional practice. A conceptual framework is offered that illustrates the vision of how insider-outsider relationships can be designed so that effective, reciprocal relationships are fostered. Four processes that can be used to promote transformation of the practices of those in the practice organisation are described.

Introduction

Practice development needs to take place within a framework that recognises the complexity of transforming organisations and bringing about large scale organisational change. In the past, perhaps because this complexity was not fully acknowledged, it was rare for academic institutions to provide support to organisations undertaking major practice development. Kitson *et al.* (1996) conclude that lack of academic links appear to have led to many failed or ineffective initiatives because staff were poorly trained, were not supervised appropriately, and had no strategic view of which problems to address first.

We believe that professional people involved in transforming practice, whether they work in health care organisations, schools or businesses, need to be skilled in facilitating change and in using research and evaluation methods in their practice organisations. In our experience, academic institutions that focus on practice development, practice development research and implementing research into practice have a significant part to play, not only in offering training and support to practitioners in the methodologies and techniques of practice development, but also in helping organisations to set strategic directions for practice development. We now present a description of how two academic institutions live out such beliefs.

Institutions with a practice development focus

The first organisation is the Royal College of Nursing Institute in the UK. Its primary focus is on the integration of practice development, research and education. For nearly ten years, it has been engaging in collaborative practice development projects with health care organisations and undertaking research into the nature of practice development. A definition of practice development in health care has been generated from a critique of this work:

> 'Practice development is a continuous process of improvement towards increased effectiveness in person-centred care, through the enabling of nurses and health care teams to transform the culture and context of care. It is undertaken and supported by facilitators committed to a systematic, rigorous and continuous process of emancipatory change.'
>
> (McCormack *et al.* 1999)

This critique has facilitated the development of conceptual frameworks for practice development (Titchen 1998, 2000; Jackson *et al.* 1999; McCormack *et al.* 1999), for practice development research (Titchen & Binnie 1993a, 1993b; Kitson *et al.* 1996, 1998), and for the implementation of research into practice (Kitson *et al.* 1996, 1998). These frameworks are located within a critical social science philosophy to achieve successful transformation at patient, organisational and strategic levels. Critical social science is a way of generating knowledge which views the world critically and seeks to redress power imbalances. Use of a critical social science philosophy, in this context, enables a rigorous approach to practice development that attempts to improve patient care by transforming the structures, roles, power relationships or cultures that hinder the delivery of the best possible care. There is an attempt to gain theoretical and practical insights and understandings, through research, debate and critique, not only about the sociohistoric, cultural and political factors that shape current practice and hinder change, but also about how to address those factors to bring about change and to better understand new practices and practitioners' ways of knowing, doing, being and becoming.

   Systematic approaches that integrate learning, development and research have been developed. These approaches are concerned not only with changing a particular practice, but also with transforming the culture and context in which care is delivered. Such a focus requires skilled facilitation imbued with a philosophy of emancipatory change. Thus participative, person-centred processes are used.

The Institute helps health care organisations to identify development needs, practice development targets, objectives and quality criteria in their business plans. It attempts to convince organisations that development staff need to be skilled and confident in the use of change management, research and evaluation techniques in specific contexts.

What is unusual about the Institute is an equal valuing by staff of practice development and research – in contrast with the tendency for academic institutions to place greater value on research. There is also a valuing of the knowledge created by practitioners in the course of their everyday work. Such values underpinned an action research study (Binnie & Titchen 1998, 1999) in which the Institute supported the successful transformation of a task-focused nursing service into a patient-centred service. Angie Titchen, an Institute staff member, worked in partnership with Alison Binnie, a senior sister and leader of the development programme in an acute medical unit. They adopted the complementary roles of actor and researcher in what they came to call a 'double act' (Titchen & Binnie 1993a, 1994) and developed collaborative, interconnected strategies (Titchen & Binnie 1993b) for:

- Facilitating organisational, cultural, practice and relationship changes
- Helping practitioners to research their own practice
- Facilitating professional learning and reflective practice
- Changing power relationships
- Generating and testing theory about how the above changes could be brought about and facilitated.

Although the organisational changes took place early in the development, it took nearly three years before a conducive culture was in place to support an ongoing developmental and person-centred environment. In this environment, creative nursing teams were shaping ward life and developing collegiate relationships with doctors, and therapeutic relationships with patients which patients experienced as healing.

Key issues to emerge from the study were the importance of ownership of the changes by staff, the creation of a learning culture, the fostering of practitioners' critical, independent and creative thinking, and learning through an iterative, reflective process in which theoretically informed ideas were put into action and evaluated. The following data give a glimpse of what this kind of ownership and participation meant to participants:

TERRY: 'I don't think I ever thought (before the development) about how I could change things or whatever, because I didn't feel I was in a position to do anything about it.'

ALISON BINNIE: 'The nurses felt that every patient should have a primary nurse ... and they said, "How do we make sure that happens?" and they came up with the solution that whoever admits the patient needs to have permission to decide who the primary nurse will be ... They negotiated the ground rules for how that would be done ... It was very much their own work.'

(Binnie & Titchen 1998, p. 96, p. 100)

The second institution that supports practice development is the University of Queensland. Two academics at the university, Jim Butler and John Edwards, who both specialise in adult development, thinking skills and action learning, worked with a mineral processing company in Australia, Queensland Magnesia (QMAG). Through a collaborative relationship with the company from 1992 to 1996, they facilitated a programme called the Action Thinking Programme.

The desired practice development was to have thinking and learning employees throughout the company. Jim and John stayed in a long-term contractual relationship with this company to ensure that they took responsibility for the outcomes of their work. They also understood the long-term evolutionary nature of practice development programmes. Their aim was always to 'design ourselves out of a job' by working with staff within the organisation to embed the programme in ways that only they could understand. They collected data throughout the programme to maintain its focus and to keep adding value. One striking measure of the value they added is the awards achieved by QMAG, four years from the commencement of the development programme:

- Queensland Exporter of the Year 1995
- Australian Mineral Exporter of the Year 1995
- Australasian Institute of Mining and Metallurgy Operating Team of the Year 1996.

An Action Thinking Programme has two central aims:

(1) To use more effectively the existing skills, knowledge and creativity of employees
(2) To develop thinking skills and continuous improvement processes.

The programme has three phases, as follows.

Phase 1

Phase 1 introduces staff to the best of current international research and practice across a range of areas: skill acquisition; professional growth; lateral, parallel and systems thinking; ways to identify root causes of underlying problems; models of change; and challenge and support structures. Each staff member designs his/her individual professional action strategy. The remainder of phase 1 focuses on action learning cycles in the workplace setting. Commitment to these iterative cycles provides the basis for ongoing professional development.

Phase 2

Phase 2 focuses on group processes and feedback loops which are seen as the major areas of leverage. Groups develop collective action plans through which they explore their personal professional performance when working in a team. There is a strong focus on identifying the differences evident in the organisation between what Argyris and Schön (1974) term espoused theories (what we say we do) and theories-in-use (what we actually do). The latest research on innovation and leading change provides ways to innovate while maintaining the impetus of our core business. The whole framework of phase 2 is situated within the context of personal responsibility.

Phase 3

Phase 3 of the programme is where the external academics (facilitators) are completely phased out and where the company takes full internal control of the programme. This involves the development of a clear vision of where the company needs to focus its energies, and generation of innovative action plans to achieve the designed performance targets. Throughout this programme, learning takes a central role.

In the business environment, practice development is most often identified with the notion of the learning organisation, a notion that is also valued in some health care organisations (e.g. Kramer & Schmalenbereg 1985). As an ideal, the learning organisation has received considerable attention from the business press and organisations alike. Despite its popularity, however, clear examples, such as QMAG, are difficult to find.

Common features in the support provided by these two academic institutions can be distinguished:

- Facilitating the acquisition/use/creation of skill and knowledge by:
    - developing critical, creative and independent thinking skills
    - setting up work-based, reflective cycles of experiential learning, i.e. action learning or action research
    - creating learning cultures
- Offering support and challenge over several years rather than months
- Facilitating decentralisation, emancipation and democracy by promoting staff ownership of practice development
- Providing structure (e.g. in the form of phases or conceptual frameworks).

A conceptual framework for transforming practice

The relationship between academic institutions and practice discussed so far contrasts with the way that most institutions in higher education relate to practice organisations, such as health care organisations, businesses, companies, manufacturers, in their attempts to develop and improve practice. The traditional relationship between the academic institution and the practice organisation is shown in Fig. 15.1. (We recognise that practice organisations participate in clinical education. This aspect is not explored in this chapter and is not identified in the Figures 15.1 and 15.2.)

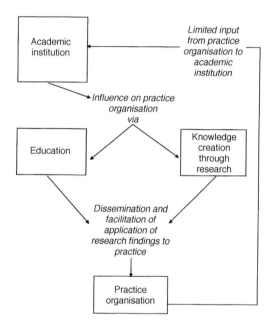

Fig. 15.1 Traditional relationship between academic institutions and practice organisations.

The traditional role of the academic institution is to develop practice through the generation and dissemination of knowledge for disciplinary practice, through professional education for beginning practitioners and through research awareness courses for professionals to help them to critique research findings and apply them to practice if appropriate. This relationship with practice organisations is not normally a reciprocal one, either in terms of knowledge creation or education, the institution being the provider and the practice organisation being the receiver. This lack of reciprocity serves to maintain the well-known theory–practice gap. Figure 15.1 shows how the practice organisation has little or no input into generating knowledge and thus, into contributing to the professional curricula delivered by the academic institution.

As well as providing educational programmes, academics have also adopted more participatory approaches, such as action research, to help practitioners apply research findings to their specific practices (e.g. Hunt 1987; Wilson-Barnett *et al.* 1990). Academics are now aware that it is often organisational and cultural barriers that prevent practitioners from transferring research into practice (e.g. Haines & Jones, 1994; Rodgers 1994). Yet working with the practice organisation as a whole, as described in our examples, is not common practice. It is rare that academics help practitioners to become more aware of and to value their own evidence, that is, the professional craft knowledge (practical know-how) they accrue through experience, or help them to test its validity. Academics may not recognise that research-based knowledge cannot be just applied 'off the shelf' in a simple deductive process. Practitioners have to make time and effort to think through the practical implications of particularising research findings, in addition to generating professional craft knowledge about how the findings can be used in the care of this particular person, situation and context (Titchen 2000).

Do academics value professional craft knowledge? Not as much as research-based knowledge, it would seem. Those driving evidence-based practice movements in Australian and British educational and health care systems (e.g. National Health Service Executive 1998) focus on helping practitioners to transfer research evidence into practice, rather than facilitating practitioners' knowledge creation and validation ability and harmonisation of the different kinds of knowledge.

We therefore propose that academic institutions that currently focus on theory development and education should take on more active roles in supporting practice development that promotes knowledge creation and validation at strategic, organisational and individual levels. We suggest that they set up the relationship shown in Fig. 15.2, which would contribute to the elimination of the theory–practice gap.

Our vision is that institutions which currently do not have a practice development focus develop conceptual frameworks, approaches and strategies for practice development (or use those that are already available). Thereby, practitioners would be helped to:

- Incorporate research into practice by critiquing research findings and developing professional craft knowledge about how to use them in particular instances
- Identify, implement and evaluate necessary structural, cultural and practice changes
- Rigorously create and validate knowledge themselves.

Moreover, knowledge could be co-created by practitioners and academics, in the process of further understanding and improving practice, about new or improved

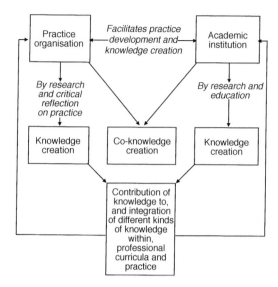

Fig. 15.2   Proposed relationship between academic institutions and practice organisations.

practices and the transformation processes necessary to get them into place. Together, the harmonisation and integration of theoretical and professional craft knowledge could be achieved through an equal valuing of each kind of knowledge and an exploration of how these different forms of knowledge interact with each other. Finally, this integrated knowledge could be used by the academic institution to re-map professional knowledge and its curricula for the preparation of practitioners.

This vision of a reciprocal relationship, in which the academic institution and the practice organisation give to and receive from each other, can be achieved by locating practice development within a critical social science philosophy and by facilitating it through a 'critical companionship' approach (Titchen 1998, 2000; McCormack *et al.* 1999). Such an approach is concerned with looking critically at the world and the systems within it with a view to changing prevailing power relationships (Habermas 1985; Carr & Kemmis 1986; Fay 1987). The academic institution, as critical companion, helps practitioners to engage in a systematic critique of their self-understandings and social practices as a precursor to determining ways of transforming the status quo. Guided by four critical social science concepts – consciousness-raising, problematisation, self-reflection and critique – staff members of the academic institute (critical companions) use a range of practical strategies, such as articulating professional craft knowledge, observing, listening and questioning, and critical dialogue.

We now turn to examine some processes that can be used by critical companions.

Processes for the transformation of practice

Creating organisational slack

The organisational requirement or condition for practice development to flourish has been termed 'organisational slack' (Schein 1995) or 'redundancy'. This concept refers to creating space for investment in development and in the future of the organisation:

> 'Redundancy is important because it encourages frequent dialogue and communication. This helps create a "common cognitive ground" among employees and thus facilitates the transfer of tacit knowledge. Since members of the organisation share overlapping information, they can sense what others are struggling to articulate.'
>
> (Nonaka & Takeuchi 1995, p. 14)

The organisation must also leave slack in the system so that innovative people do not feel oppressed by the immediate crisis of problem solving or the day-to-day pressure. The concept of lean and mean can be dangerous if it implies the removal of all slack (Schein 1995). Organisational slack can be generated in several ways. One way is by helping people to understand why many managers inhibit organisational slack, and thus organisational learning. This inhibition is created by four beliefs of managers:

- They fear innovation because they seek to avoid failure: losing present success
- They value control and therefore are unable to grant the freedom of slack: losing cohesion
- They focus on immediate productivity and thus see 'slack' as a waste: losing efficiency
- They fear loss of jobs caused by improvement: losing people.

One way forward out of these dilemmas is for the critical companion to work at the top of the organisation with the more visionary leaders and senior managers who influence policy and resource decision-making. They can be encouraged to carry out benefit/risk analyses to demonstrate to stakeholders the benefits of resourcing slack and the risks of not doing so. It can be pointed out how building in slack will enable the organisation to meet current national policies and agendas.

Another way would be for a critical companion to work with managers who hold any of the four beliefs above and help them to see the incongruence between these beliefs and those of practice development. Another is for the companion to help practitioners provide evidence of need of slack to their managers. Even when slack is provided, practitioners may still believe that they are too busy to engage in development work. In this situation, the companion can provide opportunities that enable practitioners to experience the benefit of taking time-out. This usually results in practitioners then making time.

Creating a learning culture

We have emphasised the importance of a learning culture within organisations. A learning culture can be defined as the shared vision, meanings, values, beliefs and attitudes, held by the organisation and those who work within it, that support learning at work. Within a learning culture, change is seen as possible and health/positive, and 'individuals, teams and organisations can openly discuss their practice, reflect upon what they do well and not so well, and learn from their mistakes' (RCN 1998, p. 4). There is also an attempt to bring out the best in each individual and respect and care for each person.

The first step in creating a learning culture is to foster senior management's commitment to it and then to help them and other members of the organisation to co-create a shared vision of a learning culture for their organisation through a collaborative process (see Smith 1994). It is important that people's values and beliefs about a learning culture are made explicit. Then it will be possible to determine whether there is congruence between the values and visions of different colleagues and whether there is acceptance of a particular practice development approach.

Beliefs and values can be made explicit through a values clarification exercise (Warfield & Manley 1990) in which a group of colleagues is invited to discuss the concept of a learning culture before completing the following sentences. By so doing, an individual creates a personal vision.

- I believe a learning culture is . . .
- I believe the purpose of creating a learning culture is . . .
- I believe a learning culture can be achieved by . . .
- I believe barriers to establishing a learning culture are . . .
- I believe I can contribute to creating a learning culture by . . .
- Other beliefs and values I hold about a learning culture are . . .

The sentences completed, the critical companion stimulates discussion on the similarities and differences between the beliefs and values of the group members. If there are major differences, the group discusses the reasons for them and ways in which they could resolve their differences or work together effectively despite these differences. Then the participants discuss the similarities and differences between the values they express and the practice development philosophy, exploring how they can operate in ways that are congruent with both.

Earlier, we stressed our strong focus on pointing out dissonance between Argyris and Schön's (1974) espoused theories and theory-in-use. We put the same focus on espoused values and values-in-use. So, for example, if the group agrees that a learning culture is characterised by a lively, critical community where people both challenge and support each other, but in reality the group members feel threatened and become defensive when they are challenged, the critical companion can point this out and help them to explore the historical, social, cultural or political reasons. Based on this understanding the group can discuss how they can transform themselves and their practices.

Facilitating the articulation of practice

The articulation of practice is so fundamental to the transformation of practice and to the success of an organisation and the service it provides that we devote the whole of the next chapter to it.

Enhancing the knowledge creation process by professional communities

Based on Eraut's (1994) suggestion that academic communities could develop and enhance the way professional communities create knowledge from practice, we propose a collaborative inservice education programme, informed by critical educational science and the creative arts.

In the past, inservice education in education and health has often been founded on a 'deficit' approach which does not make it easy for practitioners to recognise their own skilfulness or to feel that they have valuable expertise to share with others. It is still unusual for experienced practitioners to invite less experienced colleagues to observe and discuss their practice. To counter this trend, inservice programmes could focus on participants' strengths, that is, practitioners' professional craft knowledge and academics' knowledge creation skills, and on collaborative learning and knowledge generation. Thus, a new kind of relationship between an academic institution and a practice organisation would be set up. The emphasis would be on the two communities working *with* each other and recognising each other's strengths, rather than the more traditional approach of academics setting up programmes *for* practitioners.

As critical companions, academics could help groups of expert practitioners to surface their professional craft knowledge through story-telling, reflective accounts and creative arts media, such as paint, clay and movement, and thus access a rich source of learning for themselves. As the number of stories, accounts and expressions grows, there could be a systematic attempt to generalise by looking for recurring patterns and themes, within and between cases. This suggestion builds on the recommendations of Benner (1994) and Tanner *et al.* (1993) that practical knowledge can be extended and refined by making it public through narratives and by consensual validation. In addition, existing theory could be critiqued and tested against the emerging patterns and themes, making further knowledge available for critique, debate and testing in the field. Data collected by the practitioners during this testing would be brought to the group for analysis, critique and further debate. The critical companion would help the group to work together to seek consensus. As the group became more confident of the rigour of its findings, they could begin to share them with other groups, both inside and outside the practice organisation, again with the critical companion facilitating knowledge creation and testing.

There is likely to come a point where new insights and understandings need to be made more available for public scrutiny. When this stage is reached the critical companion could help practitioners to produce an article in paper or electronic form for critical dialogue with a wider audience. Creative arts media may be useful in helping practitioners to overcome blocks to writing, as well as offering forms of expression.

Before any of the above processes for transforming practice can be used effectively, organisations must have examined their values and identified any incongruence with the values underpinning a practice development strategy located in a critical social science philosophy. We have shown how such a strategy is imbued with a valuing of practitioner knowledge and investing in people, which means giving them time and resources for development and learning.

Conclusion

In this chapter we have demonstrated the value of academic institutions and practice organisations working together in practice development partnerships that are informed by critical social science philosophy. We have proposed a conceptual framework which re-configures traditional relationships between knowledge creation and use, offering four transformational processes that can be used to make these new relationships work. By using a critical companionship approach, the academic institution can facilitate change, at strategic, organisational and operational levels, as well as nurturing the creation of knowledge from practice that is potentially transferable to other settings. This process helps the organisation to develop a corporate vision for its development, within which individual practice developments can take place and systematic ways of collecting evidence of effective practice can be used to influence policy. It also encourages the organisation to foster development strategies and methodologies that are owned by practitioners and which enable them to critique and challenge prevailing practice ideologies.

We conclude that this new reciprocal relationship will not only improve practice and nurture growth, it will also result in disciplinary knowledge and practice being open to, and fed by, knowledge created in practice. We envisage that developing such partnerships will involve culture change in both academic institutions and practice organisations if they are to work together effectively.

References

Argyris, C. & Schön, D. (1974) *Theory in Practice: Increasing Professional Effectiveness*, Jossey-Bass, London.

Benner, P. (1994) The role of articulation in understanding practice and experience as sources of knowledge in clinical nursing, in *Philosophy in an Age of Pluralism* (ed. J. Tully), Cambridge University Press, Cambridge, pp. 136–55.

Binnie, A. & Titchen, A. (1998) *Patient-Centred Nursing: An Action Research Study of Practice Development in an Acute Medical Unit*, Report No. 18, Royal College of Nursing Institute, Oxford.

Binnie, A. & Titchen, A. (1999) *Freedom to Practise: The Development of Patient-Centred Nursing*, Butterworth Heinemann, Oxford.

Carr, W. & Kemmis, S. (1986) *Becoming Critical: Education, Knowledge and Action Research*, Falmer Press, London.

Eraut, M. (1994) *Developing Professional Knowledge and Competence*, The Falmer Press, London.

Fay, B. (1987) *Critical Social Science: Liberation and Its Limits*, Polity Press, Oxford.

Habermas, J. (1985) *The Theory of Communicative Action*, Beacon Press, Boston.

Haines, A. & Jones, R. (1994) Implementing findings of research, *British Medical Journal*, **308**, pp. 1488–92.

Hunt, M. (1987) The process of translating research findings into nursing practice, *Journal of Advanced Nursing*, **12**, pp. 101–10.

Jackson, A., Ward, M., Cutcliffe, J., Titchen, A. & Cannon, B. (1999) Practice development in mental health nursing: Part 2, *Mental Health Practice*, **2**, pp. 20–25.

Kitson, A., Ahmed, L.B., Harvey, G., Seers, K. & Thompson, D.R. (1996) From research to practice: One organisational model for promoting research based practice, *Journal of Advanced Nursing*, **23**, pp. 430–40.

Kitson, A., Harvey, G. & McCormack, B. (1998) Enabling the implementation of evidence based practice: A conceptual framework, *Quality in Health Care*, **7**, pp. 149–59.

Kramer, M. & Schmalenberg, C. (1985) Magnet hospitals: Institutions of excellence: Part 1, *Journal of Nursing Administration*, **18**, pp. 13–24.

McCormack, B., Kitson, A., Manley, K., Titchen, A. & Harvey, G. (1999) Towards practice development – a vision in reality or a reality without vision?, *Journal of Nursing Management*, **7**, pp. 255–64.

National Health Service Executive (1998) *Achieving Effective Practice: A Clinical Effectiveness Research Information Pack for Nurses, Midwives and Health Visitors*, Department of Health, Leeds.

Nonaka, I. & Takeuchi, H. (1995) *The Knowledge-Creating Company*, Oxford University Press, New York.

RCN (1998) *Guidance for Nurses on Clinical Governance*, Royal College of Nursing, London.

Rodgers, S. (1994) An exploratory study of research utilisation by nurses in general medical and surgical wards, *Journal of Advanced Nursing*, **20**, pp. 904–11.

Schein, E.H. (1995) *Learning Consortia: How to Create Parallel Learning Systems for Organization Sets*, Centre for Organizational Learning, Massachusetts Institute of Technology, Boston, MA.

Smith, B. J. (1994) Building shared vision: How to begin, in *The Fifth Discipline Fieldbook: Strategies and Tools for Building a Learning Organisation* (eds P.M. Senge, A. Kleiner, C. Roberts, R.B. Ross & B.J. Smith), Nicholas Brealey Publishing, London, pp. 312–26.

Tanner, C.A., Benner, P., Chesla, C. & Gordon, D.R. (1993) The phenomenology of knowing the patient, *IMAGE: Journal of Nursing Scholarship*, **25**, pp. 273–80.

Titchen, A. (1998) *A conceptual framework for facilitating learning in clinical practice*, Occasional Paper 2, Centre for Professional Education Advancement, The University of Sydney, Lidcombe, Australia.

Titchen, A. (2000) *Professional Craft Knowledge in Patient-Centred Nursing and the Facilitation of its Development*, University of Oxford DPhil thesis, Ashdale Press, Oxford.

Titchen, A. & Binnie, A. (1993a) Research partnerships: Collaborative action research in nursing, *Journal of Advanced Nursing*, **18**, pp. 858–65.

Titchen, A. & Binnie, A. (1993b) A unified action research strategy in nursing, *Educational Action Research*, **1**, pp. 25–33.

Titchen, A. & Binnie, A. (1994) Action research: A strategy for theory generation and testing, *International Journal of Nursing Studies*, **31**, pp. 1–12.

Warfield, C. & Manley, K. (1990) Developing a new philosophy in the NDU. *Nursing Standard*, **4**, pp. 27–30.

Wilson-Barnett, J., Corner, J. & De Carle, B. (1990) Integrating nursing research and practice – the role of the researcher as teacher, *Journal of Advanced Nursing*, **15**, pp. 621–5.

Chapter 16
Articulating Practice

Jim Butler, Robert Kay and Angie Titchen

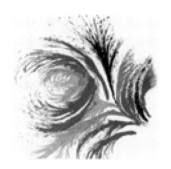

This chapter presents a critical dialogue with the process of *articulating professional practice*. On the surface this process appears to be straightforward: highly performing and innovative individuals sharing with others what they know, what they have learned. That they have the knowledge to share is proven:

> 'All research on expertise has shown that experts have a vast body of specific knowledge on which they consistently draw to generate efficient performance.'
> (Olson & Biolsi 1991, p. 241).

However, the articulation and sharing of their vast knowledge turns out to be extremely difficult and complex.

Individual knowledge is separated into 'tacit' and 'explicit' knowledge (Polanyi 1966). The distinction is described by Gopalakrishnan and Bierly (1997, p. 422) in these terms:

> 'Knowledge is explicit when it is codifiable and can be transferred from one individual to another using some type of formal communication system; tacit knowledge cannot be formally communicated and is deeply rooted in one's experience.'

Articulating practice, transferring tacit knowledge to explicit knowledge, is the focus of this chapter. The articulation process is important for two reasons. First, articulation of the individual's knowledge is an important part of demonstrating credibility and accountability of professional practice. Second, the individual as a member of a profession or specific organisation contributes to the knowledge base of this wider body. The second of these reasons is the focus of this chapter.

We argue that it is not a particular individual's knowledge that directly enriches an entire organisation or professional group, it is only the collective knowledge of the group that can transform the organisation or profession. Transformation could refer to the establishment of a 'learning organisation', the professionalisation of a group through expansion of the knowledge base and thus the credibility of the group and enhancement of the functioning of the group in terms of productivity or achievements built upon a sounder collective knowledge base. To achieve such transformation, the group, whether a specific organisation (e.g. a firm, company or institution) or a more loosely organised professional group, must constitute a collective learning system, where learning is defined as 'an insight born of experience which can be used to solve problems in the future' (Slotnick et al. 1998, p. 8). In other words, the organisation's success depends on how well its structure and culture support important learning processes. Organisational knowledge, the outcome of collective learning, is the key strategic asset (Gopalakrishnan & Bierly 1997). Such knowledge can also be referred to as the knowledge of the (professional) field.

Health care research in this field is most prolific in nursing, hence the emphasis on nursing research in this chapter. See Beeston and Simons (1996) or Mattingly (1991) for examples that address the articulation of practice less directly in physiotherapy and occupational therapy.

Benner (1984, p. 35) directly addresses the benefits of articulating the practice of an expert individual:

> 'Systematic documentation of expert performance is a first step in knowledge development, and an expert can benefit from systematically recording and describing critical incidents from their practice that illustrate expertise or a breakdown in performance. As experts document their performance, new areas of knowledge are made available for further study and development.'

This articulation can be seen as the basis of organisational knowledge development. For an organisation to develop it has been hypothesised that it must be adept at 'creating new knowledge, disseminating it throughout the organisation, and embodying it in products, services and systems' (Nonaka & Takeuchi 1995, p. 3). Articulating practice is involved in each of these three processes, but most importantly in the middle process of *dissemination.*

Perhaps the best way to address dissemination is to use the concept of 'flocking' introduced into the organisational learning literature by de Geus (1997). The concept of flocking was first hypothesised by Wilson (Wyles *et al.* 1993) to explain the accelerated anatomical evolution of primates and songbirds. The three processes used to explain fast evolution were:

- Innovation: the species has the capacity to invent new behaviour
- Social propagation: there is direct communication between the innovative individual and the wider community
- Mobility: the species flock and move en masse to new territories.

The latter two processes of social propagation and mobility were termed 'flocking'. However, it is apparent that these three processes mirror those in successful groups and organisations: innovation, dissemination and embodiment in new procedures.

De Geus in his reflections on the successful life of his organisation (Royal Dutch Shell) found that the flocking concept helped to explain its success. Learning can originate only within an individual learner (Simon 1991; Schein 1995). Therefore, for an organisation to learn in an accelerated fashion, the requirements are that the whole organisation has the capacity for the innovative individual to teach others and then for the organisation as a whole to move to a new level of performance. The organisation must be capable of taking the individual advances of innovative people and flocking in a transformative process to a new arena.

How is this flocking process institutionalised? De Geus (1997) found that the informal networking and talking with colleagues in the breaks at organisational training events resulted in intensive flocking. Thus it appears that there is an informal process of articulating and disseminating the tacit knowledge of individual practice, so that the whole organisation is enriched. It is the critical discussion of this informal as well as formal processes to which this chapter is devoted.

What is to be articulated and who is to do it?

Individuals learn by acquiring new knowledge as a basis for action. This knowledge, however, is often tacit. Organisations learn by acquiring new knowledge and embedding it in physical, process or management systems. Organisational learning, unlike individual learning, usually requires the knowledge to be articulated; that is to say, it needs to be explicit knowledge before it can be made available for action.

Within the knowledge of an individual or organisation, as well as the distinction between tacit and explicit, there is a further distinction among three domains:

'There are at least three kinds of skills and knowledge constituting this dimension of a core capability: 1. Scientific (public) 2. Industry-specific, and 3. Firm-specific. Moving from 1 to 3, these types of skills and knowledge are increasingly less codified and transferable.'

(Leonard-Barton 1995, p. 21)

It is the third kind, the highly contextual, organisation-specific knowledge, that is most in need of articulation if the organisation is to thrive and prosper.

The contemporary obsession with technical knowledge about things rather than relational knowledge about people has led to a distortion of the types of knowledge that need to be shared (Saul 1997). As Drucker says, 90% of engineering problems are psychological, and the sharing of knowledge about managing and relating to people is one of the greatest needs of organisations today (Edwards *et al.* 1997).

Life does not educate us to talk about 'our life'; it does not give us the categories to deal with who we are and how we relate. Everyone is a meaning-maker, and therefore can be assumed to possess tacit knowledge about technical and interpersonal issues. So people's articulation of their tacit knowledge requires concepts and categories which are given to them by a social process, a process of being with others (De Geus 1997).

Benner (1984, p. 32) reported an expert nurse addressing this exact problem of words and categories to articulate her practice:

> 'When I say to a doctor, "the patient is psychotic", I don't always know how to legitimise that statement. But I am never wrong. Because I know psychosis from the inside out. And I feel that, and I know it, and I trust it. I don't care if nothing else is happening, I still really know that . . . One of the things that I am doing now is getting some inservice in to talk to us about language. But all I am really trying to do is find words within the jargon to talk about something that I don't think is particularly describable.'

In general, it will be the whole range of tacit, organisation-specific, technical and interpersonal knowledge that will need to be articulated if the organisation is to achieve all that it can. The people within the organisation that most need to share are those with the most knowledge and expertise, who are most innovative, and these people are found throughout an organisation (Bruning & Liverpool 1993).

The natural language of practice

The Dreyfus and Dreyfus model of skill development (Dreyfus 1982) offers an important insight into the natural language of articulating practice. The model has five levels of skill development: novice, advanced beginner, competent, proficient and expert. As a guide, the practitioner reaches the competent stage after about three years of direct experience in the practice setting. In articulating practice we are mainly interested in the levels competent, proficient and expert, because only these levels have the performance experience that leads to a deep inner knowledge. The competent level is the first level where most performance comes from an inner understanding and personal practical knowledge (Butler 1996).

Research on the Dreyfus and Dreyfus model (Benner 1984; O'Brien *et al*. 1997) illustrates the details concerning the natural language of practice used by practitioners at each of these higher levels.

Competent

These individuals are most likely to be able to speak about their practice, because they are the ones who are most analytic, most consciously and most mentally active. They are aware of the long-range goals or plans they are pursuing. They are thinking through their practice in complex fashions. As Benner (1984, p. 27) describes this stage, 'the conscious, deliberate planning that is characteristic of this skill level helps achieve efficiency and organization'. If asked, they are generally able to articulate their practice.

Proficient

According to Benner, these people talk in maxims. They find it difficult to communicate their practice clearly because their understanding and their processing has been clumped into macro-routines:

> 'Characteristically, the proficient performer perceives situations as wholes rather than in terms of aspects, and performance is guided by maxims. Perception is a key word here. The perspective is not thought out but "presents itself" based upon experience and recent events.'
>
> (Benner 1984, p. 27)

This fact that their practice presents itself as wholes and then is spoken about in maxims leads to difficulty for proficient practitioners to articulate their practice to others less advanced than themselves. Benner (1984, p. 29) points out this difficulty in the following passage:

> 'The proficient nurse uses maxims as guide(s), but a deep understanding of the situation is required before a maxim can be used. Maxims reflect what would appear to the competent or novice performer as unintelligible nuances of the situation ... Once one has a deep understanding of the situation, however, the maxim provides direction as to what must be taken into consideration.'

This difficulty of articulating practice is also evidenced in the research of O'Brien *et al.* (1997) where a proficient accountant (trainer) was teaching a novice accountant (Jenny) in the workplace setting. The following is an illustration of the difficulties of a proficient performer teaching a novice:

> 'He (trainer) would also proffer maxims as problem solving techniques.
>> Trainer: The figures talk to you ... (and) ... You have just got to keep your ears open.
> Jenny found it difficult to use these maxims herself at the time. It wasn't until some months later, while struggling with a problem, that she began to see meaning in them.
>> I didn't know what to do ... (then) I found something. I thought this is really eerie. He tells me the figures talk to me and I laugh at him and then all of a sudden ...
> Her perception during this early time had been of feeling "lost", and waiting

for it to "click". She was concerned about her ability to handle the work when the trainer left. Jenny found it difficult to learn readily from her trainer.'

(O'Brien *et al.* 1997, p. 216)

However, as Benner states, if proficient practitioners seek to share their knowledge with proficient or expert practitioners then the maxims provide direction and disseminate knowledge.

Expert

According to Benner, these people are usually not able to articulate their practice because so much of its knowledge base is unconscious:

'The expert practitioner no longer relies on an analytic principle (rule, guideline or maxim) to connect her or his understanding of the situation to an appropriate action. The expert, with an enormous background of experience, now has an intuitive grasp of each situation and zeroes in on the accurate region of the problem without wasteful consideration of a large range of unfruitful, alternative diagnoses and solutions.'

(Benner 1984, p. 31)

As Benner says, when experts are asked to articulate why they performed such a perfect action in such a complex context, they will just say, 'because it felt right', 'it looked good'. Alternatively they may use gestures or other non-verbal methods:

'She used her hand to illustrate how the ventilatory bag feels when she is checking the lung resistance. She knows in her hands how different resistances feel, so she uses gestures to convey these differences.'

(Benner 1984, p. 19)

When this is all that experts can say there is nothing much for others to learn from such articulations. Typically, experts need quite explicit methods to achieve informative articulations. We now turn to an analysis of some of these methods.

Elicitation methods

To succeed, an organisation needs to know the strategies and tactics used by its best performers for interpreting and responding successfully and innovatively to complex and problematic situations. As argued in the previous section of this chapter, the natural language of the better performers is not likely to be formulated in a way that can be understood by the whole organisation. There is a need for more explicit methods to articulate and share the valuable knowledge attained by individuals.

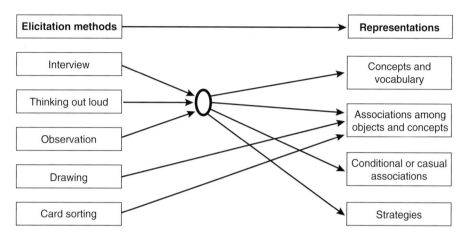

Fig. 16.1 Methods of elicitation and their knowledge representations.

Figure 16.1 is adapted from Olson and Biolsi (1991). It shows the relationships among various procedures for the elicitation of tacit knowledge and the representation of that knowledge achieved by the procedures.

To comment briefly on each of the methods:

- *Interviews.* A critical incident interview (Benner 1984) and a more general interview are the most common methods for eliciting tacit knowledge. The interviewer facilitates the expert telling 'how they do it'.
- *Thinking out loud protocols.* The person is invited to think out loud while performing the task. Thoughts and perceptions are reported during the performance.
- *Observing, listening and questioning.* Experts are observed and listened to as they go about their everyday work, then specific questions about what has been observed and the seemingly obvious are posed (Titchen & Higgs 1999; Titchen 2000).
- *Understanding the nature of tacit knowledge.* If experts are helped to develop this understanding, they are likely to be able to articulate it more readily to others (McAlpine *et al.* 1988; Titchen 2000).
- *Drawings, painting or clay modelling.* The person is asked to represent the process in any way desired, or to use mind maps, bubble maps, concept maps. The representations can reveal the different aspects of performance and the relationships between them.
- *Card Sorting.* The key concepts or processes are each written onto a separate card, then the cards are sorted into hierarchies by the expert. This method was used with success by Evans and Butler (1992) to determine experts' understanding of the welding process.

These elicitation methods evoke differing representations of the individual's knowledge. As displayed in Fig. 16.1, the representations can be in the form of concepts and their categorical and causal relationships, in verbal or nonverbal expressions. Each expression adds its contribution to the articulation of practice, and has its strengths and weaknesses. In addition, they can be limited in their applicability due to the difficulty experts often have in accessing their fleeting perceptions or inferences (Olson & Biolsi 1991).

Conditions for articulated practice disseminating within an organisation or profession

As stated above, the purpose of articulating practice is to disseminate innovative technical and interpersonal tacit knowledge for the good of the organisation or profession. This dissemination process needs various conditions to be operating within the organisation if it is to be successful. These conditions will be met if the culture of the organisation values knowledge and believes in the centrality of knowledge to performance. As Leonard-Barton (1995, p. 19) said so well:

> '*Values and norms:* These determine what kinds of knowledge are sought and nurtured, what kinds of knowledge-building activities are tolerated and encouraged. There are systems of caste and status, rituals of behaviour, and passionate beliefs associated with various kinds of technological knowledge that are as rigid and complex as those associated with religion. Therefore, values serve as knowledge-screening and knowledge-control mechanisms.'

We now present a brief overview of some of the values and beliefs that need to characterise the culture of the knowledge generating and sharing organisation.

A radical constructivist dissemination process

According to the radical constructivism of von Glaserfeld (1989), individuals construct their experience of an event through the structure of their nervous system. Although each individual's constructions will be different, over time and the continuation of similar experiences, commonalities develop in the understanding and interpretation of events and issues. It is these commonalities that are often described as the transfer of tacit knowledge. It is perhaps more accurate, however, to suggest that tacit knowledge is not transferred but recreated in each individual.

Maturana and Varela (1992) use the notion of a consensual domain of language to describe this phenomenon. As the individuals within a team or organisation continue to have similar experiences, congruencies arise in the way they make meaning out of those experiences. In order to describe and give order to these experiences, new distinctions in language develop. Idiosyncratic words, anagrams and slang develop to allow shared interpretations of events. Others outside this consensual domain require time and recurrent experience with those inside it before they may make similar meanings out of their experiences.

Within an organisation, the central notion that can be drawn from this discussion is that the organisation must value the creation of interpersonal interaction and congruent experiences because they are vital to the transfer of knowledge. The example of de Geus (1997) already provided in this chapter once again applies.

Shared world view and vision among the individuals within the organisation

Transmitting and receiving knowledge involve people's world views and belief systems (Argyris 1982; Butler 1996). Research (Langfield-Smith 1992) has demonstrated the need for shared collective cognitions. This research shows that within a group collective cognitions are transitory phenomena, changing in response to circumstances. However, over time and many episodes, a greater overlap in shared belief systems is an outcome.

Knowledge can be effectively shared by two people only if they share a similar interpretive framework (Argyris 1982). This shared framework, or world view, will allow their ladders of inference to transmit and receive similar messages. Shared frameworks are important because most organisations are run by teams rather than by individuals. The collective knowledge of the group can be more than the sum of the individual knowledges, due to the synergies within the group:

> 'Innovations with tacit knowledge are difficult to share with others outside the community-of-practice because they will not understand the terminology and basic principles associated with the knowledge. It is harder to integrate tacit innovations into other knowledge areas. This makes the development process more difficult to manage and costly, compared to explicit innovations.'
>
> (Gopalakrishnan & Bierly 1997, p. 423)

A practice field within the organisation that is valued, resourced and supported

An organisation always has innovators, people who wonder why things are as they are. These people will never flourish and give value to the organisation unless they are listened to and supported. To provide this support, organisational slack (explored in Chapter 15) and organisational space are required.

To return to the concept of flocking, de Geus (1997, p. 97) has the following advice for managers:

> 'Innovation and flocking require *organisational space* – freedom from control, from direction, and from punishment for failures. Experiments must take place with relative safety. Conversation must be free and candid, without fear of reprisal.'

To achieve this practice field is difficult in an organisation where the production imperative is always in competition with the learning imperative. However, these difficulties can be overcome. For example, in the patient-centred nursing innovation (Binnie & Titchen 1999) discussed in the previous chapter, one of the key reasons for the project's success was that senior nursing management created a structure and culture in which innovative practitioners had space and authority to experiment and develop. The practice orientation, investment of time, education and climate of support for innovation attracted able, creative practitioners. However, Binnie and Titchen found that merely providing this organisational space was not enough; a new practice culture had to be created. Nurses had to be explicitly given permission and helped to develop relevant practical and thinking skills so that they could take control over their working lives and experiment with their practice. Moreover, they needed help not to expect reprimands for admitting weakness or failure and to be honest and open with each other.

Acceptability of error, feedback, and learning from experience

People do not automatically learn from failure, so 'organisational slack' in which people experiment and practice will not automatically lead to learning. It is necessary to design the culture and the processes so that people learn to 'fail forward', to articulate what they have learnt. The culture must contradict the assumption that

> failure = learnt nothing = achieved nothing = waste of time = useless.

Rather the culture needs to assert that success and failure are both rich learning outcomes, necessary to the enterprise that promoted the experimentation and slack.

Feedback is a significant process in the articulation of practice. It is a way of making clear to the self what the self knows; it reveals personal practical knowledge, or professional craft knowledge as referred to in Chapter 15. Performance without feedback is blind, unconscious and unarticulated. Feedback makes the consequences of actions visible and indirectly makes the performance itself visible and therefore able to be articulated.

In this sense, feedback always involves 'articulating practice', because to give feedback about performance one must, at least in some minimalist way, say something about practice. To be informative feedback must provide an incremental increase in knowledge for the recipient (Ilgren *et al.* 1979)

Performance or human actions need feedback in order to make clear the relationships and the correlations between variables that are the very currency of articulating practice. Personal performance or work or practice is based on correlations: if action A is carried out, consequence B (which is desired) follows.

This personal practical knowledge is the essence of the 'action schema' which are central to articulated practice.

Timeliness of knowledge

One of the greatest challenges for organisations, as they attempt to maximise the value of the knowledge existing within them, is access to that knowledge at the right time and place. In large organisations it is not always possible to meet face-to-face with other people; timetables do not match, and quite often those who would value their input do not know they exist.

To address this issue, organisations have spent inordinate amounts of money on information technology, particularly databases and e-mail, in order to connect the people within the organisation to each other. Sadly, these investments often fail to provide the financial and organisational returns that had been envisaged. Problems with software incompatibility, technical breakdowns and most often user error have shown that although information technology can do much to increase the efficiency of communication within organisations, it does not represent a fix-all in terms of knowledge management.

The difficulty in addressing this issue is that it is impossible to know what knowledge will be useful, for whom it will be useful and when they will want it. Notions such as *useful*, *timely* and *meaningful* are not innate characteristics of the information but rather judgements that the practitioner places upon the information. As such, if knowledge and its timely use is the focus for improvement it is necessary to recognise where it is: not in a database but in people's heads or bodies.

It follows that it is less important to have information about a topic on a database than it is to have information about where to get more information or tap into the knowledge. The information system acts as a signpost to the knowledge, not a repository of it.

Conclusion

This chapter has emphasised learning and articulated knowledge in the service of action. This triad is essential to the development of organisations and professions, because as Leonard-Barton (1995, p. 8) said,

> '*Activities* – not goals or financial rewards or even skills (until they are activated) – create a firm's capabilities.'

Individuals learn and organisations can learn from the individuals within them. The process requires the dissemination of individual knowledge. This dissemination process typically requires the articulation of individual, tacit, organisation-specific knowledge by expert innovative people within the organisation. The articulation process does not always require language use by the individual who possesses the knowledge; the knowledge can be learnt by others within the same context and shared and disseminated through social cognition processes and creative arts media.

Knowledge is the treasured value within organisations. It is in people's minds and bodies. If an expert leaves an organisation, a huge store of personal practical knowledge, essential to the organisation, leaves. It is imperative that that knowledge is left within the organisation. Elicitation methods are helpful in this regard, but so also is the organisational culture which needs to understand where the essential knowledge resides.

Since some of this knowledge has no mental representation, people need help to transform it into collective cognitions through recurrent interactions. The work of researchers such as Benner (1984), McAlpine *et al.* (1988), O'Brien *et al.* (1997) and Titchen (2000) has given us the clues in how this help might be given.

The implications of this research are that the organisation needs to provide support to help expert practitioners and innovators to tell and interpret practice stories (thus sharing collective perceptions and cognitions), then, through a process of critique, to seek consensual validation and subsequently to share this expert knowledge with others in the organisation. A further implication is that the organisation needs to ensure a structure in which expert practitioners work alongside the less experienced to provide recurrent interactions, and have time in the working day for the articulation and critique of their knowledge.

References

Argyris, C. (1982) *Reasoning, Learning and Action*, Jossey-Bass, San Francisco.

Beeston, S. & Simons H. (1996) Physiotherapy practice: Practitioners' perspectives, *Physiotherapy Theory and Practice*, **12**, pp. 231–42.

Benner, P. (1984) *From Novice to Expert*, Addison-Wesley, Menlo Park, CA.

Binnie, A. & Titchen, A. (1999) *Freedom to Practise: The Development of Patient-Centred Nursing*, Butterworth-Heinemann, Oxford.

Bruning, N.S. & Liverpool, P.R. (1993) Membership in quality circles and participation in decision-making, *The Journal of Applied Behavioral Science*, **29**(1), pp. 76–95.

Butler, J. (1996) Professional development: Practice as text, reflection as process and self as locus, *Australian Journal of Education*, **40**(3), pp. 265–83.

de Geus, A. (1997) *The Living Organisation*, Longview Publishing Ltd, Boston, MA.

Dreyfus, S.E. (1982) Formal models vs. human situational understanding: Inherent limitations on the modeling of business expertise, *Office: Technology and People*, **1**, pp. 133–65.

Edwards, J., Butler, J., Hill, B. & Russell, S. (1997) *People Rules for Rocket Scientists*, Samford Research Associates, Brisbane, Australia.

Evans, G. & Butler, J. (1992) Expert models and feedback processes in developing competence in industrial trade areas, *Australian Journal of TAFE Research and Development*, **8**(2), 13–32.

Gopalakrishnan, S. & Bierly, P. (1997) Organizational innovation and strategic choices: A knowledge-based view, in *Academy of Management, Best Paper Proceedings 97* (eds L.N. Dosier & B. Keys), pp. 422–6.

Ilgren, D.R., Fisher, C.D, & Taylor, M.S. (1979) Consequences of individual feedback on behaviour in organisations, *Journal of Applied Psychology*, **64**, pp. 359–71.

Langfield-Smith, K. (1992) Exploring the need for a shared cognitive map, *Journal of Management Studies*, **29**, pp. 349–68.

Leonard-Barton, D. (1995) *Wellsprings of Knowledge: Building and Sustaining the Sources of Innovation*, Harvard Business School Press, Boston, MA.

Maturana, H. & Varela, F. (1992) *The Tree of Knowledge: The Biological Roots of Understanding*, Shambala, Boston, MA.

Mattingly, C. (1991) Narrative reflections on practical actions: two learning experiments in reflective storytelling, in *The Reflective Turn: Case Studies in and on Educational Practice* (ed. D. Schön), Teachers College Press, London, pp. 235–57.

McAlpine, A., Brown, S., McIntyre, D. & Hagger, H. (1988) *Student-Teachers Learning from Experienced Teachers*. The Scottish Council for Research in Education, Edinburgh.

Nonaka, I. & Takeuchi, H. (1995) *The Knowledge-Creating Company*, Oxford University Press, New York.

O'Brien, J., Houldsworth, B., Butler, J. & Edwards, J. (1997) Learning in the restructured workplace: A case study of a novice, *Education + Training*, **39**, pp. 211–8.

Olson, J.R. & Biolsi, K.J. (1991) Techniques for representing expert knowledge, in *Towards a General Theory of Expertise* (eds K.A. Ericsson & J. Smith), Cambridge University Press, Cambridge, pp. 240–85.

Polanyi, M. (1966) *The Tacit Dimension*, Anchor Day, New York.

Saul, J.R. (1997) *The Unconscious Civilisation*, Penguin, Ringwood, Vic.

Schein, E.H. (1995) *Learning Consortia: How to Create Parallel Learning Systems for Organization Sets*, Centre for Organizational Learning, Massachusetts Institute of Technology, Boston, MA.

Simon, H. (1991) Bounded rationality and organizational learning, *Organization Science*, **2**, pp. 125–34.

Slotnick, H.B., Kristjanson, A.J., Raszlowski, R.R. & Moravec, R. (1998) A note on mechanisms of action in physicians' learning, *Professions Education Researcher Quarterly*, **19**(2), pp. 5–11.

Titchen, A. (2000) *Professional Craft Knowledge in Patient-Centred Nursing and the Facilitation of Its Development*, University of Oxford DPhil thesis, Ashdale Press, Oxford.

Titchen, A. & Higgs J. (1999) Facilitating the development of knowledge, in *Educating Beginning Practitioners* (eds J. Higgs & H. Edwards), Butterworth Heinemann, Oxford, pp. 180–88.

von Glaserfeld, E. (1989) *Knowing Without Metaphysics: Aspects of the Radical Constructivist Position*, SRRI No 208, University of Massachusetts.

Wyles, J.S., Kimbel, J.G. & Wilson, A.C. (1993) Birds, behavior and anatomical evolution, *Proceedings of the National Academy of Sciences*, **90**(7), 232–4.

Chapter 17
Knowledge and Practice in the Education of Health and Human Service Professionals

Fran Everingham and Jude Irwin

The quest to understand knowledge in the context of practice in the health and human services inevitably raises questions about the education of practitioners. In particular, issues are raised about the types of curriculum design and teaching that might best promote student learning and encourage students to draw appropriately on knowledge to use in practice situations. In this chapter we identify some of the dilemmas that confront academics and practitioners in creating opportunities for students to develop, articulate and apply their knowledge in diverse sites of practice. We explore issues that need to be addressed in curriculum development and teaching to assist students in beginning to become 'expert' practitioners in the health and human services.

Education for professional practice in the health and human services (e.g. health, welfare, community and social work) is the preparation of students for employment in a complex, diverse and rapidly changing world. An integral component of many of the human service education courses is the practicum which students undertake. This is the site where it is often claimed that the integration of theory(ies) and practice should take place and be 'tested' out. It has been argued that it is the emphasis on theory and its application that separates the professions from other skilled occupations (Curry & Wergin 1993). Eraut (1994) challenges the notion that theory can be applied in a straightforward way, arguing that practitioners use it interpretively and associatively, employing much more complex processes than mere application. It is perhaps from a lack of understanding of these complex processes that dissatisfaction is commonly voiced as either student failure to integrate theory with practice, or failure to transfer learning from the classroom to the real world.

Theory is a contestable domain. Modernist theorists have drawn on science and rationality to develop general and widely applicable explanations for particular phenomena. For practitioners in the health and human services these theories have been utilised to attempt to bring order and predictability into practice. They enable practitioners to observe, describe, explain, predict, plan and enact change (Howe 1997), and if the 'rules' of a theory are applied then 'good' practice will ensue. Most recently postmodernists have critiqued the use of these grand theories and their broad-based or universalising explanations and change strategies. Instead, they argue that small scale theorising, building on the unique experiences of individuals and recognising different realities, can provide rich sources of knowledge on which professionals in the health and human services can draw.

We argue that the linking of theory and practice is not a linear process, but as Candy and Crebert contend, 'actually consists of spontaneous improvisations on the basis of an "epistemology of practice" rather than on an application of simple rules and formulae to complex, unique and real life problems' (Candy & Crebert 1991, p. 579). We also argue that integration is the product of learning, experience and maturity and in this sense it is the product of lifelong professional learning, not merely the endpoint of a student preparation programme. If this is accepted there are numerous reasons for students to struggle with 'integration' or what we have termed the nexus of learning.

Factors that can inhibit integration

We have identified six often interrelated factors (set out in this section) that contribute to the (dis)integration of theory and practice. The complex interaction of these factors often makes it unrealistic to expect students to understand or articulate a theory-practice link. Ways of overcoming these inhibiting factors are discussed later.

Content discourse or traditional knowledge structures

In professional education the terms 'theory' and 'knowledge' tend to be used interchangeably, both terms commonly referring to propositional knowledge alone rather than the broader constellation of knowledges that are relevant to effective practice. Recognition of different types of knowledge and how these interact in professional life is a comparatively recent development. Knowledge may variously refer to the content of academic disciplines on which a specific profession draws, the theories and professional practice models or approaches of the profession, professional craft knowledge, and personal knowledge. These all intersect on a daily basis to refine professional knowing and action. Thus the perceived 'gap' in student learning might reasonably be viewed as the omission of certain types of knowledge from the curriculum; that is, it is the curriculum that is failing the student, rather than the other way around.

Contributing to the narrow view held about professional knowledge in the curriculum is the unfortunate discontinuity between propositional knowledge and professional craft knowledge created by the comparatively recent move of some health professional education from practice settings to the academy (e.g.

nursing). Legitimating professional education within the academy was done by promoting propositional knowledge from the disciplines as the basis of professional education. Curricula were organised around the traditional disciplines, with the assumption that skills practice should follow didactic exposure to theory in the classroom (Barnett 1990). Field education became an 'add-on', rather than being recognised as a significant learning context where authentic learning can occur.

Contextual complexity

The second factor contributing to the perceived gap is the context for learning. It has been found that the context of learning seems to be more important than the curriculum design (Titchen & Coles 1991). The ideal context appears to be the real one in which the student will use the knowledge, that is, the practice setting. It has also been argued that this setting is where the convergence of knowledges occurs: 'There is no getting away from the fact that the nature of professional knowledge is embedded in the job itself' (Candy & Crebert 1991, p. 580). Despite its sometimes marginality within the academy, field education generates a unique experience for students. Fundamental to the compelling journey of the practicum is its power to shape attitudes, values and professional identity through the opportunities it affords for learning. Within the practicum the application of knowledge and skills is essential, as is the capacity to contribute to collective goals and to establish webs of interpersonal relationships to get the job done.

However, despite the practice setting being the best context for the nexus of learning to be facilitated, contextual complexity can be an inhibiting factor, for example, disparate field settings, variation if not conflict in the functional and procedural requirements between institutions, political complexity and interpersonal dynamics. Nevertheless, it is these very phenomena that enable students to experience the reality of professional thinking in action (Schön 1983), to truly confront the thorny realities of uncertainty and learn to respond to the unexpected. Also contributing to the perceived failure of students to harness the opportunity effectively may be the contrast in learning conditions between the academic and practice setting. In addition, the disciplines 'may not map well onto the fuzzy presentations and phenomena that practitioners encounter in their work. Professional practice problems don't come labelled by their contributing disciplines' (Curry & Wergin 1993, p. 351).

Student maturity

Landmark work on the developmental nature of students' conceptions of knowledge suggests that students move along a continuum from believing that all questions have indisputable answers to the position that few problems in the real world have simple solutions (Perry 1970). This implies that initially, students may have neither the breadth of knowledge nor the perspective to generate sophisticated, well-reasoned, highly defensible arguments, the generic basis of most professional thinking. It is possible, however, to build the conditions under which such thinking might be facilitated, as discussed later.

Curriculum design

The way curricula are designed may also contribute to difficulties in communicating knowledge appropriately to students. There can be what has been referred to as 'slippage', if not total fragmentation, when links are not made between different aspects of study units. Not surprisingly, Perkins and Saloman (1992, p. 208) describe the 'disconnected curriculum': one in which the subject matter 'does not connect well to anything else but the class in which it is taught'.

Central to the problem of fragmentation is the tension which exists between the imposed structure of curriculum in the academy and the nature of professional practice in the workplace. The learning about practice is taken out of the social context of the workplace and reconceived within the regulative structures of the academy, with the consequence that students focus on passing examinations rather than on their development as practitioners. The classic ordering of curriculum is often into 'segmented time-tabled blocks [where there is] more emphasis upon the content of the material presented than on the process of learning with understanding' (Candy & Crebert 1991, p. 579).

The Tylerian objectives model approach to curriculum development and documentation, which compartmentalises and simplifies outcomes into knowledge, skills and attitudes, is a further culprit in the separation of theory from practice, not to mention causing the artificial separation of emotion from cognition and action. Design attempts to redress this situation include basing curricula around professional processes (such as the nursing process and the clinical reasoning process) or structuring curricula that utilise experienced-based learning and the processing of meaning from this experience. The efficacy of process-inclusive designs is suggested by Titchen and Coles' (1991) finding that students in a problem-based physiotherapy curriculum adopted more desirable study approaches than students in a subject-centred curriculum.

Underdeveloped pedagogies

In the move to the academy for the health professions, practice-based pedagogy was largely dismissed as vocational training and continues to be undervalued. In any event, such pedagogy was mostly directed at skill development rather than at theory construction, thus having some distinctive shortcomings in the academy. Meanwhile, underpinning professional education with the disciplines inevitably brought with it an academic teaching culture, sanctioned as superior and imbued with traditional didactic pedagogy that in its own way poses limitations. In considering relevant pedagogy, we support styles of facilitation and types of mechanisms that help map, legitimise and thus communicate the interrelationships between different types of knowledge and facilitate the processing of meaning and student construction of understanding.

The academic and clinical or practice teacher duality

There are several issues that contribute to reinforcement of a duality between academic practitioners and field/practice teachers. First, values about the focus of learning may differ, in that academics may emphasise research and higher order thinking while field teachers may focus on tasks, techniques, interaction and the interpersonal, including the act of caring. Second, power and status are unequally distributed between academics and field teachers, with the perception that a hierarchy of credibility exists, whereby academics who generate theory are more credible than teacher practitioners. Third, field/practice teachers report having little opportunity for input into the curriculum, and argue that it is often out of touch with current practice (anecdotal evidence from practitioners). Obviously, the relationship between academic and professional communities will influence the extent to which knowledge and practice are separated. Two ways to tackle this would be to reduce any perceived or real 'social and intellectual distance' (Barnett *et al.* 1987, p. 62) between academic and field/practice teachers, and to build mutuality of concern for the integration of theory and practice.

The use of process in curriculum

In the previous section we argued that a number of factors make it difficult for students to see the connections between theories and practice. How, then, do we create opportunities for students to begin the process of becoming professionals and specifically to begin to use the knowledges which 'expert' practitioners draw upon? Throughout this chapter much of our argument is based on an understanding that knowledge is acquired through a set of learning processes which are embodied in professional practice. We argue, therefore, that in order to promote learning and the connections between theory and practice, curricula should be process-inclusive or process-orientated. What do we mean by this?

In its simplest form, *process* in the context of learning refers to the variety of procedures surrounding the acquisition and utilisation of knowledge, whereas *content* refers to the mass of information transferred to the student (Parker & Rubin 1966). Furthermore teachers, in their role as facilitators, frequently use the act of 'processing' to help learners attribute or construct meaning from their learning experiences.

The term *process* is also used to refer to professional ways of thinking and working. Barnett (1992), Eraut (1992) and Titchen and Higgs (1995) offer overlapping analyses of these processes and their place in curricula for professional preparation. Eraut (1992) proposes that professional practice is defined by a set of processes that constitutes a form of knowledge in its own right. Process knowledge consists of knowing how to utilise the many processes relevant to a particular profession, including how to make use of propositional knowledge and act on the basis of procedural knowledge. Other examples are acquiring information, skilled behaviour, deliberative processes, giving information, and controlling one's own behaviour. Cognitively demanding deliberative processes include planning, problem-solving, analysing and evaluating and decision-making. These processes 'require unique combinations of professional knowledge, situational knowledge and professional judgement' (Eraut 1992, p. 110). Eraut advocates that initial professional training 'must be performance based . . . (and) . . . process knowledge of all kinds should be accorded central importance' (Eraut 1992, p. 117).

In Barnett's view, the transcending professional capacity is the process of critical reflection on one's own practice. He recommends methods that engage deep approaches to learning and that give students 'insight into their own learning strategies (metacognition)' (Barnett 1992, p. 206). Thus Barnett would contend that the key to connecting theory and practice is the process of critical reflection. Reflection is a process increasingly associated with professional education and professional practice. It is valued as a means to help find clarity in what might otherwise remain perplexing. Thus the reflective practitioner undertakes 'engaged listening, seeking to understand, and being open to all possibilities' (Diekelmann 1990, p. 301). For Barnett the presence of practice in the curriculum 'must be justified in terms of opportunities it affords for the students' critical reflection' (Barnett 1990, p. 159). With this assertion Barnett is proposing that all students should be reflective practitioners, coming to understand their 'theories-in-use', and from this act they will be empowered and liberated as learners.

Within the health professions, Titchen and Higgs (1995, p. 315) pose clinical reasoning as the key for integration of different types of knowledge, where 'the relationship of sources of knowledge is seen as interdependent, rather than hierarchical, and the whole person, and the contexts of practice are taken into account'. In some respects, this is contextualising learning by teaching ways of reasoning that are relevant to the professional practice models of a profession. This is explored in more detail in the next section.

Process-based curriculum

Current curriculum designs that are congruous with emphasis on either or both learning processes and professional processes can be termed 'process-inclusive' or 'process-based'. Candy and Crebert refer to a shift from content-based to process-based education in which peer evaluation, consultation and collaboration feature strongly (Candy & Crebert 1991, p. 584). Process-based designs attempt to articulate the relationship between curriculum structure and the professional practice model in the particular profession. Professional practice models reflect the ways in which a particular profession undertakes its professional processes. In addition, the curriculum must be *congruent* in terms of the planned learning experiences that enable learners to develop the capability to use such processes. Furthermore these processes must be made visible by explanation and modelling, built into modes of assessment, and also elicited through debriefing. Bruner (1966) described the 'process model' for constructing a curriculum. His view was that each discipline has a set of processes which determine the way in which knowledge evolves or is produced within it, and that curricula should mirror these processes in order for students to learn to work with knowledge rather than merely accumulate it as a product. The teacher's role is that of facilitator rather than transmitter of a body of predetermined information.

The development of process-based curricula requires consideration of a range of issues. The relationship between academic and professional groups, as already discussed, will influence the extent to which knowledge and practice are separated. So, given the critical link forged by the field teacher between the student and the curriculum, collaboratively designed curricula (in which shared theories and practice are negotiated and made visible by all parties involved) might contribute toward overcoming any territoriality and reducing the confusion for students about theoretical approaches. Other development issues include (Everingham & Bandaranayake 1999, p. 268):

> 'the rapid growth of knowledge, avoiding the temptation of content coverage through an overcrowded curriculum, illuminating the cognitive processes required for critical thinking and clinical reasoning, building the effective interpersonal skills that are pivotal in all the caring professions, acquiring skills and values that underpin the desire and capacity for continued education, and developing generic transferable skills that increase career flexibility.'

Two process-inclusive curriculum designs that attempt to locate professional education more strongly in the workplace are now described.

Problem-based and issue-based learning

Problem-based learning, as originally conceived for the McMaster Medical School, is intended to enhance clinical decision-making through the use of purpose-designed, realistic problem simulations. The aim is to overcome the increasing irrelevance of the undergraduate curriculum in its capacity to address the real world and to do this using real problems as a means for integrating learning.

The objectives of the approach (to be addressed simultaneously) include:

- The acquisition of a knowledge base (propositional knowledge) that is organised in a more useful way, more easy to recall in the clinical context, and easily extended through self-study
- Development of scientific or analytical reasoning skills (problem-solving)
- Development of self-directed learning skills
- Encouragement of independent and critical thinking
- Sensitivity to all of the patient's needs
- Encouragement of the integration of information from the various preclinical sciences.

(from Barrows 1986)

Problems selected for study define the basis of the curriculum. Choice is determined by the prevalence of the health problem in the population. The focus of learning includes clinical logic, urgency, treatability and interdisciplinarity. The utility of problem-based learning is its potential to promote deep approaches to learning (Engel 1991). Notice, in the objectives above, the mix of processes to do with both learning and professional ways of thinking. Not surprisingly this curriculum innovation has spread to other professions.

Issue-based learning is similar to problem-based learning in that its starting point is a particular issue. An issue-based learning curriculum was introduced in 1996 to the Department of Social Work Social Policy and Sociology at the University of Sydney, after it undertook a major curriculum review of the professional years of the Bachelor of Social Work (that is, the final two years of a four year course). The reasons for this change primarily arose from the context, expectations and demands of social work practice in a rapidly changing world and from the existence of some of the factors, discussed earlier, that inhibit the integration of theory and practice.

Whilst the new programme shares many of the pedagogical principles of 'problem-based' learning, the term 'issue-based learning' was chosen to encapsulate the idea that social work and social policy address personal and social issues (George & Napier 1997). These principles include the integration of interdisciplinary knowledge such as social policy and practice, attention to process as well as product, the transferability across contexts of practice of generic skills (for example, analysis and communication), and adult learning where students' prior knowledge is acknowledged and drawn on and learning is to a large extent self-directed. The curriculum is located within a critical social science perspective, with social justice and social change being a central focus (George & Napier 1997).

Issue-based learning units are constructed in ways that reflect the complexity of the social world, focusing on the interrelatedness of issues, thus reinforcing integration rather than separation. Much of the learning is done in small groups where students are presented with real practice situations and are expected to collaborate with their student colleagues in responding. The development of partnerships with agencies is critical, since many of the practice scenarios are generated by experienced practitioners in those agencies. Practitioners are also involved in class situations on appropriate occasions.

Small group learning is supported by lectures, workshops, skills classes and field education placements. Assessment involves a range of activities including debates, student presentations, critical reading and analysis exercises, peer assessment, reflective journals, learning portfolios and group projects. Students are helped to be self-directed in their learning, although they find it difficult at times because of previous experiences of traditional education (including the first two years of the social work programme). This innovative approach to social work education is still in its early days, but initial evaluations by practitioners have been positive, particularly in terms of preparing students for field education.

Process-based pedagogy

Having argued for the relevance of process-based curricula to the integration of theory and practice, we now examine the pedagogy that is congruent with such curricula.

Nurturing intellectual maturity

Perry's (1970) work suggests that learners move from a simplistic notion of amassing and reproducing facts to the ability to critically interrogate knowledge and operate effectively in full cognisance of its inadequacies. Candy proposes that it is not enough simply to tell learners that knowledge is more complex and tentative than they might have considered. Rather, individuals need to 'confront the inadequacies in their present conceptions' (Candy 1991, p. 296) and to be autonomous in evaluating their practice epistemologies. Candy flags many useful mechanisms for nurturing intellectual maturity and self-direction, including bibliographic instruction to enable learners to explore and evaluate information. This is facilitated by a systematic introduction to the knowledge framework of the field, demonstrating the processes through which knowledge is created and used in the particular field and how it has evolved historically. The identification of rules that are used to judge knowledge in the field, issues that are at the forefront of current thinking, and the provision of cognitive apprenticeships also aid this process (Brown *et al.* 1989).

Central to this mix of design and facilitation is engaging deep approaches to learning, building student confidence in learning, and increasing independence of students from the teacher, particularly in relation to managing work-related learning (Candy & Crebert 1991). While these mechanisms would need to be embedded in curriculum, separate studies in the history and philosophy of science offer students a salient litany of confronting uncertainty, struggling with conflicting truths and the transient nature of knowledge. From Barnett's perspective, all would be directed towards extending students into new territories by creating shifts in their perception of knowledge and by developing their capacity for critical reflection (Barnett 1990).

Peer support and accountability groups can be used to assist in the development of intellectual maturity (Carson 1998). Such groups comprise three or four students who meet on a regular basis. They act as a support network in the process of evaluating and reflecting on their practice during the practicum/field placement. These groups ideally incorporate components of action/research/learning. Important practice skills to be learned include supporting others and evaluating the effectiveness of one's own practice, using feedback and evaluation from others. When conflict develops, the group must learn to deal with it. This is also a way of learning to take responsibility for working in a team (Irwin & Napier 1998).

Reducing setting discontinuity

Although the classroom and the field offer distinctive and valuable learning opportunities, one key to creating the nexus of learning is to reduce the discontinuity between ways in which students are asked to learn in both these settings. The aim is to increase the authenticity of learning by reducing the gap between the ways professionals learn and work after graduation and the ways student learning is promoted in the field and classroom. In our examples of problem-based and issue-based learning we have shown how this might be achieved by basing learning around real problems, issues and cases. Here the emphasis is on evidence-based reasoning and assessment that goes beyond cramming for batteries of multiple choice exams, towards asking students for analysis of the theoretical dimensions of a problem and exploration of solutions that are anchored in the constraints of a real situation. As presented earlier, these assessments might be pursued using reflective journal reports, portfolios of achievement, negotiated assessment, peer consultation and evaluation and team projects. Such assessments encourage the formation of connections between classroom learning and placement, planting the idea of lifelong learning and preparing the student to identify and articulate learning.

Contextualising learning

The value of learning in the workplace is the opportunity to contextualise learning in a chaotic, vague and unpredictable world, where decisions may be influenced as much by resource constraints and political pragmatism as by theory. Student preparation beforehand and debriefing during and after the experience are common models of teaching. Boud and Walker (1991) offer a unifying model for learning from experience, from the classroom to the field and back again, which involves preparation, observation, action and reflection. Structures used to support learning where observing and acting are simultaneous include prompts to thinking and practice, such as learning agreements and workbooks; mirroring ways of working through team work, peer learning and feedback; and nurturing critical reflection of personal theories-in-action or issues such as power relations through journal writing, for instance. Given the clashes between classroom ideals and the contradictory conditions and political com-plexity often experienced within the practicum, the student's critique of the context would constitute an empowering tool with which to further interrogate experience and discover knowledge.

Bridging the theory/practice gap

Bridging the gap is achieved by provoking connections to other potential contexts using techniques such as *brainstorming* to apply the new knowledge in other contexts. Hodgson examined the experience of students in lectures and found that relevance is activated by lecturers who are enthusiastic about a topic and who are able to offer a 'vivid example or illustration'. Students are thus enabled 'to go beyond the outward demands of the learning situation and make connections between the content of the lecture and their understanding of the world around them' (Hodgson 1997, p. 171). The value of bridging the gap needs to be stressed to students; they may need to be encouraged to keep notes concerning the examples given. The gap can also be reduced by simulating or replicating the other environment.

Replicating the authentic environment

Strategies that replicate the real context involve using learning methods which generate the kind of internal dynamics that mirror thinking and working in the real world of work, in particular, the more socially shared context of learning (Candy & Crebert 1991). Techniques include simulation games, role play and mental rehearsal. Problem-based learning falls in this category because the study problems not only are drawn from the context in which the learning will be applied but also require real problem-solving processes.

Utilising the sanctuary of the classroom

Within this pedagogy, the classroom still has value as a significant place of sanctuary from which to examine the field experience. The novice can examine problems in a more modest formulation, allowing analysis of critical evidence at a pace that supports the level of experience of the student; here, also, the symbiotic relationship between knowledges of practice can be explored in 'slow frame', using questioning and learning conversations to probe issues, examine depth, ponder uncertainty and negotiate meaning.

Engaging the interpersonal dimension

A curriculum that engages process also demands new ways of teaching that promote useful student encounter with the affective domain. Such methods incorporate an interpersonal dimension in learning, unlike those that entrench study isolation. The teacher 'becomes an explorer of meaning and significance with students' (Diekelmann 1990, p. 301); the meaning and complexity of the context are negotiated through interaction, the quality of which is enriched by the capacity of the facilitator to establish an authentic relationship, to be a trusted guide on a challenging journey. Galbraith describes facilitation as a 'trans-actional process' involving 'collaboration, support, respect, freedom, equality, critical reflection, critical analysis, challenge and praxis' (Galbraith 1991, p. 3).

To help students explore the affective domain, particularly in relation to 'difficulties' in their work with clients, they can be encouraged to identify a situation with a client (or colleague) where they had some concerns about their intervention. They audiotape their account descriptively, detailing the parts of the interaction that concerned them most. They give the recording to their supervisor (without any analysis), for analysis in supervision. The supervisor encourages the student to tease out and confront the issues that may be hindering practice development and to understand the complexities and interpersonal dimension of the professional role.

Utilising a dialogue-based dynamic

One role of the teacher is to create a discussion environment which nurtures the critique of ideas, within a milieu of tolerance intended to engage students in critical dialogue. In this dialogue the cognitive processes of both the teacher and the student are the learning material. The key is open-ended questioning, seeking to lift and extend student thinking in the context of a learning conversation. This dialogue-based dynamic is designed to:

- Illuminate theory that was embedded in practice but not consciously observed by the student
- Evaluate practice from a theoretical perspective
- Anticipate or predict action in the light of theory
- Challenge, question and reveal theory that underpins thought or action
- Analyse the adequacy of action or solution in the light of relevant theory
- Model processes of thinking that draw on theory and reflection
- Model how practitioners theorise

- Elicit competing theories that practitioners use in situations
- Examine the choice of one theory over another (including professional craft knowledge).

Portraying the value of knowledge

'The value we put on knowledge will profoundly influence the experience that we offer students in encountering and participating in knowledge' (Barnett 1990, pp. 43–4). Barnett's point is that knowledge is not value-free, although we do not always acknowledge the values we have for knowledge. If we cannot articulate the relationship between academic and practice knowledge or communicate the value of practice knowledge, then there is little hope of the student making the connection. If we portray knowledge as a process of acquisition, a drudgery, a job to be done, a threat, a punishment, then the nexus will not be achieved. Rather, we should communicate knowledge as a vehicle for self-understanding (Barnett 1990, p. 43).

Implications for teachers

The examination of process-based pedagogy has implications for the teacher. Whether academic, clinician or practitioner, the teacher must be a *facilitator* with the capacity to:

- Challenge thinking through learning conversations
- Facilitate students' engagement with the affective domain in a mutual journey of increasing complexity
- Harness emotion as a legitimate bridge to critiquing the experience of the practicum
- Be comfortable in displaying and engaging the relational dimension that is a feature of these professions
- Traverse the field of certainty and uncertainty in a way that builds student capacity for professional judgement
- Nurture courage in the face of the unfamiliar and support risk-taking
- Create from an individual's story relevance for the group, while at the same time attending to the uniqueness of the experience
- Work with learning as a dynamic process that is responsive to opportunity
- Be flexible in response to burgeoning maturity and experience of the beginning practitioner
- Portray and prompt reasoning processes embedded in the practice models of the particular profession
- Facilitate critical thinking and reflection
- Support and encourage independence.

Conclusion

For each profession, the ways in which to organise the curriculum will be different. As Grundy (1987) observes, curriculum is not governed by laws, but is a cultural construction reflecting values and beliefs about how people interact in the world. Thus curriculum choices will vary between the professions. The challenge is in reconceptualising the classroom as a place to learn about practice, and the practicum as a place to learn about theory, thus creating the nexus that will enable students to begin to develop the mix of knowledges required for expert practice. Process, in its many forms, appears to be the mechanism for facilitating this complex and deep learning.

References

Barnett, R. (1990) *The Idea of Higher Education*, Society for Research into Education and Open University Press, Buckingham.

Barnett, R. (1992) *Improving Higher Education: Total Quality Care*, Society for Research into Education and Open University Press, Buckingham.

Barnett, R., Becher, R. & Cork, N. (1987) Models of professional preparation: Pharmacy, nursing and teacher education, *Studies in Higher Education*, **12**(1), pp. 51–63.

Barrows, H. (1986) A taxonomy of problem-based learning methods, *Medical Education*, **20**, pp. 481–6.

Boud, D. & Walker, D. (1991) *Experience and Learning: Reflection at Work*, Deakin University Press, Melbourne.

Brown, J., Collins, A. & Duguid, P. (1989) Situated Cognition and the Culture of Learning, *Educational Researcher*, **18**(1), pp. 32–42.

Bruner, J. (1966) *Towards a Theory of Instruction*, Harvard University Press, Boston.

Candy, P. (1991) *Self-direction in Lifelong Learning*, Jossey Bass, San Francisco.

Candy, P. & Crebert, R. (1991) Ivory tower to concrete jungle, *Journal of Higher Education*, **62**(5), pp. 570–92.

Carson, L. (1998) *Peer support and accountability groups*, unpubl. paper, Department of Social Work, Social Policy and Sociology, University of Sydney.

Curry, L. & Wergin, J. (1993) Setting priorities for change in professional education, in *Educating Professionals: Responding to the Expectations for Competence and Accountability*, (eds L. Curry & J. Wergin), Jossey Bass, San Francisco, pp. 316–28.

Diekelmann, N. (1990) Nursing education: Caring, dialogue and practice, *Journal of Nursing Education*, **29**, pp. 300–5.

Engel, C. (1991) Not just a method but a way of learning in *The Challenge of Problem-based Learning* (eds D. Boud & G. Felleti), Kogan Page, London, pp. 23–33.

Eraut, M. (1992) Developing the knowledge base: A process perspective on professional education, in *Learning to Effect* (ed. R. Barnett), Society for Research into Education and Open University Press, Buckingham, pp. 98–118.

Eraut, M. (1994) *Developing Professional Knowledge and Competence*, The Falmer Press, London.

Everingham, F. & Bandaranayake, R. (1999) Teacher education programs for health science educators, in *Educating Beginning Practitioners: Challenges for Health Professional Education* (eds J. Higgs & H. Edwards), Butterworth-Heinemann, London, pp. 263–70.

Galbraith, M. (1991) The adult learning transactional process, in *Facilitating Learning: A Transactional Process*, (ed. M. Galbraith), Kreiger, Florida.

George, J. & Napier, L. (1997) *Contestable concepts in the social work curriculum*, Paper presented at the Australian Association of Social Work and Welfare Education Conference, Canberra, September.

Grundy, S. (1987) *Curriculum: Product or Praxis?*, Falmer, Sussex.

Hodgson, V. (1997) Lectures and the experience of relevance, in *The Experience of Learning*, 2nd edn (eds F. Marton, D. Hounsell & N. Entwistle), Scottish Academic Press, Edinburgh, pp. 150–71.

Howe, D. (1997) Relating theory to practice', in *The Blackwell Companion to Social Work* (ed. M. Davis), Blackwell, Oxford, pp. 170–6.

Irwin, J. & Napier, L. (1998) *(Re)forming field education*, Paper presented at the National Conference of the Australian Association of Social Work and Welfare Education, Cairns, September.

Parker, J. & Rubin, L. (1966) *Process as Content: Curriculum Design and Application of Knowledge*, Rand McNally, Chicago.

Perkins, D. & Saloman, G. (1992) The science and art of transfer, in *If Minds Matter*, (**1**) (eds A. Costa, J. Bellanca & R. Fogarty), Skylight, Illinois, pp. 201–8.

Perry, W. (1970) *Forms of Intellectual and Ethical Development in the College Years*, Holt, Rinehart and Winston, New York.

Schön, D. (1983) *The Reflective Practitioner: How Professionals Think in Action*, Basic Books, New York.

Titchen, A. & Coles, C. (1991) Comparative study of physiotherapy students' approaches to their study in subject-centred and problem-based curricula, *Physiotherapy Practice*, **7**, pp. 127–33.

Titchen, A. & Higgs, J. (1995) Facilitating the use and generation of knowledge in clinical reasoning, in *Clinical Reasoning in the Health Professions* (eds J. Higgs & M. Jones), Butterworth-Heinemann, Oxford, pp. 314-25.

Chapter 18
Parallel Journeys in
Professional Practice

Sue Radovich and Joy Higgs

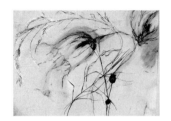

The stories of our lives often meet with other people's stories in everyday settings. In this chapter we explore professional practice in one such everyday setting, the school classroom. The chapter focuses on Sue Radovich's professional practice journey as the central thread and weaves around this thread the journeys of several groups of people who participate together in a common venture (the facilitation of effective learning and communication) in this venue. We incorporate several sources of data into the central story of Sue's professional doing, knowing, being and becoming, and the related stories of her fellow journeyers. The first source is several pieces of written material that Sue has prepared recently to plan for, market and reflect upon her professional practice. The second is an interview conducted by Joy Higgs in which Sue explored her own professional practice and the experiences of participants in the programme. This chapter presents Sue's story and also provides commentary (indented text) in the form of reflections/asides to examine journeys occurring in parallel to the primary story and consider broader issues about professional practice journeys.

Three categories of school teacher are mentioned in this chapter. To clearly differentiate their roles they are referred to as the 'classroom teacher' (or simply the 'teacher'), the 'support teacher learning difficulties', and the ESL or 'English as a second language teacher'. To avoid confusion we systematically use the word 'children' to refer to the primary school pupils, and 'students' to refer to the university student speech pathologists participating in clinical placements at the primary schools.

My journey begins (Sue's Story)

Ten years ago I began work in a unique kind of setting, a special education support centre, where I was employed as a speech pathologist. This context was unusual in that my employer was the health department but I worked predominantly in educational settings. Through this centre, I worked in primary schools alongside teachers with special roles in addressing children's learning difficulties. My role was to work with children who had learning difficulties or specific reading difficulties and it was my job to determine to what extent and in what ways oral language contributed to these problems. During this time I worked with special needs teachers from the Catholic school system and an educational psychologist with a school counsellor background. Working with this team and with the many schoolchildren involved shaped my love for working with that population.

The traditional speech pathology education provided in New South Wales at that time did not prepare me for the breadth of work involved in this school context. Instead I learned through a trial by fire, working hard to develop some unique skills and professional knowledge needed for this job. I spent several years investigating, researching and developing clinical skills and at the same time developing a real passion for working in this area. I had reached a point where I felt quite confident in saying that the techniques, strategies and therapy that I had developed, worked and worked well with this population.

It was during this period that I developed many of the dimensions of my current approach to speech pathology in schools. I found that the usual speech pathology model (involving the withdrawal of individual children from the classroom with the goal of intensive one-to-one therapy in a 'clinical'-type set-ting) was unsatisfactory for the children and unsatisfying for me. Traditionally, speech pathology has developed out of a medical model of intervention; 'with-drawal therapy' reflects this management of speech disorders. This traditional medical model of intervention implies that the speech pathologist has sole responsibility for the diagnosis and intervention used with the child. By com-parison, the concept of a wellness model is the promotion or enhancement of optimal health and well-being, in this case communication competence. In this approach the natural classroom environment is the ideal setting for therapy; this therapy is not an isolated activity but is incorporated into normal classroom life.

I had seen therapies and ways of working emerge from my creative experience and critical self-appraisal, that I do not believe I could have developed as an individual working with the child one-to-one. Withdrawal is a sub-optimal approach in that it does not sufficiently draw on the opportunities that the natural classroom environment provides to involve school teachers and special needs teachers in the therapy process and to incorporate the participation of other children (without learning difficulties) in activities which foster learning development for both the children targeted in the therapy and also the assisting children. In addition, working in the classroom allows children to work on their communication skills within the context of everyday conversations and activities.

The next step – developing a collaborative systemic model

Apart from my conviction about the strengths of this approach and my obser-vation of the efficacy of a collaborative classroom approach to the management of learning difficulties, my other motivation to move to this model was the satisfaction I found in working with other adults in a team. Together we were able to provide a consistent and more comprehensive approach to address the children's needs. Further, my role as a therapist was extended. I learned to value the collaboration of developing resources together with the teachers, of exploring different ways of working, and also I came to deeply appreciate my role as a teacher in my facilitation of learning and sharing my knowledge with the other adult members of the team.

Professional journeys

A characteristic of professional journeys as reflected in Sue's experience is the dynamic nature of effective, successful journeys. Moving from one work role context to another involves framing and re-framing one's professional identify, activities and work relationships.

Branching out into private practice

Changes in the funding system and in my family commitments led me into private practice. I created a practice, called Educational Speech Pathology, based in schools. This practice involved the negotiation of contracts with individual schools to provide speech pathology services for the children. This involved the application of a systemic approach in several schools.

I describe my 'systemic approach' to school-based (speech) therapy as one which:

- Adopts a comprehensive and holistic model of therapeutic assessment (Larson & McKinley 1995)
- Acknowledges and cultivates the positive influences of speech pathology beyond the clinician–child relationship into the wider school environment
- Instigates measures of the influences of speech pathology within the school, not only in terms of the actual intervention programmes but also in terms of the professional development of staff, speech pathology students and changes in workplace practices.

Sue's journey

As Sue's journey progresses we see the transition of novice to expert. She takes her pre-graduation learning (largely theoretical and propositional knowing, plus traditional clinical roles and skills) into a less familiar environment. Her personal knowledge base, values, visions of people working together, and skills in problem-solving and interpersonal interactions, along with her professional entry 'doing and knowing' abilities, are combined to confront the challenges and opportunities of this new environment. She learns the power and liberation of this combination and her doing, knowing, being and becoming (both personal and professional) are enhanced by this growth experience. In the ten years of working in this context Sue has extended, challenged and refined her knowledge and skills to a high level of expertise and she has re-defined what expertise means in this setting.

My overall goals in implementing this programme were:

- To provide speech pathology services within the school setting which reflect my commitment to systemic intervention
- To provide functional, naturalist intervention for school-aged children experiencing language-based learning difficulties within the communicative context of their school life
- To ensure that the intervention has a sound speech pathology research and practice base, is linked with the appropriate speaking and listening aspects of the K-6 (Kindergarten to year six primary school years) English curriculum and, where possible, to the current classroom themes
- To ensure that appropriate and agreed measures for accountability are included in all aspects of service
- To provide an opportunity for 'collaboration in practice', encouraging the mutual upskilling of both speech pathology students and teachers.

The teachers

At this point the second journey commences. Classroom teachers, even support teachers for children with learning difficulties, and ESL teachers have traditionally regarded speech pathologists as school visitors who withdraw children for therapy sessions, then return them to the classroom. This traditional medical model approach focuses on the treatment of 'curable' conditions. It fails to recognise the pervasiveness of the impact of learning and communication difficulties on every aspect of children's lives; the lost opportunities that classroom-based, team-provided therapy programmes could provide. As the health professions and the community continue to seek relevant models of health care, support for health care models or approaches which reflect social ecology practices (similar to the system-wide, holistic and collaborative, interactive approach in Sue's model) is increasing (Higgs *et al.* 1999).

Developing a philosophy of teaching – crafting an approach to doing and knowing

Initially the collaboration in my practice involved myself (as clinician), the teachers and the specialist teachers. This was an important step because it led to establishing the credibility of the programme (to others and to myself). I needed the teachers, schools and parents to see me as first and foremost a clinician working for the children's good, not primarily as a business person, a teacher or an administrator. This level of confidence was important before proceeding to the next phase (involving speech pathology students in the process), so that the strategies for language and learning enhancement could be tested, developed and owned by the participants and so that the teachers and the school system could be sure that the priority of the therapy activities would be the schoolchildren, not primarily the benefit of the university students.

It was also at this stage that I realised that I was actively seeking out new fields of knowledge particularly in the areas of linguistics, TESOL (teaching English as a second language), qualitative research, clinical education, and business and marketing research, to inform my practice and clinical education interests. This had a powerful effect on increasing my conviction that I was reaching the same conclusions and experiencing many shared (but new to me) discoveries with a larger unseen body of people (researchers). I felt justified and strong in my directions because I could back arguments up with 'the literature', which seemed to be expected and mandatory in my liaisons with the universities. By comparison, the schools wanted to be shown, and emphasised what they saw as, the 'practical' applications. I learned that I needed to have two language systems when negotiating, because each party respected different forms of knowing.

The teachers' journey – changing perspectives

Alongside Sue's own journey of discovery about teachers, schools and teaching, the teachers needed to acquire a knowledge of the nature and scope of speech pathology and an understanding of the benefits of different models of service delivery. Together with Sue they developed a shared language to better work together.

The administrators' journey

There are many complex factors involved in the participation of therapists in schools. Suffice it to say (in this chapter) that the schools participating in this programme needed to come to terms with a new way of operating if they were to take advantage of the positive opportunities that the programme provided. The school's administrators (e.g. principals) needed to gain knowledge about speech pathology so that they could make informed decisions when negotiating their employment contract. Sue has seen that a part of professional responsibility is to ensure that an agreement with potential employers considers clearly the needs and expectations of all key stakeholders (children, parents, teachers, school, students, university and therapists), and to discuss goals, roles, strategies, numbers of clients/children, therapy venue, timetables and resources. This, again, is a reflection of the need for active participation and negotiation among the various programme stakeholders.

The children

A fundamental argument underpinning the systemic model is that isolating children for therapy fails to recognise that communication and learning are essentially social activities influential in the children's emerging self-identity. I do not believe that separating development (or remediation) from the natural context of its use is congruent with the essence of language (i.e. as a social tool). For these children, a key social and language context is school life and the daily social and learning tasks in which they engage. Children need language and learning skills for their life roles/tasks, so they should learn in this context. For optimal generalisation of therapy to occur, I believe language should be facilitated within the child's familiar everyday environment with practical and demonstrable generalisation built in. While there may be periods of withdrawing children and working on certain skills, the overall systemic programme should include periods of generalising those skills where they need to be used.

The children's journey
The children involved in the programme began with communication disorders. They emerged with enhanced communication, learning and social skills, which improved the quality of their lives and that of their families.

Passing on knowledge and skills to the next generation

Along with my evolving practice model came a rich enthusiasm for teaching; my next step was to seek involvement of university speech pathology students (initially from the School of Communication Sciences and Disorders at the University of Sydney) in my school-based practice. I based my teaching approach on my first-hand knowledge of the difficulties associated with integrating speech pathology systemically in primary school environments. In planning my approach to clinical education, I believe I understand where the student is coming from, in that I can remember clearly the challenge and the uniqueness of working in this population in this way.

My goal for the students was to provide them with opportunities to:

- Develop their skills in identifying speech and language needs within the school-aged population
- Develop and implement intervention programmes that have a curriculum focus
- Develop an awareness of the multitude of facets of school life and the various curriculum expectations
- Appreciate the diversity of children in mainstream educational settings.

I wanted to help the students learn about the satisfaction that comes from a collaborative strategy and from reaching out beyond the clinical therapy approach to explore a broader range of goals and therapeutic/educative approaches. I knew for them this would be a journey of discovery – discovery of themselves, their potential, and of a team strategy where the product is greater than the sum of people working on it.

> ### Framing the students' journey
> From the richness of her own journey Sue has spent much time, energy and vision framing a context and opportunity for students to pursue their own journeys of doing, knowing, being and becoming. Each of these journeys is unique; each brings its rewards and challenges for the students and for Sue as clinical educator and mentor.

As part of their experience of school-based therapy, students need to come to understand their role in the school and the perceptions of this role. Schools and teachers often place the speech pathologist in the role of the expert. Students, coming to terms with their professional identity, can approach their teaching role in different ways, perhaps over-confidently, perhaps tentatively. Learning to balance the role of student, novice clinician, professional role model and team member is a challenging task. The students also need to learn to deal with the incongruences they find between their theoretical learning and their practice experience, between the service delivery model(s) to which they are committed (or are advocating) and the approach needed by the school. Some students enter the school setting like crusaders, convinced of the value of going in and withdrawing certain children (for therapy) without knowing how to generalise the developing skills in a broader way to group work or class-rooms.

> ### Professional journeys – multiple dimensions
> Sue's journey into professional expertise and the students' journeys as they enter their professions can be seen as journeys into:
> - Reality (of expectations, accountability, responsibility and holistic care)

- Wisdom (practice wisdom, which is deeper and richer than learned professional knowledge)
- Professional identify
- Integration of personal and professional selves
- Team work
- Creativity and new practice visions.

The teaching-learning model – systemic collaboration in action

Figure 18.1 portrays the teaching-learning model I have developed. It illustrates my various selves in action: self as individual, self as clinician, self as clinical educator and self as programme manager. All of these selves are brought to the role of the clinical educator.

Related models

In a related model the multi-faceted roles of educational programme manager were categorised as task manager, group manager, individual development manager, environmental manager and overall programme manager (Romanini & Higgs 1991). Denshire (2000) identified the importance and value of bringing self into clinician/educator tasks in terms of authenticity and enhancement of the professional role. Similarly, McAllister and Higgs (1998) have explored the various selves (self as person, self in relationship with others, self as educator) brought into the role of clinical educator. Peer and collaborative learning is variously portrayed by Ladyshewsky (2000) in clinical education, by Amies and Weir (2000) in their strategy for peer facilitated practice development, and by Cohen and Sampson (1999) in their exploration of peer learning.

Reflections on the journey into professional artistry – melding doing, knowing, being and becoming

In reflecting on my professional journey over the last ten years particularly, and on the creation of the model of school-based practice (systemic collaboration) presented in this chapter, I recognise the various selves that I and other professionals bring to our practice. A journey into professional artistry is one of transition and melding. The transition involves taking one's self as an individual with life experience and aspirations (being) and as a novice professional with an entry level of knowledge (knowing) and practice skills (doing), and growing into areas of potential strength (becoming). We learn to value and meld our personal and professional strengths in our professional roles. And we learn to use the benefits and recognise (and where possible diminish) the limi-

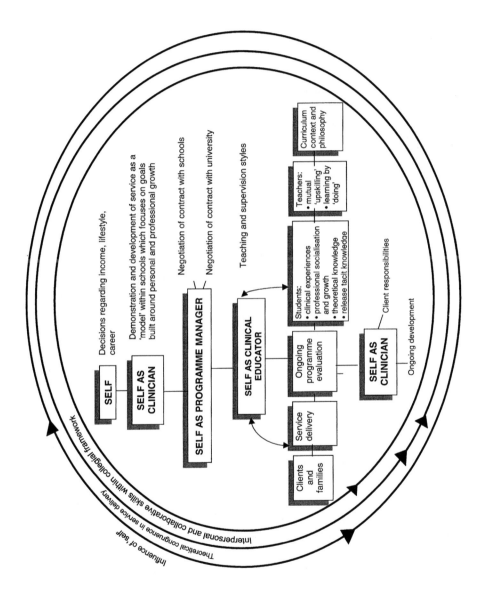

Fig. 18.1 Parallel journeys in action.

tations of the art, craft and science of our professions and our individual professional capacities.

> ### Sue's journey – reflections
>
> Yet professional artistry is greater than *more*, as in more knowledge, more skill, more understanding. In talking about transition we are talking about perspective transformation (Mezirow 1981); an evolution where we build on our strengths, using self-direction and critical appraisal as we take responsibility for our competence and quality of care. In addition, professional development is about confidence. Through ongoing and rigorous testing and refinement of our practice we gain conviction about the quality and sound basis of our professional interventions, about the creative approaches we adopt and about our programmes which continue to push the boundaries of what we have previously known and what is current practice. We learn to be inventive in the face of uncertainty, to be risk takers in the face of confusion and time/resource pressures, and to be reflective thinkers in the face of our needs for challenge and career fulfilment. All these activities and developments (both personal and professional) are amalgamated into the heightened level of critical self-awareness, the refined capacity for professional inventiveness and responsiveness to contextual circumstances and the openness to growth and learning, which comprise professional artistry.

Conclusion

Professional practice is not limited to the therapeutic role of the health professional. It involves various participants, each of whom has their own perspective on the process and outcomes of the practice intervention/interaction. Further, professional practice is an evolving phenomenon as reflected in the interrelated journeys of the players in this programme.

References

Amies, C. & Weir, S. (2000) Using reflective group supervision to enhance practice knowledge, in *Practice Knowledge and Expertise in the Health Professions* (eds J. Higgs & A. Titchen), Butterworth-Heinemann, Oxford.

Cohen, R. & Sampson, J. (1999) Working together: Students learning collaboratively, in *Educating Beginning Practitioners: Challenges for Health Professional Education* (eds J. Higgs & H. Edwards), Butterworth-Heinemann, Oxford, pp. 204–11.

Denshire S. (2000) *Imagination, occupation, reflection: Ways of coming to understand practice*, MAppSc(OT) thesis, The University of Sydney.

Higgs, C., Neubauer, D. & Higgs, J. (1999) The changing health care context: globalization and social ecology, in *Educating Beginning Practitioners: Challenges for Health Professional Education* (eds J. Higgs & H. Edwards), Butterworth-Heinemann, Oxford, pp. 30–7.

Larson, V.L. & McKinley, N. (1995) *Language Disorders in Older Students: Preadolescents and Adolescents*, Thinking Publications, Eau Claire, WI.

Ladyshewsky, R. (2000) *A quasi-experimental study of the effects of a reciprocal peer coaching strategy on physiotherapy students' clinical problem solving skills*, PhD thesis, Curtin University of Technology, Perth, Australia.

McAllister, L. & Higgs, J. (1998) *What's it like to be a clinical educator? Stories from the coalface*, paper presented at annual conference of Speech Pathology Australia, Perth.

Mezirow, J. (1981) A critical theory of adult learning and education, *Adult Education*, **32**, pp. 3–24.

Romanini, J. & Higgs, J. (1991) The teacher as manager in continuing education, *Studies in Continuing Education*, **13**, pp. 41–52.

Chapter 19
Developing Creative Arts Expertise

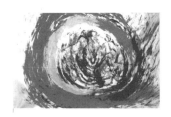

Joy Higgs, Ian Maxwell, Ian Fredericks and Lyn Spence

On First Looking into Chapman's Homer
Much have I travell'd in the realms of gold,
And many goodly states and kingdoms seen;
Round may western islands have I been
Which bards in fealty to Apollo hold.
Oft of one wide expanse had I been told
That deep-brow'd Homer ruled as his demense;
Yet did I never breathe its pure serene
'Till I heard Chapman speak out loud and bold:
Then felt I like some watcher of the skies
When a new planet swims into his ken;
Or like stout Cortez when with eagle eyes
He star'd at the Pacific – and all his men
Look'd at each other with wild surmise –
Silent, upon a peak in Darien.

(John Keats (1795–1821), *Potetical Works*, 1884)

Keats was so moved by the power and liveness of Chapman's translation of Homer that he wrote this sonnet after spending all night reading Homer with a friend. The poem expresses the intensity of Keats' experience; it also reveals how passionately he cared about poetry. To communicate how profoundly the revelation of Homer's genius affected him, Keats uses imagery of exploration and discovery. In a sense, the reading experience itself becomes a homeric voyage, both for the poet and the reader. (Poem analysis provided by the State Library of New South Wales.)

In Keats' verse, above, we see many of the players and elements which comprise this topic of developing creative expertise. Here the poet, artist and actor combine to create and perform a work of sublime artistry to the delight and awe of the art consumer.

> ### Reflective notes
> *An important consideration in exploring the topic of expertise in the creative arts is the need to differentiate between the act of creation which characterises the role of the composer, the painter and the writer and the act of creative performance which characterises the role of the actor, the singer and the dancer. While the distinctions between these roles are neither complete nor totally desirable, we found, in our deliberations, that it was important to recognise that creativity in the creative arts included both the birth and realisation of creative vision (e.g. playwrighting, music composition, painting), and the creative interpretation of existing visions (e.g. musical scores, plays, songs).*
>
> *Perhaps we could consider these two (overlapping) roles as being the artistic creator and the creative performer.*

To create this chapter we sat down together for an intellectual creative improvisation discussion in the style of a jazz session. Drawing on our knowledge and past experiences, and on our capacity for creating and realising visions, we engaged in a loosely orchestrated, free flowing debate on the topic of expertise in the creative arts. We employed the depth of knowledge and frames arising from our backgrounds in drama, music composition, singing and writing, improvising back and forth as we wound our way inside this topic, examining both the apparent and the meta-levels of this absorbing discussion. To reflect these different levels we employ the device of 'reflective notes' to illustrate the 'player's guide', the 'artist's vision', the 'writer's muse' and the 'scholar's interpretations'.

So, on to the goal. What is expertise in the creative arts? After much deliberation we came to the conclusion that 'it depends': on the point of perspective of the decision-maker and the field of operation of the creative artist. In our discussion we pondered this question: If you were asked to sum up expertise in creative artists using three characteristics how would you answer?

For actors (by Ian Maxwell)

I would offer watchability, availability and reliability. Watchability is simply the capacity to command an audience's attention. We might say of an actor, 'I couldn't take my eyes off him, even when he wasn't the focus of the scene.' This capacity, the ability to draw the focus and engage the attention of an audience, facilitates the creation of a belief that the scene portrayed is happening even though it is not real: it literally *fascinates*. Availability is a similar notion, in that it can involve making oneself accessible to the audience; additionally, however, it denotes the actors' capacity for engaging with suggestions from the text they are working with, from their colleagues, their director, and, of course, from their own range of experience and training. Actors might talk in terms of 'not being precious', of being 'open', and of being willing both 'to run with an idea', and, just as importantly, 'to let go' of something that 'isn't working'.

Reliability is the capacity to produce on cue, night after night; to reproduce the accuracy of performance but without doing it mechanically; to achieve a blending or tension between structure and inspiration, structure and anti-structure. This was the great insight of the director, teacher and actor Constantin Stanislavski: for theatre to be an *art*, the work of the actor had to be 'inspired'. Stanislavski understood inspiration as coming from a deep subconscious store, the spirit. Only when actors are tapping this resource can their work be real, genuine – an art. The actor's task, then, is to have the technical skill of accessing his or her subconscious on demand, Stanislavski's cardinal principle being that through conscious means we reach the subconscious. Actors are only artists when their craft is powerful enough to release the inspirational wellspring of the spirit; that craft, however, is fundamentally rational, systematic and disciplined, and is the product of an intense, sustained period of training of the body and mind.

The emphasis on craft as the means to achieve the end of inspiration has been the cornerstone of a range of non-western performance practice for centuries, illustrated, for example, in Zeami's treatises on the Japanese Noh theatre, written in the fifteenth century. To this day, the Noh theatre actor will train from childhood for a particular character-type in a given repertoire of plays, learning 200 plays by rote, essentially playing the same character every time. The aesthetic of Noh demands an almost exact reproduction for every performance; performances will be essentially identical each time: the craft mechanism is in place. However, what will distinguish one performance as being superior to another are moments of pure inspiration or beauty: a tiny, transcending moment of inspired difference within sameness which, to the Japanese audience, represents the outstanding performance.

For composers (by Ian Fredericks)

My three characteristics for experts are transparency, persistence and altered consciousness. The artist creating the work strives to make the mechanics of the craft transparent or invisible to the audience. At the same time this craft is meant to be transparent or explicit to peers and other experts in the specific field, who will recognise master craftsmanship as the composer 'makes it seem easy'. The composer is at once a creator and a technologist, understanding and being technically competent in the use of the capacities, limitations and nuances of the instruments (of composition and presentation) which will enable the composer to realise his or her vision. Composers need to know themselves, to be in touch with their internal reality and to be open to the creative moment, forgetting everything, both extraneous matters and technical considerations; to throw away former barriers and limitations. For ages, nothing may happen; creativity may be stalled. It is like gazing into an abyss. Then all of a sudden it happens: a kind of gestalt shift in perception, a transcendental experience or rather, a spiritual awareness, which permits the realisation of a dream or vision. Indeed, a new universe is created or liberated by the composition.

We can think of this expertise of the artistic creator as requiring creative intelligence because the act of composition is one of conceptualisation, of creating something from nothing. Practice and technical expertise is only a vehicle, a tool for creation which, of itself, is insufficient. Without the creative spark the creation cannot occur. The creative genius is somebody who aims at and achieves something nobody else can see. The outstanding artistic creator realises (makes manifest) the creative vision (or target) in a way that others cannot achieve and at a higher level than others can effect.

Above all creation is an act, not a process, although it occurs through a process that has to be trusted and allowed to go its own way. The creative act is characterised by *decision-making* and the courage to accept one's own decisions and abide by them. Such a commitment is paramount. In addition, this creativity results from transcending and abandoning established procedures and existing visions, and creating new visions through insight, persistence and courage. This is 'the creative way'.

> ### Reflective notes
> *An interesting consideration in the context of this book (which deals with the health sciences and education as well as the creative arts) is the way creativity can occur (and indeed is necessary) in science in the same way that technology (and science) is utilised in the creative arts. We live in changing and interesting times when the dominance of science in the science arenas is supported by demands for evidence-based practice in the professions, but this dominance is being challenged by calls for people-centred practice. In the art arenas the enormous advances in science and technology are challenging the historical craft and artistic traditions of the arts. Technology in the arts is a tool to enhance artistic techniques, an amazing new means of critical appraisal and development and, indeed, a whole new means of artistic expression.*
>
> *Ian Fredericks commented in our discussions that this blending of science and art occurs in both of his 'alter egos': engineer and composer; the former a hard science, the latter a creative role. His observations led us to articulate, as an emerging trend, a growing cross-disciplinarity in these and in other professions, between the 'creative' (extrapolation) and the 'precision' (focus) dimensions arising from art and science.*

In choreography

Creativity involves inspiration and vast imagination, knowing the capacity of the dancers (for whom the dance is designed) and having the ability to work with people to translate the vision into performance.

> 'Because I loved the music so much and it made an impact on me, I thought it would be a great one to do (choreograph). It's Piano Sonata no. 7, by Prokofiev. I've been working on it for a couple of years . . . First of all, I envisage a theme, images in my mind, rather than people actually dancing around. I put it into a story in my head. I think of movement in combination with that, rather than just movement alone . . . Everyone gets inspiration in different ways . . .
>
> Jiri Kylián opened up a whole new world. . . . He came from Czechoslovakia, and has a strong attachment to the past. The deep longings he has for his homeland come out a lot in his work. He'll come in, very inspired by the music. He'll immediately start working with two or three people, and experiment with movement. He'll move around himself, and the people behind him will imitate him or come up with something of their own he likes, and he'll use that, and go on from there. It's giving and taking . . .'
>
> (Tim Gordon, cited in Munday 1987, pp. 88–9)

For singers

Expertise is attained when everything about the singing is right; it 'pings'. The sound has resonance, brightness and colour and it is wonderfully easy. It feels right to actually produce the sound. The whole effect is greater than the parts. The sensation for the listener is that the sound seems to float. They will also be aware of the 'ping', a clear, full and resonant sound.

Expertise in singing evolves from training the voice to produce a consistently pleasing sound, and from developing the singer's musical and dramatic ability. When singers have mastered the mechanics of voice production they must combine this craft knowledge with skills in musical interpretation (understanding the genre) and dramatisation (comprehension of the song). It is the combination of these three factors which enables singers to demonstrate their artistry, to create a mood or characterisation that reveals meaning in a song to the listener.

The singer/musician and the composer have a curious and sometimes uncomfortable interdependence upon each other. Singers rely on the composer's notation as a platform from which to demonstrate their skill. The composer will claim the kudos for the inspirational spark and technical knowledge inherent in the creation of a musical score. However, 'a musical score is not equivalent to a musical work . . . Musical notation is a written artefact without musical properties, although it provides necessary limits to interpretation' (Edlund 1996, p. 367). Without the expertise of the performer to realise the composition, the score has no musical identity, but even the most talented musician can do little with a poor composition.

For visual artists (painters, sculptors)

Expertise involves technical excellence and a truth to the chosen genre. But to draw ahead of honest craftsmen and women the outstanding artist moves beyond the known or current limits of that genre. Like composers the true artist creates an expression of a unique vision. And the artist communicates this vision to the audience. Or perhaps the artist creates a vision and encourages observers to dream their own dreams or hear their own messages from the artwork.

The painter or sculptor, the poet and writer demonstrate excellence by revealing new aspects of the world. Whether this goal is personally driven (reflecting 'the creative conceit of genius') or seeking to enlighten, expose, inspire or communicate new understandings, these creative artists exhibit the capacity to reveal an otherwise unrevealable world. The poet, for instance, as in our introductory lines, can take the reader to new heights of awareness and new depths of understanding.

For musicians

Performance artistry or a sublime performance demands virtuosity. But this is not just technical excellence. The outstanding musical performance should communicate to the audience, should touch the audience. Expert musicians manifest their love for their art in the performance. And musicians should have the capacity to infuse the music with something ineffable, whether this is humour, irony or a more sublime understanding of the musical piece than the audience has yet achieved. There is something else too, in creative performance; the outstanding performer can be someone who has the courage to be bold, to drink the elixir of audacity and extend the art, to take risks and re-create the creations:

> 'When you drill down to the roots of creativity, you will see that its most important factor is courage. This, in turn, demands audacity – involving boldness and daring. Audacity is a marvellous elixir. It has the power to shatter barriers ... Audacity requires a break with tradition and a deviation from one's normal decorum.'
>
> (Nader 1999, p. 124)

Achieving the 'ping', the perfect moment in a creative performance, is a beautiful idea that has haunted western metaphysics for centuries. This is the idea of an absolute 'presence of the moment' where everything comes together. It is the absolute dream of western music and art critics. In anthropology, the work of Victor Turner (1982) on ritual performance (and its subsequent elaboration by

Richard Schechner into a generalised theory of performativity encompassing theatrical forms in addition to ritual) suggests that the power of ritual practice derives from its capacity to generate a sense of continuity between and within participants, a quality Turner labels *communitas*, and which might be thought of as providing the basic material for building a sense of society. For Schechner (1976), theatre practice represents a secularised (and, arguably, somewhat diluted) version of this same transcendence of self: boundaries are dissolved and reformed in a state of heightened, communal engagement; the individual is reconstituted as part of a greater whole reflected in the heightened and extra-ordinary experience of the participants.

The creative artist who is in this state of heightened creativity or performance perfection appears to be performing effortlessly, to be acting without making decisions, and to be unconscious of all prior learning. Yet this refined level of performance is neither as simple as a reflex reaction nor as innate as intuition. Instead it represents a unique blending of the imagination and artistry of the individual, the refined decision-making of the expert and the learned, polished and largely automatic, ingrained skill characteristic of all highly skilled athletes and technical experts.

The expert creative artist has an appreciation of the situation, an intense concentration and context awareness which make the artist capable of planning uniquely for the audience or setting. In addition, the outstanding creative artist demonstrates the capacity for within-performance calibration, the ability to perform micro-adjustments, to assess and raise the level of performance in response to, or raised by, the mood of the audience. The artistic creator, similarly, has the capacity to assess the emerging creation mid-development and adjust, discard, enhance and re-create this artistic product. Creation of an artistic product requires a kind of honesty, a critical self-knowledge and self-appraisal which sets high standards and does not give up till these goals are attained.

A singular dimension of creative artistry is the unique contribution made by individual artists to their creative works. This ineffable 'something' raises indi-vidual performances to a greatness that is unforgettable. Rubens, for instance, was 'an unsurpassed master in the handling of colour' (Murphy & Devapriam 1979, p. 94).

Reflective notes

In the above discussion several issues emerged, beyond the frames of the different artistic media. One of these was the notion of balancing structure and technicality with creativity and inspiration, yet recog-nising that creative acts tend to require the suspension of focus on technique to allow the created universe to direct its own way.

A second meta-idea was the question of transparency of the craft of the artist. This term was used to represent the idea that the craft is the means to achieve the artistic outcome (the presentation or creative product) rather than the visible centrality of the art. Success and expertise was seen to occur when the art hid the process, the perfection of the technique or the toil of the training and practice. Yet the expert observer can appreciate both expertise and artistry. The most successful artist, athlete, craftsman, is the one who 'makes it seem easy' to an onlooker.

Thirdly, expertise is located within the traditions and conventions of the particular genre chosen by the artist. The criteria for judging jazz differ from those used for classical music. Similarly, Impressionism and abstract art, opera and popular songs, live theatre and movie acting, differ in expectations.

Another commonality in expertise across the creative arts is a capacity for self-evaluation, which, beyond intellectual reflectiveness, and beyond responsiveness, is a heightened awareness that amounts to transcendence of the ordinary.

Finally, we recognised the experience of the sublime performance. It has been described as 'being on song', 'a sweet spot', 'a ping', 'being on top of the performance', 'being at one with the audience', 'the presence of the moment', 'when everything clicks'. At the same time this high level self-perceptiveness is associated with a sense of detachment where the artist can stand outside of self as well as being immersed in actual or potential self and being connected to vision, art, inspiration and technical perfection.

The audience may comprise experts, peers, informed consumers and people who 'just know what they like when they see or hear it'. So what do we want these people to experience through the creative arts? How would they perceive a superior performance or artistic creation?

Our team responded:

- I would want the music to knock the socks off the audience.
- The special performance will be truly impressive. In acting the sublime performance can achieve in the audience a collective gasp as the absorbed watchers recognise something essentially exquisite. We want to create an impression of beauty, enjoyment, awe or appreciation which lingers long after the performance. The performer needs to know the audience, to respond invisibly and effortlessly to the different needs and expectations of different audiences; to be just as convincing with a children's group as an audience of critical peers.
- While the expert audience may appreciate the technique, they want the art to transcend it. We want to convey the skill to our peers. Average consumers, on the other hand, want to appreciate the (extraordinary) performance occurring before them, not needing to know or see what has gone into making that

spontaneous creative explosion, the 'ah', the 'wow', the unforgettable experience.

In 1973 Kelvin Coe and Marilyn Rowe won silver medals at the International Ballet Competitions in Moscow and an award for the best partnership. Kelvin reflected on this experience:

> 'The fact we used the stage like Russian dancers was singled out, and they were intrigued with the "little" choreography they'd almost forgotten: the filigree dancing with little beats and little footwork . . . I don't think anybody was more surprised than we were when we got the medal . . . The biggest shock was that in the first thing we did, the pas de deux (from *La Fille Mal Gardée*) and the variations, the place just erupted. It went bananas!' Marilyn added, 'They'd never seen anything like the choreography . . . the Russian dancers in the wings thought it was entrancing.'
>
> (Munday 1987, p. 58)

> Nureyev danced at a performance of the Kirov ballet in Paris. 'The effect was sensational. He was given extra performances (and received) . . . dramatic acclaim.'
>
> (Bland 1976, p. 20)

The outstanding performance, the expert creative artist's legacy, has an enduring dimension. Long after an outstanding artistic performance, the publication of a great novel or music composition, the opening night of an exceptional new play or ballet or the showcasing of the superb talents of a painter, there is an enduring legacy, an acknowledgement that something exceptional has been produced:

> ' "Truly his coming was . . . an exemplar sent by God to the men of our arts, to the end that they might learn from his life the nature of noble character, and from his works what true and excellent craftsmen ought to be."
> This quotation comes from the Life of Michelangelo written by his friend and fellow artist Giorgio Vasari. Although the book was published more than four hundred years ago the fundamental point is still true today: that Michelangelo possessed, to a degree rarely equalled and certainly never surpassed, creative ability so outstanding and wide ranging as to command universal admiration, both during his own lifetime and ever since.'
>
> (Daniels 1981, p. 6)

> ### Reflective notes
> *We thought long and hard about the essence of expertise as well as the characteristics of expertise. The essence of expertise in creative artists (in both roles, i.e. creative performers and artistic creators)*

could well be summed up in the word 'sublime', inferring the achievement of a product or performance of outstanding creative excellence, a pure or beautiful example of the genre, a state of altered being in the construction or presentation of a creative vision, a realisation of that which others cannot see, or an exquisite creative performance with the tools of body, mind and imagination. And for creative artists themselves, the sublime extends to the experience of delight, of passion personified in the creative work. We have attempted in this composite, to explicate the almost nameless essence of creative expertise, the 'je ne sais quoi' which distinguishes the brilliant artist from the above average one.

The key characteristics we could look for in expert artistic creators and creative performers are inspiration, transcendence beyond the ordinary, impact on an audience or history, technical superiority, completeness, passion, commitment, adventurousness, self-knowledge, a unique perspective and a capacity to open windows to other vistas.

How is expertise in the creative arts acquired? Or is it inherent?

When you are absorbed as performer or artistic creator in a heightened focus on the experience or a creative act, it is as though you are playing a piano with notes that are so big that you could not fail to hit the right one each time. Or if you are a singer you hit the perfect note throughout the entire performance. We are very inclined in those moments to use terms like 'innate', 'instinct', 'feeling'. But if the artist relies only on a kind of spontaneous genius, this is an extremely fragile thing. The perfect moments are actually hard won; in reality they are commonly the pay-off of years of dedicated training, along with a certain type of creative focus, a certain kind of artistic disposition. But in that perfect moment all that preparation disappears and all you have is the absolute imminence of the experience. It is very easy to talk about that as something pure, unformed and effortless, but in helping the novice *creative performer* prepare for these glorious experiences, the emphasis is on the training, on reflective realisations and on helping these artists to learn what it is like to recognise, understand, experience (and hopefully repeat) these moments. For the *artistic creator* the preparation takes various forms which may emphasise learning and extending the theory and techniques of the form of art and appreciating the essence of creative genius. Yet for some artistic creators the key to promoting the experience of 'the glorious moment' is to encourage freedom of expression at any time 'the muse' demands.

How can we help students of creative arts to experience the 'sweet spot', the shift in reality, the change in perception? Perhaps educators can describe their own experiences, or promote the students' confidence and exploration, and encourage them to believe that this emergence to another level of creativity and realisation *will* occur. We can help the novice to recognise the 'ping' when it does arrive.

Another approach is to engage students in experiential exercises. For instance, an exercise for students of jazz is to 'play on only one note' to achieve a focus on rhythm. For composers (and jazz players), an exercise to achieve the 'sweet spot' experience is 'free form improvisation'. This is music that is free of rhythm, free of harmony and free of melodic considerations. The object of the exercise is to listen to what is happening, to play off the 'absent one' (i.e. the missing *fifth player*) and especially in a group situation to listen to the other members in the group and to *play off one another*. Freeform improvisation is such an important training exercise that it has become an art in itself in both jazz and neoclassical music, featuring in many concerts and in many recording sessions. This kind of exercise encourages nonconformity and a complete departure from *normal practice*, which is the essence of *the creative act*.

Creative artists need to spend time learning to understand their instrument deeply, whether it is their body, their voice, their violin, their computer or their palette. To achieve this understanding the artist may turn scientist, learning the knowledge and skills of acoustic engineering, anatomy, biomechanics and chemistry. The artist may spend hours perfecting the skills of voice production, bodily control, physical flexibility and acuity, brush handling finesse and computer programming. In addition artists need to learn about the ways of knowing, being and doing within the artistic genre, medium and community they have selected.

Reflective notes

Expertise in the creative arts requires a seamless blending of the art, craft, theory and science of the chosen artistic medium, genre and community.

Consider the process of 'the getting of practice wisdom' and the development of professional artistry in the creative arts. One of the few truly great masters of world art was Rembrandt van Rijn:

'His early pictures show that he was still dependent on the style of his teacher Lastman . . . However, even here we can perceive the distinguishing features of the future master: his special interest in biblical themes, his close attention to moving psychological movements, and his search for new means of expression. His acquaintance with the works of the followers of Caravaggio in Utrecht enabled him to enrich his images with strong contrasts of light and shade, and to use light as an ethical force to differentiate between good and evil . . . (In the 1640s a rift between artist and patrons/society began to appear, linked to Rembrandt's unwillingness to make concessions to the demands of changing fashions) ... Rembrandt reached the height of his maturity as an artist in the 1650s. His main focus of concerns in this period is man and his spiritual state. It is a time when the artist deploys his great abilities to the full. The content of his paintings becomes more profound and sublime, his technical skill bolder and more versatile, and *chiaroscuro* [the treatment of light and shade, a variety of light and shade] his chief means of expression.'

(Murphy & Devapriam 1979, p. 80)

> ### Reflective notes
> *In this cameo we see many elements to the getting of expertise in the creative arts: the natural propensity, the passion and the dedication which the artist brings to the task; the training, critique, mentors and fashions which provide external influences; the strength of personal goals, self-identity and passions which frame the artist's direction.*

So what does the person bring to the art?

'One of the aims of classical dance training is to impose an impersonal uniform discipline, and many good dancers become little more than anonymous illustrations of academic virtues. Nureyev has never been that kind of dancer. (His dancing broke the conventions of classical propriety.) His approach is invariably human, warm-blooded and personal. His qualities as a dancer are inseparably connected with his character ... the most immediately noticeable characteristic is an exceptional singleness of aim, coupled with a range of natural gifts which seems specially designed to achieve it. Drive and flexibility (two hallmarks of his dancing) are perhaps his greatest assets.'

(Bland 1976, p. 42)

On a final note, there is a fascinating contradiction, or paradox, at the heart of the expert creative artist. Within the uniqueness of great performances or creations, artists may experience themselves both inside and outside the work they are creating, as simultaneously being both more themselves than they usually are, and being not themselves at all. Instead, they may have the experience of being 'inspired', 'flowing' or 'swept away'. Self is transcended while at the same time being reinstated and reaffirmed in a complex, wonderful reflexive synergy that is the mystery of creativity.

Acknowledgement

Thanks to Josh Fredericks and Henry Bialowas for their thoughtful insights.

References

Bland, A. (1976) *The Nureyev Image*, Cassell & Collier Macmillan, London.

Daniels, J. (1981) *Michelangelo*, Octopus Books, London.

Edlund, B. (1996) On scores and works of music: Interpretation and identity, *The British Journal of Aesthetics*, **36**(4), 367–81.

Munday, R. (1987) *The Australian Ballet: 25 Years*, Australian Consolidated Press, Sydney.

Murphy, B. & Devapriam, E. (1979) *USSR: Old Master Paintings*, Australian Gallery Directors Council, Sydney.

Nader, J.C. (1999) *How to Lose Friends and Infuriate People: A Controversial Book for Thinkers*, Plutonium, Pyrmont, Australia.

Schechner, R. (1976) From ritual to theatre and back, in *Ritual, Play, and Performance* (eds R. Schechner & M. Schumann), The Seabury Press, New York.

Turner, V. (1982) *From Ritual to Theatre: The Human Seriousness of Play*, Performing Arts Journal Publications, New York.

Further reading

Brook, P. (1968) *The Empty Space*, MacGibbon & Kee, London.

Bryan, M. with Cameron, J. & Allen, C. (1998) *The Artist's Way at Work*, Pan Books, London.

Castaneda, C. (1971) *A Separate Reality*, Penguin Books, Ringwood, Australia.

Caudill, M. (1992) *In Our Own Image*, Oxford University Press, New York.

Diderot, D. (1957) *The Paradox of Acting* (translated by Walter Herries Pollock), Hill & Wang, New York.

Nearman, M. (1984) Feeling in relation to acting: An outline of Zeami's views, in *ATJ*, **1**(1), 40–51.

Penrose, R. (1995) *Shadows of the Mind*, Oxford University Press/Vintage, London.

Reanney, D. (1994) *Music of the Mind – An Adventure into Consciousness*, Hill of Content, Melbourne, Australia.

Rink, J. (1995) *The Practice of Performance: Studies in Musical Performance*, Cambridge University Press, New York.

Roach, J.R. (1985) *The Player's Passion: Studies in the Science of Acting*, University of Delaware Press, Newark.

Stanislavski, C. (1937) *An Actor Prepares* (translated by Elizabeth Reynolds Hapgood), Eyre Methuen 1980, London.

Storr, A. (1997) *Music and the Mind*, HarperCollins, London.

Chapter 20
Weaving the Body, the Creative Unconscious, Imagination and the Arts into Practice Development

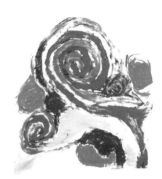

Emma Coats

This chapter describes a holistic approach to personal and professional development, which weaves together the unconscious, our imaginative, physical, and rational self with the use of the creative arts to guide and illuminate practice. I have likened the sections that form the chapter to the four seasons of the year:

Part 1: Beginnings, could be compared to winter, the growth that goes on beneath the ground. It is a short review of the origins of my work, and the key ideas that I am concerned with.

Part 2: Coaching a fellow professional, is analogous with spring. It contains a description of my first project in health care in March 1998, when I coached Angie Titchen in preparation for her use of the creative arts at the writers' retreat in Australia – the event which was the seedbed for the ideas that gave birth to this book.

Part 3: Facilitating the use of the body and the creative arts with health care professionals, is like summer, the first fruits of a joint collaboration with Angie Titchen. It is an account of a workshop which we co-designed and facilitated on the theme of 'giving voice to intuition', for the 5th Reflective Practice Conference, at Robertson College, Cambridge in June 1999.

Part 4: The Epilogue, is like autumn, the harvest. It is a poetic reflection on this work as I write this chapter over July–September 2000, and pointers to the future.

The narrative continues now with the seeds or deeper work that led to the emergence of my approach.

Part 1 – Beginnings (winter)

Background journey

I use the metaphor of winter as an allegory for a quest I was engaged in over a three year period (1997–99), about new work I wished to do. Four particular influences informed this period of 'winter' growth: my experience of working in business for over 18 years up to 1996; my deep interest in the creative arts which I have been exploring since 1988; my personal and professional development through various forms of depth psychotherapy, and in neurolinguistic programming; and my training over the past five years in a Certificate in the Therapeutic and Educational Application of the Arts, at The Institute for Arts in Therapy and Education in London.

Personal inquiry

My quest began to resolve when I engaged in a reflective inquiry into the different realms of my experience in 1999. I had felt split while involved in the contrasting worlds of business, psychotherapy and the arts, and I saw that split generally reflected in organisational life. It seemed to me that the deeper world of the self and the depth of our expressiveness were valued and encouraged within the realms of therapy and the arts, but were mostly left out of working life.

I wanted to achieve two things which interwove with each other: to discover a way of transposing the richness of the imaginal and the expressive from the realms of therapy and from art into the wider world of work; and to create a new career as a facilitator of professional development using the various languages of the creative arts.

Emergence of my approach

I immersed myself in a process of autobiographical writing, artistic expression and archetypal ritual. Gradually a personal paper emerged in which I articulated a model for professional development which explored the integration of the creative unconscious and the imagination with verbal methods of problem solving, using a variety of creative arts methods (Coats 1999). I tested the paper with a number of practitioners and researchers in Britain including Angie Titchen, a personal friend. This slowly led to the launch of my professional practice as a facilitator in organisational settings, in the realms of health care, education and in business.

Strategies and applications

The aim of this approach is to engage in a process of creative consultancy with the whole of ourselves, learning from other dimensions of our being, using creative forms of knowing. Strategies include a range of arts processes – paint, clay, movement, image theatre (dynamic gestures portrayed through the body), music, poetry and creative writing. The information (or knowing) that arises through these methods may be expressed in metaphors, images or in art works as a result of exploring the phenomenology and wisdom of the body, the creative unconscious and the imagination.

The information that emerges is then worked with using dialogue and critical reflection to support, challenge, guide or transform our experiences in organisational life. The overall intention is to help navigate the turbulent worlds of complexity and uncertainty in our professional lives, or our being and becoming, whether we are exploring roles, tasks, relationships or organisational strategies. Parts 2 and 3 of this chapter illustrate some of the ways of realising these aims in practice.

Part 2 – Coaching a fellow professional in the use of the creative arts (spring)

The context

In 1998 Angie Titchen asked me to coach her in preparing for her role as co-facilitator of the writers' retreat in Australia. I liken this section to spring, as it was the first practical manifestion of my emerging quest. Angie wanted to introduce the creative arts into the retreat as processes to support participants to 'move into unfamiliar territories and different ways of thinking'. Although familiar with using arts processes in her personal life, she had not worked with them before in a professional setting. In the account I describe methods I used for the coaching session, which include the use of rational and unconscious knowing, the imaginative domain, and enactment or role play.

Preparation: rational and unconscious knowing

I wanted to achieve a rational understanding of the different dimensions or complexity of the context Angie would be engaged in. So in advance of the session, I questioned her about practical information: number of participants at the retreat, types of work people do, the nature of the environment in which sessions would be run, the timing of sessions, what would happen before and afterwards; and the personal: her assumptions about participants' likely experience of the creative arts and her concerns and needs about her role and intentions as facilitator.

Then I worked with unconscious knowing to support myself in creating a strategy. I gave space and time to my creative unconscious to generate ideas, having 'flooded' my mind with information. I spent some time in my local park, in a process of reverie, musing and contemplation.

Strategy

A variety of thoughts and two key metaphors emerged out of this process as a pathway for the session. I wrote them up in the form of an appreciation of Angie's needs, focused on a series of questions:

Thoughts

(1)   Identity and roles: who am I, who are they?
(2)   Desired results: what do I want to achieve for myself, what do I want to achieve for others?
(3)   Intended behaviours: what am I going to do, what do I want others to do?
(4)   Capabilities: how am I going to do x, how are others likely to do x?

The aim of these questions was to stimulate both my and Angie's thinking about her intentions, and also to consider and learn from the imagined perspective of her fellow participants. This would generate much richer learning about her role than if we stayed just within her own viewpoint.

Metaphors

The metaphors acted as meta-frames for holding the overall purpose of the session, and the essence of my role. The first metaphor, a triple helix (my invented term – see Fig. 20.1) was a crystallisation of the three interwoven routes which I thought we needed to cover, for Angie to arrive at her desired outcome of gaining an embodied sense of introducing the creative arts into the writers' retreat, and to work confidently with them.

The second metaphor was that of a bridge; it helped me to think about the purpose of my role. I saw it as supporting Angie to expand her identity and to surface issues and doubts by co-creating new knowledge and experiences. In

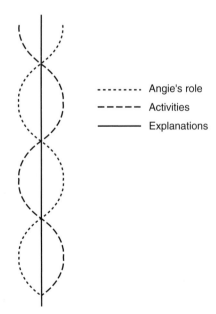

----------- Angie's role
– – – – – Activities
———— Explanations

Fig. 20.1   The triple helix.

particular, the knowledge encompassed knowledge about herself in relationship to the retreat participants and how she communicates (explanations), knowledge about working with creative arts processes (activities), and knowledge about her identity over the duration of the retreat (role).

Embodied sense of working with the arts

My intention was for Angie to acquire practical knowledge of introducing the creative arts and the issues that may arise, as a result of the processes we would engage in. I hoped that her knowing would become embodied, as opposed to purely intellectual without experience to support it. After discussing the strategy I had proposed, we then took a day for the coaching session itself.

The coaching session

Internal and external attention to what is figural

I begin by paying attention to how Angie is, noticing what she says, her energy, and concerns, and staying aware of what comes up in me in response to my observations. I take my cue from her. I do not know what our first step is going to be, and by keeping an awareness on my internal state I use myself as a resource to support the coaching process.

The previous work now provides background support, as Angie and I engage in the actual process of journeying together towards her desired outcomes. The preparation has become the foundation or groundwork; now she and I attend to what is figural or of immediate concern.

Angie is focused on how people at the retreat might respond to working with dance or painting (see Chapter 3) to explore ideas, which may be a very unfamiliar process. This parallels her need to increase her confidence in facilitating such methods. As she talks, I remember a conversation I have had about potential reactions to a new process being likely to fall within three broad realms: enthusiastic, ambivalent or defensive.

Spatial sorting to help differentiate issues

I suggest we assume responses at the retreat might fall into similar categories. Angie concurs, and we divide the space we are working in into three, to represent each of these responses. I learned about this method of using space from my training in neurolinguistic programming. It helps to separate out aspects of a complex task or role, and is useful for keeping track of different feelings and responses to particular issues.

Use of enactment to enrich learning

We then engage in a role play, enacting these responses ourselves, entering each of the three spaces and role-playing both facilitator and participant, using our imaginative powers. My aim is for Angie to acquire experiential insight into what it might be like to receive a combination of these responses, and how she would manage herself. She will gain further insight by putting herself into the participant roles, with me playing her role. I encourage us to play with the enactment, doing it as truly as we can, so that it is meaningful and results in useful guidance.

Angie discovers that she needs to experiment with her role repertoire as facilitator, allowing herself flexibility rather than staying in one mode of being, and to find ways to support herself in answering responses experienced as difficult or challenging. Her role play as a participant experiencing the different types of reactions has given her a deeper understanding of what might be motivating such responses, and thus clarifying how she could respond more effectively to them.

Archetypal imagery in support of role repertoire

As we reflect on this part of the session, I remember Angeles Arrien's model of the Four-Fold Way (Arrien 1993): the archetypes of warrior, healer, teacher and visionary. This model views the self as embodying these four aspects, each encompassing a different way of being in the world. The model is based on indigenous people's perspective on the self, and is drawn from native traditions from around the world.

I suggest we experiment with it as a means of developing the exercise. My aim is for Angie to explore alternative ways of being, and to discover a felt sense of congruence in terms of her intention, what she says and how she says it.

Role play as diagnostic and as rehearsal for becoming

This second role play is the equivalent of the actor's rehearsal. The first was more diagnostic, discovering what needed to be worked on. Of course the reality of actual participants at the writers' retreat will be different, but this rehearsal begins to make the unfamiliar more known, and to serve as a resource that Angie can draw on. She takes on the different archetypal roles while I play the range of 'participant' responses. I use my experience to discover what most motivates me when Angie introduces the arts and talks about different activities, and to notice how I feel about her responses to me as participant.

Conflict

There is one point where we get stuck, when I push Angie too hard to move through a difficult aspect of responding to very challenging responses. I learn, my constant learning, to go more slowly, and to keep a sense of attunement to what is happening. I lost contact with her process at that moment, because I became fixed on what I thought needed to happen, rather than staying with her process. After some discussion we move through. Later when we reflect again on this moment, Angie shares that although it was difficult, it was also revealing in terms of how people at the retreat might feel, if they felt pushed into doing something that was too much of a stretch.

Endpoint

By the end of the day, Angie tells me that she feels a strong sense of purpose and clarity about her new role, in terms of her confidence, how to introduce creative arts processes, and the different types of issue she may need to engage with. From the writers' retreat she sends a postcard saying, 'the creative arts really worked – not only was creativity released, but the openness, warmth and caring facilitated both personal and professional transformation ... My preparation with you was absolutely key.' I am delighted.

For me this confirms that working with the whole self, engaging rational and unconscious aspects of ourselves, and exploring the power of the imagination through enactment has proved very useful. Spring, representing the emergence of my work, and my support of Angie's becoming, has turned into summer, a flowering of her potential, and an affirmation of my emerging practice.

Part 3 – Facilitating the use of the body and the creative arts with health care professionals (summer)

Background

This account is drawn from a workshop that Angie and I offered at the 5th Reflective Practice Conference. I have traced the journey of the workshop to illustrate what we did and my intentions, together with descriptions of people's experiences as witnessed by me or reported by participants. I think of this section as analogous to summer, because it represented further growth for this work, and was the first fruits of a joint facilitation between Angie and me in working with the creative arts.

The context

The conference was jointly organised by The Holistic Practice Group at Luton University and the Royal College of Nursing. It was attended by health educators, researchers and practitioners from Britain and overseas. Our workshop, Giving Voice to Intuition, was offered within the remit of one of the conference themes, 'valuing intuition as the core of personal knowing'.

Eleven people came to the workshop, which was two hours long. Prior information had been given through an abstract in the conference programme. The intended learning outcomes were:

(1)   Identifying and listening to intuitive knowing
(2)   Responding to and unfolding intuitive knowing through a variety of creative processes
(3)   Articulating and transforming intuitions into meaningful action in the world.

The workshop setting

Imagine now that you are by a stream in the beautiful gardens of a Cambridge college, in mid-summer, in England. Laid out around you on the grass are large tarpaulin mats with jars of water, brushes, sheets of paper, tubes of brightly coloured paint, and paper plates as palettes. Under a large oak tree is a plastic bowl holding a slab of terracotta clay, with a couple of knives for cutting it.

Stage 1: Introduction and warm-ups

We begin by gathering in a circle on the grass. My heart is beating fast, and I am anxious. I do not know how people are going to respond. Angie and I introduce ourselves, and frame the workshop as a journey of discovery, exploring intuition with our rational and creative capacities. I invite everyone to work at their own pace, respecting the fact that if something feels too uncomfortable not to do it, and to ask questions at any time. The group is attentive. No questions are asked at this point.

We start with a couple of warm-up games. The aim is to bring out more of ourselves, and to begin to build a sense of community within the group, creating energy and connections amongst us. This is the third day of the conference, so everyone is full of the general hubble and bubble of conference culture, which has focused primarily on intellectual engagement with research presentations. However our intention is for knowledge creation to happen via an interplay between the different aspects of ourselves, not just through our intellects.

Angie leads a centring exercise: everyone shuts their eyes, focusing first on the sounds outside the garden, then the sounds inside the garden, then the sounds inside themselves. It is a technique of gradually focusing into the moment, and letting go of external concerns, in order to become more present.

Engaging our bodies through gestures

I invite everyone to open their eyes, and to allow a gesture or stance to emerge of how they are now. I ask Angie to demonstrate this process, and then together we unfold our personal stance or gesture. We let it go, and then create a new one to represent how we would like to feel by the end of the workshop.

Everyone participates, and a variety of gestures are created, a snapshot would show arms held high in the sky, or out in front of the body, some legs and feet close together, others more apart, and the upper body in open or curved body postures. Some heads look up, others forward towards the front, or down towards the ground.

My intention is to bring an awareness of our bodies into the workshop from the beginning, and to learn from our gestures how we are. It is a direct form of knowing, which may arise out of a thought, or intuitively without prethought. The first gesture marks our being, or where we are now, and the second our becoming, or where we want to be.

Perhaps as you are reading this, and if you are in an appropriate place, you might like to experiment with allowing yourself to move into a body gesture, or stance, about how you feel reading this, or about something that is important to you, and simply notice what happens, and what you discover . . .

Stage 2: Making connections

We find our own space, and Angie leads us in a movement exercise walking around the grass and saying 'hello' to each other through our feet. I can see that some people are more self-conscious than others but everybody takes part and seems willing to try it out. Once we have all said hello in this way, Angie asks each person to shake hands with one other, then to sit on the grass together, and share reasons for coming to the workshop. There is a buzz of energy, and talk.

We are moving now from the physical domain back to the rational, to begin the next stage of the workshop. The warm-up games have supported the group to form in an unusual way, that attends to more of ourselves than if we had simply sat down and had a discussion. Energy has been stimulated, and new ways of relating engaged in, which underpin future stages of the workshop where we will work again with the use of gesture to explore intuitive knowing.

After people share why they have come, we invite everyone in their pairs to discuss two experiences of their use of intuitive knowing in their professional practice. One instance should be where they had acted effectively on the intuition, and one where for some reason they had not, but later wished they had.

Physical expression as critical reflection

The pairs spend ten minutes discussing and reflecting on the two different experiences they have chosen. We then explore the physical experience of the events each person has described. Angie demonstrates this first, by recalling a time when she did not act on her intuition, and lets that memory be evoked physically through a gesture. She adds a repetitive movement to her gesture, and whatever word is at the top of her mind that is true to the essence of her experience. She then dissolves the gesture.

I invite the group to do this together, in their pairs, making physical their experience of when they did not act on their intuition, adding a word and repetitive movement if they feel comfortable enough. When one half of the pair is engaged in the process, the other acts as a witness. I ask each pair to reflect with each other on what they discover.

My intention is to draw out or make explicit the tacit knowing about that experience as it is held in the body, in order to generate learning about what happened. Everybody takes part, and there is an animated discussion within the pairs about the experience.

Group use of physical expression

Angie invites the pairs to form two small groups. In their groups she asks them to form a gesture or stance of their experience of acting on their intuition. Both groups create gestures, and there is a general picture of body postures that are open, expansive in space.

This picture contrasts with the physical expression of experiences of not acting on intuition, where many body postures in the pairs were contracted or tight, with heads focused down, arms held close to the body or head. I invite each group to witness the other groups' gestures of acting on their intuition, and after the witnessing to reflect on the experience within their groups.

During this activity I was asked why I had invited one group to go first. I replied that I did not know, I had made a purely spontaneous choice. The person said it had been uncomfortable for them to watch the others, and so I invite them to share that reflection with the whole group.

Sitting on the grass, we have a discussion about the experience of being seen. Some people found it acceptable, others had felt self-conscious, and parallels were made with people's practice about the vulnerability of their patients in being seen. A comment was also made that health care practitioners are more used to representing difficult experiences than positive ones – 'perhaps we don't show enough of our joy in nursing'.

The use of physical expression to reflect on experience has been powerful. Insights have been evoked, and the use of the body for expression in enhancing professional awareness has surfaced deeper feelings and thoughts about practice.

Stories from research

Following our discussion, Angie invites participants to listen to some stories from her research work on the use of intuition by an expert nurse in patient-centred care. I add a short reading from Ferruci's *What We May Be* (1982) about his views on intuition, the relationship between intuition and the mind, and the potency of internal imagery. These stories act as support for the validity of intuition, which may often be challenged in a climate of evidence-based health care. The intention is also to point forward to the next stage of the workshop, which focuses on the imagination and the power of creative imagery.

Stage 3: Engaging the creative unconscious

The readings lead to the midpoint of the workshop. We have been together for about 45 minutes and have an hour and a quarter left. I now invite participants to create an image, using paint or clay, which in some way represents their intuition, or themselves acting effectively on it. I suggest people may wish to allow the image to emerge, or to ponder it before creating.

Image making

Participants divide into the two groups which had formed earlier. Each group chooses a tarpaulin mat to sit on. There is an air of expectancy. People begin to explore the paints, and everyone works individually within the group. The atmosphere is one of lightness, and involved concentration. The groups spend about 15 minutes creating their images. A myriad of paintings emerge; some have scenes from nature – trees, butterflies, landscapes – others are more abstract, with different shapes and forms of colour.

The imaginative domain as critical reflection

Angie and I sit with a group each, inviting participants to talk about their image, what it evokes, the meanings it inspires, and any influence it may have on the individual's future practice. A person who wants to ask for comments from other members of the group may do so.

We start, and in both groups a wealth of information is shared about the images and their personal and professional meanings. The process has been effective in surfacing learning or previously unknown viewpoints from the deeper self, as a guide to enriching or changing practice. People express surprise about what has surfaced through the images, wonder at the process: 'I don't know where it came from, shows my doubts and my expansion', and the importance of valuing intuition: 'we analyse and rationalise everything, I am going to go back and trust my intuition more'.

Stage 4: Ending through physical embodiment and rational reflection

Angie and I invite our respective groups to find a way together to create a group sculpture, using gestures to act as a summary of the workshop. Each group experiments with what they want to express, and then takes it in turn to show their group sculpture. There is a greater sense of presence, spontaneity and physical freedom than in the group use of gesture earlier in the workshop. Something profound has happened. I think a community of trust has evolved, a valuing of expression, and a sense of new connectedness within the self and between group members.

The two groups join together and we sit in a circle for feedback and to share reflections on the workshop. One person talks of realising 'how important it is to use my body'. Another participant says, 'this was the workshop to come to'. Someone else tells how 'it was difficult at the beginning because of my awareness of the windows overlooking the space'. One of the group says, 'I am so amazed that I was able to do a painting, I am going to put it on my office wall'. Another adds, 'I am going to get my staff to try some painting – it was so powerful'.

After the reflections, Angie leads a grounding exercise. Then we all say goodbye. The workshop is over, it has been a good summer's day. The use of the body and of symbolic imagery has illuminated people's relationship to their intuition and to wider aspects of practice, while demonstrating the surprising richness of engaging with other aspects of the self.

The final section is a poetic reflection on this way of working, with issues and pointers to the future.

Part 4 – Epilogue (autumn)

Untitled

It has been a long time journey arriving at this place in the chapter, and this point in time
forty years in fact
And I am not sure what to say.
How to critique what I've done
The issues that are important,
directions I'd like to see evolve.

What do you think?

Perhaps I can start with what feels right, then what needs to change...
It feels right to emphasise our wholeness, our deep creativity,
what's hidden inside, and the wisdom of the body,

but issues can emerge,
of embarrassment, self doubt,
resistance, fear of failure,
mistrust of creativity,
of the imaginal world within.

Assumptions need to be checked out more,
at the beginning of a workshop
about how people feel,
and on messages received about their creativity.
Making things explicit, that get in the way
of daring to be more of who we are.

I would like to see
long-term studies of this kind of work, looking at its impact in day-to-day life.
I would like to see
the emergence of creative arts 'studios' in every practice setting
where people can explore their being and becoming...

Would you?

(Emma Coats, September 2000)

References

Arrien, A. (1993) *The Four-Fold Way*, Harper, San Francisco.
Coats, E. (1999) *An Emerging Meta Model for Developing Workplace Practice*, unpublished paper, London.
Ferrucci, P. (1982) *What We May Be*, Turnstone Press, Northamptonshire.

Further reading

These books discuss different ways of working with our creative capacities and/or of coming into relationship with our deeper selves.

Allen, P. (1995) *Art Is A Way of Knowing*, Shambhala, Boston, MA.

Dilts, R.B., Epstein, T. & Dilts, R.W. (1991) *Tools for Dreamers*, Meta Publications, Capitola, CA.

Fritz, R. (1994) *Creating*, Butterworth-Heinemann, Oxford.

McNiff, S. (1992) *Art as Medicine*, Piatkus, London.

McNiff, S. (1998) *Art Based Research*, Jessica Kingsley, London.

McNiff, S. (1998) *Trust the Process*, Shambhala, Boston, MA.

Morgan, G. (1993) *Imaginization*, Sage Publications, Newbury Park, CA.

Part Four
Reflections

Chapter 21
Professional Practice:
Walking Alone with Others

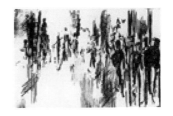

Joy Higgs and Angie Titchen

Reflections on Being a Professional

We sat around, we walked and talked about professional practice.
It's easy to talk about doing – what nurses do, what teachers do,
what actors and musicians do.
As observers and performers in each of these fields we can say,
more or less informedly, what it is that we do,
even if how we do what we do is less explicit.
Knowing is less visible than doing
but much is written about knowing – at least the public knowing.
Our embodied knowing, our spiritual knowing is more mysterious.
But Being, . . . does that have a place in professional practice?

What have we learned from our teachers about Being?
. . . to distance and thus protect self from the pain of others' suffering,
. . . to maintain credibility and authority through professional attitudes
    . . . not by chance do 'clinical' and 'academic' sound remote
. . . to portray the role, to be true to the creator's intent
    . . . not to present self in every performance.

'Professional' . . . is unequal, is it not?
A difference in need and capacity to provide or serve . . .
A difference in knowledge and expertise.
But perhaps we need to abandon the sterile notion of equity
and replace it with complementarity.
The professional's service, performance or role
requires the client's need or appreciation or use,
just as the client's expectations and needs
vindicate the relentless demands of education, critique and
professional development.

Being for the client's being
is to confront new challenges.
Shall we just 'develop rapport' with our patients

to aid data acquisition and treatment compliance?
Is 'creating a climate conducive to learning'
a skill to be learned in Basic Classroom Teaching 101?
And is it enough to perfect our craft's techniques
to perform or create an artistic work?
We have explored the human face of professional artistry
and have found these old ways wanting.

We may think, instead, of returning full circle,
sacred circle, sacred hoop, medicine wheel, yin and yang,
to the traditional healing ways
to the magic and awe of creativity
to the notion of engagement with those we serve, and
to the creation of meaningful interchange;
...or we may seek to understand the new expectations
of a knowledge-rich, time-poor society
as we harness the strengths of the wonders of our sciences,
the dependability of our crafts
and the artistry of our creative possibilities.

Yet, Being is beyond the client's being.
It is also the professional person,
not just the knowledge and technical competence,
or even the skills in human interaction,
of the professional practitioner.
So, first, this being with values, attitudes, faults and foibles
creates a singular stamp on the performance.

Each journey, for client and professional,
is a journey alone
to live and go on with oneself.
Being and needing to find ease with being oneself.
Yet, Being is also walking alone, with others.
Sharing the endeavour, the outcomes and the journey.
There is an exchange
a gaining and getting, not just a giving.
In all, strengths, weaknesses, gains, losses,
pain, hurt, pleasure and joy.

(In the above we use the term 'client' to reflect the participative rather than passive role we are advocating for our partners in professional practice: the patients, students, learners, audiences, critics, groups, organisations and communities.)

In seeking to move beyond the recent Western traditions of professional practice, through reflections on long past healing, teaching and arts traditions and through exploring other cultural traditions and emerging trends in society, many different ideas about 'being' in professional practice have been drawn into this book. Our individual and collective inquiry has brought realisations and given voice to several key messages which are reflected in the poem above.

In particular, we emphasise the inseparability of self and professional role and indeed, the desirability of their integration, both for the enhancement of the service that professionals provide and for the enrichment of their own journeys. As Denshire (2000, pp. 3–4) relates:

> 'When the "new professionals" (Corbett & Corbett 1999, p. 111) adopt without question potentially alienating structures, such as the separation of the professional from the personal, their behaviours can increase professional distance and reinforce inflexible boundaries in the name of efficiency and techno-rational practice (Fish 1995). One feature that … critiques of contemporary life appear to share is a shift toward breaking down dichotomies or unhelpful dualisms, which can be seen as paradoxical or ambivalent, in order to reach a more integrated understanding of human existence (Marginson 1998). In human-related professions there is a gradual recognition of the flow of experience between various roles that people take on in their daily lives. To some extent, people's inner and outer experiences are seen as connected rather than as compartmentalised, and the multiple and enfolded nature of what people do is starting to be acknowledged.'

We recognise the importance of understanding and acknowledging self as part of employing a critical social framework for professional practice. Self-knowledge is a precursor to achieving the goal of transforming self and helping others to empower themselves; 'we need to take the risk of seeing ourselves as we truly are, coming to know ourselves through experience' (Freshwater 1998, p. 179).

> 'My own understanding is the sole treasure I possess and the greatest. Though infinitely small and fragile in comparison with the powers of darkness, it is still a light, my only light.'
>
> (Jung 1990, p. 107)

Jung describes self as a mysterious and paradoxical totality, centre of both consciousness and unconsciousness. To gain self-awareness, we have to struggle to understand the contradictions, conflicting opposites and paradoxes that we are, and to dip into our unconscious and raise it to consciousness. When we more fully understand our contradictions, we can transform ourselves and help others to do so:

'Enlightenment of our own path leads the way to further paths. But we also learn that when we seek out our own light and shine it, it actually helps illuminate the path for others to see their way. However, just as the bright light casts a shadow, so our own light will also illuminate our own and other people's shadows ... How do we know where, when and how to begin? Perhaps the answer is to begin where we end – truly unifying our experience of the opposites.'

(Freshwater 1998, p. 183)

We also recognise that there are two kinds of self, the authentic self and the false self that we can bring into professional practice:

'When we remember who we are, we bring our authentic selves forward. Many times, however, we are forced at an early age to hide our true selves in order to survive. At some point, this hiding becomes unnecessary, yet we find it hard to break the habit. Every day we choose anew whether we will support the authentic self or the false self ... Among some native cultures of the Americas, the term "Sacred Hoop" is synonymous with the term "authenticity", or being connected with one's spirituality. These peoples say that whenever we have the experience of being ourselves, we are "in our Sacred Hoop"; and when we have come home to who we are, we "sit inside our Sacred Hoop".'

(Arrien 1993, p. 80)

If we can express our authentic selves, then we can access our creativity and through that realise our life-dreams.

We see our being as deep at the centre of ourselves, as a harmonisation of our intellectual, physical, emotional and spiritual energies. Given that we also recognise that our body is our self, we encourage professionals, when these energies are out of balance, to return to the body to harmonise them. Movement can be a beginning, a way into balance and self-understanding (Cooper 1996).

We promote a greater understanding of the changing views of society and the need for individual professionals to play a part in social responsibility as the relevant price for professional privilege:

'Professional entry tertiary education serves several key goals: the general goal of higher education to develop independent learning, thinking and problem solving skills, the professional socialisation of students into their designated profession, the acquisition of knowledge and skills which are discipline specific and the acquisition of life skills within the context of social responsibility.'

(Higgs & Hunt 1999a, p. 230)

We seek to replace rigid concepts of professional autonomy as authority over others, with the notion of client–professional partnerships in which complementarity rather then equity is emphasised, given the vulnerability of some clients. This is portrayed in the following description of such a partnership created by and with 'interactional professionals':

'Interactional professionals will be equipped with generic skills (including skills in communication, problem solving, evaluation and investigation, self-directed learning and interpersonal interaction) which will enable them to engage in lifelong learning and professional review and development, as well as responsible, self-critical autonomous practice of their professional role. They will be capable of interacting effectively with their context in a manner which is transformational, facilitative, interdependent and symbiotic (i.e. both influenced by and influencing that environment).'

(Higgs & Hunt, 1999b, p. 15)

In walking alone with others we need to understand our own frames of reference (our cultures, spirituality, professional roles), to understand other people's backgrounds and seek reconciliation between these various frames. This is vividly illustrated in the following report about a group of professionals collaborating on a research project investigating women in medicine:

'A major theme of the discussions by the women in the re-search groups was the re-conciliation and the healing layers of meaning; the healing of the fundamental split between the practical and the mythological – the practical being emphasised by the feminist approach of the validation of experience (the stories told by the women), and the mythological (the stories of women over aeons of time); the healing of the splits in medicine – between the science of disease and the arts of health; and the importance of the re-conciliation between the feminine and masculine principles in our society.'

(Bridgman 2000, p. 11)

Finally, we identify the value of affirming and supporting other participants in collaborative professional journeys. This is reflected in the following poem written by one of our authors and a participant in the writers' retreat.

Paired Flying

Exploring self-expression alone
Apparent differences in expression
Assumptions, beliefs,
Growing understanding
Meeting and confluence
Magic moment of freedom
To be together
Shared understandings overwhelm the

apparent differences
The relationship soars and bursts
Paired flying
Gang-Gang Cockatoos.

(written by a participant in the writers' retreat)

References

Arrien, A. (1993) *The Four-Fold Way*, Harper, San Francisco.

Bridgman, K.E. (2000) *Rhythms of awakening: Re-membering the her-story and mythology of women in medicine*, PhD thesis, The University of Western Sydney, Hawkesbury.

Cooper, D. (1996) Beginning with the body, in *Discovering the Self Through Drama and Movement* (ed J. Pearson), Jessica Kingsley, London, pp. 17–26.

Corbett, K.C. & Corbett, J.C. (1999) The new professional: The nexus of healthcare trends, *Canadian Journal of Occupational Therapy*, **66**(3), 111–15.

Denshire, S. (2000) *Imagination, occupation, reflection: Ways of coming to understand practice*, MAppSc(OT) thesis, The University of Sydney.

Fish, D. (1995) *Quality Mentoring for Student Teachers*, David Fulton Publishers, London.

Freshwater, D. (1998) The philosopher's stone, in *Transforming Nursing Through Reflective Practice* (eds C. Johns & D. Freshwater), Blackwell Science, Oxford, pp. 177–84.

Higgs, J. & Hunt, A. (1999a) Preparing for the workplace: Fostering generic attributes in allied health education programs, *Journal of Allied Health*, **28**(4), 230–9.

Higgs, J. & Hunt, A. (1999b) Rethinking the beginning practitioner: 'the Interactional Professional', in *Educating Beginning Practitioners: Challenges for Health Professional Education* (eds J. Higgs & H. Edwards), Butterworth-Heinemann, Oxford, pp. 10–18.

Jung, C.J. (1990) *Memories, Dreams, Reflections*, Fontana, London.

Marginson, S. (1998) Playing monopoly on the side-lines, *Australian Universities Review*, **2**, pp. 52–6.

Chapter 22
Towards Professional Artistry
and Creativity in Practice

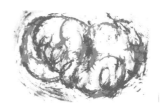

Angie Titchen and Joy Higgs

Strands of colour spiralling in a helix
Represent different knowledges,
Equally valued,
Informing, complementing and clarifying each other.
As these parallel strands move and swirl forward, they fall
Into the maelstrom of the 'fertile void'.
(written by Angie Titchen at the writers' retreat about the picture shown here)

In this book we have explored the nature of professional practice and how professionals cope with and respond to change both from without and within the professions. Contributors have examined the nature of professional artistry and have established the key role of professional artistry and creativity in seeking quality in professional practice and in responding to and creating change.

This chapter builds on the consideration of knowing and doing in Chapter 1 and being in Chapter 21, and on the exploration of innovative ways of becoming in professional practice. The chapter reflects themes and arguments presented by the various authors in the book. It focuses on the link between becoming and creativity. While we recognise the enormous value in professional development of cognitive reflection and discourse, we focus in this chapter on the role of creative arts in the development of the individual professionals and their practice. We offer a vision for the development of professional artistry and creativity in practice. The vision includes the use of creative arts such as movement, music, sculpture, painting and drama as valuable and powerful media for nurturing growth of self, professional self and the profession through research, education and practice development. (In the creative arts professions, practice development may be better conceptualised as development of the genre or artform.) Our approach to becoming and its facilitation brings together ancient and contemporary wisdom. It builds on our experience and research and opens up new ways of knowing, doing and being in practice. We offer it as a 'model for creative and critical becoming'.

In this model we recognise the opportunities that creativity and creative arts strategies provide for generating and optimising change in professional practice and in society more generally. Given that contemporary professional practice takes place amidst uncertainty and constant change within society and within our practice, academic and professional organisations, we need change to be a positive force. In the midst of imposed change we can choose paths that see us immersed in chaos, either being reactive and victimised or being proactive as agents or reframers of change. This reframing could be facilitated by creativity and a critical social science perspective. Thus creative arts strategies would be imbued by a critical social science philosophy and its processes of enlightenment (leading to perspective transformation), empowerment and emancipation. Thereby, we see creativity as both an end and a means of positive change.

Understanding professional artistry

What do we mean by professional artistry and creativity in practice? We suggest the following definitions (Higgs *et al.*, in press).

Professional artistry is the meaningful expression of a uniquely individual view within a shared tradition. It involves a blend of:

- *Practitioner qualities* – for example, connoisseurship, bodily intelligence (Merleau-Ponty 1962), emotional intelligence (Goleman 1996), spiritual intelligence (Zohar & Marshall 2000)), emotional, physical, existential and spiritual synchronicity, passion, adventurousness, courage, ability to let go and trust the intelligence of the creative process (McNiff 1998a) and attunement to self, others and what is going on. Bodily intelligence is the wisdom of the body or embodied knowledge. Emotional intelligence gives us awareness of our own and others' feelings, facilitating empathy, compassion, motivation and appropriate responses to pain or pleasure. Spiritual intelligence enables us to address and solve problems of meaning and value and place our actions, lives and pathways in wider, richer meaning-giving contexts. It gives us our moral sense and allows us to discriminate, to aspire, to dream and to uplift ourselves. While bodily and emotional intelligences allow us to work *within* the boundaries of our situation and be guided by the situation, spiritual intelligence lets us work *with* the boundaries and shape and transform the situation. Spiritual intelligence is the intelligence of the soul which we use to heal ourselves and make ourselves whole. We call upon it when we are creative, using our deep, intuitive sense of meaning and value to guide us when we are at the boundary of order and chaos, that is, at the very edge of our comfort zone.
- *Practice skills* – for example, expert critical appreciation, ability to disclose or express what has been observed, perceived and done, and metacognitive skills used to balance different domains of professional craft knowledge in the

unique intervention with each client, and to manage the fine interplay between intuition, practical reasoning and rational reasoning and between different kinds of practice knowledge.

- *Creative imagination processes* – for example, imagining how we can transform ourselves, others, organisations, professions or the outcomes of personalised, unique interventions and creative strategies to achieve them.

By using cognitive, intuitive and sense modes of perception, professional artistry enables the practitioner to:

- Mediate propositional, professional craft and personal knowledge and bodily, emotional and spiritual intelligences in the use of applied science and technique in the messy world of practice through professional judgement
- Realise practical principles
- Use the whole self therapeutically, facilitatively and creatively.

Practice wisdom is the possession of practice experience and knowledge together with the ability to use them critically, intuitively and practically. Including characteristics of clarity, discernment and caring deeply from an objective stance, practice wisdom is a component of professional artistry.

These qualities, skills and processes and their blending are built up through extensive introspective and critical reflection upon, and review of, practice.

Preparing: the chrysalis

Just as the emergence of a butterfly from a chrysalis is preceded by intensive preparation, so too preparation is needed to foster professional artistry and creativity in practice. In Chapter 19 the authors consider the development of expertise in the creative arts professions, introducing two forms of professional practice: the artistic creator and the creative performer. We can relate these occupations to creativity in other fields of professional practice where professionals can be artistic creators of new practices and creative performers of existing practices.

Creativity in practice is defined as the ability of the professional to be inventive and imaginative:
(1) In creating new practices and contributing to the development of new kinds of professions and
(2) Alongside the routine skills of everyday practice.

In this chapter, we argue that becoming as individual professionals, as organisations and as professions often means facing the uncertainty of the dark abyss (or the unknown) which was referred to in Chapters 6 and 19. Leaping into this abyss is a means of enhancing professional artistry and creativity in practice. Perhaps we need to undergo transformation, for artistry and creativity to emerge, for the challenges of the unknown to be met, for the butterfly to break free from the chrysalis. We need courage to jump in, to abandon the safe route of unquestioning compliance with established rules, procedures and proven models. Fortunately, there are a number of factors (not mutually exclusive) that can prepare the way for this leap into the dark and for the use of creative arts within a critical social science approach. These factors can include the following.

Recognition and equal valuing of different types of knowledge
This requires:

- Individuals and organisations recognising and valuing professional artistry and creativity in practice
- Willingness of organisations to explore creative art works as educational and research products
- Willingness of universities to broaden assessment procedures to include creative art works.

An openness to explore new relationships between theory and practice
This requires:

- Practice and academic organisations collaborating in knowledge creation for practice
- Understanding that knowledge is a treasured organisational value
- Recognising that knowledge is both cognitive and embodied
- Re-conceptualising how and where people learn, understanding that both classroom and workplace are venues for learning about practice and theory.

Learning and empowerment cultures in the workplace
These involve:

- Recognising that professional work demands integration of personal and professional self and thus, examination of professionals' beliefs, perceptions and actions
- Promoting freedom to experiment and take risks in practice, controlled by professional responsibilities and ethical considerations
- Legitimising lateral, creative or 'blue skies' thinking
- Facilitating a philosophy of 'working with' and 'learning alongside' each other, rather than 'doing to' or 'telling', with expectations of compliance.

Transformational leadership and liberating structures

These involve:

- Providing organisational flexibility, resources, support, release from professional duties and physical space for using creative arts and engaging in critical dialogue
- Preparing staff for critical companionship roles in which the critical companion uses a wide repertoire of critical and creative arts skills for facilitating professional becoming, practice development and practice research. This is an example of our model of critical and creative becoming in action (see below). (Critical companionship is a metaphor for a facilitative relationship in which a more experienced practitioner accompanies a less experienced practitioner on an experiential learning journey (Titchen 2000).)

Willingness to reconceptualise professionalism as

- Being comfortable with the uncertainty inherent in professional practice
- Challenging implicit social practices and political agendas
- Working within person-centred relationships in which clients become enlightened, empowered and emancipated
- Doing or using research and contributing to knowledge base of the profession
- Involving continuous change, transformation of self, organisation and profession.

Transforming: a model for creative and critical becoming

We have chosen a Celtic knot as the metaphor for the creative and critical becoming of individuals, organisations and professions (see Fig. 22.1). The Celtic knot is based on an ancient geometric form often referred to as the 'seed of life'. It is created, in our model, by an interwoven pattern of four circles, representing:

- The four human aspects of knowing, doing, being and becoming
- Four theoretical perspectives: humanism, spirituality, phenomenology, critical social science
- Four 'players' in the new professional practice model (see Chapter 6)
- The four-fold way of the warrior, healer, visionary and teacher operating within the critical companionship model and creative arts media.

The four circles weave together to portray wholeness, flow and dynamism, but always return to the point of balance at the centre. The balance, a point of tension, represents professional artistry and creativity in practice. The space at the centre symbolises the act of becoming, reflecting *the dark* or the abyss; a fertile void or uncertainty into which we have to leap if we are to engage in creative and

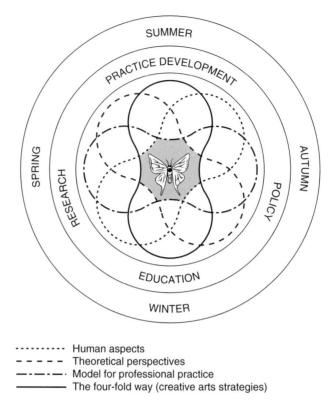

Fig. 22.1 legend:
- ·········· Human aspects
- − − − − − Theoretical perspectives
- —·—·—· Model for professional practice
- ———— The four-fold way (creative arts strategies)

Fig. 22.1   A model for creative and critical becoming. In developing our symbol, we were influenced by a painting by Jody Bergsma, entitled *Wings of Transformation* Artcard #3579.

critical becoming and *the light* or the transformation or new life and direction that we attain through professional artistry and creativity. The space also expresses the fifth or absent 'player' of the new professional practice model and 'no beginning and no end', only a change of worlds (represented by the life cycle of a butterfly, emerging from a chrysalis to spread wings of brilliance and colour).

The outer concentric rings embrace the four by four interwoven circles and represent the contexts of the model, that is, research, practice/genre development, education and policy. The seasons of the year reflect the changing seasons in our professions and professional practice. The seasons hint at the relationship of our model to the universe and the spiritual aspects of becoming.

Dimensions of the model

In this chapter, we focus our discussion on the theoretical perspectives and on the four-fold way within the four contexts of research, practice development, education and policy.

The human aspects

The human aspects of the model represent professionals as people doing, knowing, being and becoming as they go about their everyday work with clients and development work.

Theoretical perspectives

The model is underpinned by four theoretical perspectives: humanism, spirituality, phenomenology and critical social science.

Humanism

Humanism is linked with existentialist philosophy and the analysis of the nature of human existence. This existence is seen as a dynamic process of becoming, rather than a temporary state of being. This philosophy in our model emphasises professionals' ability to rise above cultural, social, historical and political influences, to transcend mundane reality and to realise their true human potential in their work. The model is concerned with human freedom, with showing people that they are free to choose 'not only what to do on a specific occasion, but what to value and how to live' (Warnock 1970, p. 2). Existentialism's concern with the uniqueness of the human individual and with the meaning and purpose of human life is also assumed in the model. Becoming is therefore related to developing maturity as a person and with person-centred practice.

Spirituality

We have deliberately chosen the Celtic knot or 'seed of life' metaphor for our model to allude to the Celtic spiritual tradition with its close association with the natural world. (We have been influenced here by Irish philosopher and poet John O'Donohue (1997).) Hence our likening the seasons of the year to seasons in the growth of professions and in a professional's practice or career.

Winter is a time for pruning back and cutting away dead wood. Some aspects of our personal and professional selves and our professions have to die to make space for new life, growth, and possibilities. It is also a time for resting, consolidating, incubating and preparing for new life and growth. The winter solstice marks the return of the light, as underground growth and shooting begin.

Spring is a time for sowing the seeds of new ideas, images, practices and world views, grafting new onto old, nurturing tender young plants, protecting them against the frost.

Summer brings a flowering and blossoming of new ideas and inspirations. We water and feed plants to sustain their vigorous growth. The summer solstice marks the diminishing of the light and reminds us that more clearing and underground work will be necessary in its time.

Autumn brings harvesting, enjoying and celebrating the fruits of our work, but with an eye on winter approaching.

As with the wisdom of other indigenous peoples, the Celtic tradition was not burdened by the duality which has caused us to separate humans from the natural world, mind from body and spirit, left brain rational thinking from right brain imagination, intuition and creativity. In our model we seek to undo these dualities within contemporary contexts and milieux. We are trying to bring ancient wisdom and practice wisdom into 21st century mainstream professional knowing, doing, being and becoming: a confluence of artistry, craft and science.

Phenomenology

Based on the methods of phenomenology, the model puts emphasis on people's perspectives of their experiences and on seeking understanding of the meaning and interpretation of these experiences (e.g. Schutz 1970; Gadamer 1975).

Critical social science

We have incorporated the following key ideas from critical social science in our model (see Habermas 1972; Mezirow 1981; Freire 1985; Fay 1987; Carr & Kemmis 1986):

- The transformation of self and practice through illumination, empowerment and emancipation with simultaneous generation of new knowledge. This includes knowledge about the nature of old and new practices, how to transform old, unsatisfactory, inadequate practices, how to overcome cultural, social, historical and political obstacles to change, and how to develop new practices.
- Making visible regimes of truth that oppress some groups, and opening up space for other ways of being in the world
- Cooperative knowledge generation through critical dialogue, contestation and debate.

The professional practice model

In Chapter 6, Lee Andresen and Ian Fredericks offer us a new model of professional practice which, we suggest, is firmly located in the four theoretical perspectives above. In this model, professional artistry and creativity in practice are generated through conversation or improvisation between five different players and between intuition, the unconscious and imagination (see Fig. 22.2).

Professional artistry transcends each separate player in the conversation and represents synergy between the four standard players and the fifth player, creativity. Like expertise in the creative arts (explored in Chapter 19), innovative practice which is unique to each professional practice situation requires audacity, courage, risk-taking and a kind of (professional) love. Based on the inquiry which produced this book and on research carried out by Titchen (2000), we propose that this view of professional artistry and creativity in practice is the hallmark of professional expertise.

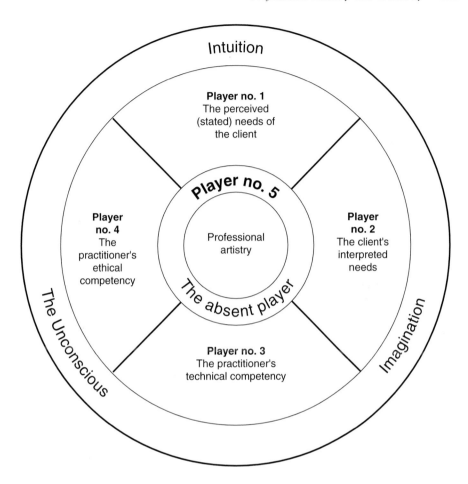

Fig. 22.2   The professional practice model.

A four-fold way approach

Various approaches could be adopted to develop professional expertise. One such approach is the four-fold way, an innovative, creative arts approach to furthering our understanding of professional artistry and creativity, and their development. This approach is offered within the framework of critical companionship.

Finding the balance of knowledge, imagination and intuition and achieving harmony within ourselves so that we can be innovative, creative and facilitative is complex and requires extreme maturity. In developing an approach to help professionals find the point of balance, we have been influenced by Angeles Arrien (1993), an anthropologist and educator who has explored the bridges between cultural anthropology, psychology and comparative religions. Her work shows how the wisdom of indigenous peoples around the world is relevant to our professional lives and our relationship with the Earth and in restoring the balance within ourselves and the natural environment.

Aztec poem
The mature person:
heart firm as a stone,
heart as strong as
the trunk of a tree.
Noble face, wise face:
owner of his/her face
owner of his/her heart.
the mature person:
noble face, firm heart.

(Arrien 1993, p. 51)

We experience strong connections between Arrien's four-fold way and Celtic spiritual wisdom in which each human being is seen as an artist and where reverence for nature is seen as helping us along pathways of discovery about ourselves and our relationships with others and the world.

> 'In order to keep our balance, we need to hold the interior and exterior, visible and invisible, known and unknown, temporal and eternal, ancient and new together. No one else can undertake this task for you. You are the one and only threshold of an inner world.'
>
> (O'Donahue 1997, p. 14)

The four-fold way includes the four archetypes of warrior, healer, visionary and teacher:

- *The way of the warrior*. Showing up and choosing to be present allows us to access the human resources of power, presence and communication.
- *The way of the healer*. Paying attention to what has heart and meaning opens us to the human resources of acknowledgement, love, gratitude and validation.
- *The way of the visionary*. Telling the truth without blame or judgment maintains our authenticity and develops our intuition and inner vision.
- *The way of the teacher*. Being open to outcome, not attached to outcome enables us to recover the human resources of wisdom and objectivity.

We agree with Arrien who suggests that because these archetypes are shaped by 'the deepest mythic roots in humanity, we too can tap into their wisdom' (Arrien 1993, p. 1). People can choose to adopt these four ways and sets of behaviours in an endeavour to address the factors outlined above as they prepare the way for critical and creative becoming.

The warrior archetype
The way of the warrior is useful when introducing innovative ideas and approaches. For example, colleagues or students might require convincing about

the acceptability and credibility of a new practice approach if it is seen as weird, subjective or 'flaky'. An empowering and inspirational communication of a proposed innovation could result from the right choice of words, tonality, non-verbal body language, timing and context. The way of the warrior means taking risks; if we fail it means taking them again. It also means using our power in ways that empower ourselves and others. For example, Charles Higgs (Chapter 9) has taken a stand against the corporate ideology that is infiltrating education to the detriment of humanism. Dawn Best and her co-authors (Chapter 8) argue against government policies that are limiting resources and threatening close, colla-borative relationships between clients and practitioners. Cathy Charles (Chapter 5), Colleen Mullavey-O'Byrne and Sandra West (Chapter 4) have challenged the policies that support an unrealistic aspect of evidence-based health care, that is, a quest for certainty.

The healer archetype

The way of the healer may be articulated through looking after ourselves as well as those for whom we have professional responsibility, and through caring for our work environments and making them healthy places. Expressed also through love for our colleagues and through professional or 'moderated' love (Campbell 1984) for our clients, healing involves reciprocity, the ability to give and receive gifts of care, concern, wisdom and love. Healing is also creativity which can be facilitated by journeying, imagery and creative visualisation, self-affirmation or self-esteem work. Complementing the intellectual, emotional, psychological and metaphysical journeying in critical companionship is the mythological journeying supported by the healer archetype; a journeying to upper worlds (where we go for guidance and healing, analogous to the 'Greater Self' (Gibran 1926)), middle worlds (day-to-day reality in our work, relationships and so on) and lower worlds (to reclaim lost parts of ourselves and empower ourselves with the help of allies and power animals). Wherever we go in a journey and through the imagery we may discover there, we will find what we need to become healing agents and change makers. The way of the healer will also help us to overcome our addiction to the need to know, to attain certainty, through reliance on propositional knowledge alone. This way is beautifully illustrated by Sally Denshire and Susan Ryan (Chapter 12) as Sally heals the rift between her heart and head and her personal and professional domains through autobiographical narrative and reflection. It is also visible in Sue Radovich's story (Chapter 18) of nurturing the journeys of her fellow travellers in the classroom, and Anne Cusick's and Dorothy Scott's chapters (Chapters 10 and 11) on becoming new kinds of knowledge creators.

The visionary archetype

When we walk the way of the visionary, we act from our authentic selves, are truthful and honour four ways of seeing: intuition, perception, vision and insight.

Holding fast to our visions for becoming new kinds of professions and professionals magnetises opportunities for doing so and opens up our creative spirit or purpose. To be able to tell the truth without blame or judgement means that we have to be open to alternative viewpoints; this means being open to the four ways of seeing in this archetype.

Giving voice or 'singing up' the truth is key in this archetype. Debbie Horsfall, Hilary Byrne-Armstrong and Rod Rothwell (Chapter 7) tell us the truth without blame. We can feel their authenticity through their choice of words and imagery. They encourage professionals to sing up the relationship between power and knowledge as part of their ethical responsibility. Different ways of seeing are shown in Lee Andresen's and Ian Fredericks' dialogue (Chapter 6) which inspires us to tackle our blind spots and fixed perspectives. In Chapter 19, the team provides a vision of excellence and expertise in the creative arts professions. Arrien (1993) points out the ancient wisdom of spontaneity, childlike curiosity, humour, laughter and forms of play as ways of opening up our viewpoints. How often do we allow ourselves to play and to laugh at ourselves at work?

The teacher archetype
The way of the teacher expresses the human resource of wisdom. Earlier, we defined practice wisdom as having the characteristics of clarity, objectivity, discernment, flexibility and caring deeply from an objective stance. This way is a practice in trust. Trust provides the container for practice wisdom qualities to grow. Joy Goodfellow and her co-authors (Chapter 13) show the positive and negative effects for students when relationships with supervisors are based or not based on trust. The teacher archetype helps us to learn to trust and to sit comfortably with uncertainty and states of not knowing. By being open to outcome and not attached to particular outcome(s), the teacher archetype encourages us to balance our attachment and nonattachment, and to avoid any tendency to control rather than trust. Through nonattachment we can express our practice wisdom. An unattached stance helps us to accept our experiences as they are and then be creative with them. Proactive professionals who seize on changes from outside and turn them into opportunities for positive change are expressing the way of the teacher. The classroom practice model discussed by Robyn Ewing and David Smith (Chapter 14) illustrates a proactive approach to practice development.

Walking the four-fold way – using creative arts to facilitate professional and practice development
Holding the four archetypes in balance, as illustrated by Emma Coats (Chapter 20), we see the four-fold way as a means to experiment with the use of creative arts media to develop professional artistry and creativity in practice. We have conducted workshops exploring use of the creative arts to expand and enhance

our doing, knowing, being and becoming in professional practice, education, research and practice development. Such activities help participants to take a fresh look at how we learn and reflect on our practice. They allow risk-taking and experimentation in a safe context, allow access to and use of bodily, emotional and spiritual intelligences and release creativity.

Creative arts can be thought of as:

(1) The media of artistic and imaginative expression, e.g. paintings, clay models, poems, creative writing, story-telling, body sculptures, dramatic representations, landscape art
(2) The human skills and creative imagination processes involved in expressing an image in one of those media
(3) Professional roles in their own rights.

Table 22.1 provides an overview of forms of creative arts media which can facilitate professional becoming. McNiff's (1992; 1998a) work might be helpful here.

Table 22.1   Creative arts media in professional becoming.

Musicality/making music
Musicality refers to taking musical ideas and using them in professional contexts for exploration and growth, e.g. writing in jazz improvisation mode, getting in touch with the aesthetics of practice, opening the mind to creative visualisations.

Enactment/embodiment
The enactment/embodiment strategy facilitates both access to our bodily intelligence and the internalisation of our cognitive knowing. Putting the knowing into action can be achieved through dance, drama, perspective positioning, body sculpture, role play and spatial sorting.

Narrative and imagery
Stories or narratives can depict lived experience or they can be symbolic using word imagery. In addition, word imagery can be used to convey more than the words themselves express. Metaphors, for instance, can powerfully communicate a nexus of ideas, meanings and symbols. As conceptual and aesthetic containers, they allow us to grasp, remember and share meanings in a kind of shorthand. Poetry writing is another way of conveying symbolism and meaning. Other effective forms of imagery include painting and sculpture.

Critique
It can be useful to help professionals combine creative arts experiences with the more familiar territory of critique through critical dialogue. Opportunities are made to reflect critically on experiences and the emotions, visions, insights, understandings and knowings that have emerged in engagement with creative arts media. Thereby, professionals are encouraged to bring cognitive, rational aspects of themselves together with their creative, bodily, emotional and spiritual intelligences.

The purposes for which the activities associated with creative arts can be used are:

- Knowledge creation and refinement
- Exploring the integration of knowledge, intuition, imagination, innovative and creative practice, i.e., professional artistry
- Visioning new practices and how we can make the journey towards them
- Developing team-work
- Changing world views
- Challenging contemporary discourses that disempower and silence voices and working together to enlighten, empower and emancipate ourselves (professionals and clients)
- Inspiring and rehearsing political action
- Developing positive ways to sit with uncertainty
- Supporting change and transformation.

By making the ordinary become exotic, creative arts can reveal professionals' tacit knowing, insights, practice and wisdom and make them available for public scrutiny, verification and validation, contributing to practice knowledge development, if found to be credible. They can also be used to help research-sensitive practitioners and practice-sensitive researchers face and overcome the many dilemmas that face them, such as practical problems, emotional responses, personal, political and ethical dilemmas, differences in interpretation, obstacles relating to collaboration with stakeholders in research, informed consent with vulnerable groups, researching artistry and rationality and how they work together, and deriving research questions that are pertinent to practice.

Creative arts can be seen as both means and ends in practice and in research (McNiff 1998b). Research findings and expressions of practice can be represented through linguistic art and nonlinguistic forms such as sculpture, painting, stained glass art, dance, or disseminated through multimedia presentations, film, music and pictures to provide opportunities for evocative comprehension. This kind of comprehension entails what we begin to understand about the phenomenon in question through what the artwork evokes in us, our response to it, how it makes us feel, what we see, how it makes sense to us, what it reminds us of, and what we imagine.

Spreading wings and flight: professional artistry and creativity in practice

The art of becoming

As with all forms of creativity, the art of becoming as a professional, becoming more or different, requires us to let go old ways of knowing, doing, being and becoming. It requires the ability to relax in the face of uncertainty and 'to trust that the creative intelligence will find its way' (McNiff 1998a, p. 3).

'The discipline of creation is a mix of surrender and intitiative. We let go of inhibitions, which breed rigidity, and cultivate responsiveness to what is taking shape in the immediate situation. The creative person, like the energy of creation, is always moving. There is an understanding that the process must keep changing.'

(McNiff 1998a, p. 2)

When we go with the creative flow we cannot know in advance what will happen or appear. Its magic is unpredictable. Influenced by McNiff, we suggest that ideas or mental images are the seeds of creation which come into the physical world through a partnership with the physical qualities of art making. Sometimes, however, we have no mental images at the outset; they emerge through the creative act, whether it is a piece of creative art or practice itself. We are aware, however, that the constant practise of skills, use of all kinds of professional knowledge and critical reflection on practice, over many years, are also necessary for the development of professional artistry. Although creation and creativity often apparently occur magically, they are built on a foundation of focused exercise and preparation, often following frustrating periods when nothing seems to be working or happening. McNiff encourages us to persist in our creative efforts, explaining that surprising resolutions of the practice problems confronting us will occur when we are not expecting them. Creative discipline involves staying open and being responsive to new ideas and approaches. This openness and dynamism are inherent in our Celtic knot model.

'The (creative) "process" has an intelligence that can be trusted, and the gift of creation is the ability to work with it. Envisioning the basis of creation as spontaneous movement suggests that the most fundamental discipline involves keeping the channels for expression open and responsive to what is moving within us and within our environments.'

(McNiff 1998a, p. 21)

We have come to recognise that conflict and uneasiness are part of the creative process and that transformation often occurs when we have lost our way and find new ways of returning. Critical companions may set out with professionals to unknown destinations, nearly always embarking on these journeys with a lack of certainty as to how they will eventually get there. Companions can use a range of skills to help professionals find new paths, interact with creative arts media and transform themselves in the process, like the butterfly emerging from its chrysalis. Then, like the butterfly, they are ready to take flight and spread wings of brilliant colour to practise in new ways, in new places and at new heights. The flight of the butterfly-professional is synergy, synchronicity, balance, interplay: a dance. And from this flight the cycle begins again, just as the seasons of the year take us through the life-death-life cycle.

Conclusion

The key message of this chapter and, indeed, of this book, is that professionals practise in an uncertain and ever-changing world and that they need to develop creative, innovative and proactive approaches to professional practice. Professionals who work in public services need to reinvent their professions and transform themselves in every generation or they will become obsolete. Change, especially imposed from outside, can be difficult: professionals may resist change and new ways of knowing, doing, being and becoming. They may feel reactive rather than proactive, victims rather than change makers.

Among the foci in this book have been professional practice as a creative journey and the exploration of creativity, innovation and the act of creation. We have talked about the need to step into the unknown for the processes of creation and transformation to occur, and some of the nurturing and enabling factors that will help us to take this step. We have emphasised the courage it takes to leap into the dark abyss and to trust the process of creativity, going with the unexpected and previously unimagined as we journey towards surprising and new outcomes that can occur when we trust the process. To help us learn how to trust and to take this risk as we begin to shape new research, practice, education and policy landscapes, we have offered a model for creative and critical becoming. The model uses creative arts media as a supported way for experiencing the leap into the dark and the magic that ensues when the creative spirit and process find their own way. The creative arts, used within a framework of critical companionship and the four-fold way, teach us to persevere with the anxiety, turbulence and discomfort of the unknown and to start on a journey with an unknown path and destination. Learning to trust the process will increase our confidence as we seek to be creative in our practice, in our relationships with clients and colleagues, in order to bring about change and transformation.

We suggest that many professionals who are open to trying out the creative arts will need skilled facilitation. The way that we have developed in our work uses the four-fold way (Arrien 1993) as described above in the framework of critical companionship (Titchen 2000). A critical companion deliberately adopting the warrior, healer, visionary and teacher archetypes can support and challenge professionals to let go of old fears and socialisation; to have the courage to use the creative arts as a means to develop their professional artistry and creativity in practice. There will also be other applications that we have not considered here; for instance, educators who have used medical humanities approaches (see Thow

& Murray 1991; Darbyshire 1994) or creative arts with patients or students could transfer their skills to these new contexts.

The dark abyss, the journeys and the unending cycles are captured in our Celtic knot. There is balance, interplay and connection between four human aspects, four theoretical perspectives, four players in the professional model and the four-fold way – the use of creative arts within critical companionship.

There is transcendence in the form of the fifth player in the professional model, the Muse, the Greater Self, spirituality, soulfulness. There is evolution of professional practice and the professions through research, practice development, education and research and through seasonal cycles. And at the heart of the model is professional artistry, creativity in practice, light and transformation emerging from darkness.

This model helps us go back to our roots, to the time before human beings divided and compartmentalised knowing and knowledge; to the time when art, craft and science were one. Integrating ancient and contemporary world views and wisdom, we envisage a new kind of professional practice that brings art, craft and science together to enable powerful practice to occur. However, many questions remain for practitioners, educators, researchers and practice developers. Does the model work in different professions, in different contexts? Is there a distinction between the professional artistry and creativity of artistic creators of new practices and that of creative performers of existing practices? Are there steps in creativity? Does each profession have its own aesthetic? How can creativity and professional artistry be facilitated in novices? And so on . . .

References

Arrien, A. (1993) *The Four-Fold Way*, Harper, San Francisco.

Campbell, A.V. (1984) *Moderated Love*, SPCK, London.

Carr, W. & Kemmis, S. (1986) *Becoming Critical: Education, Knowledge and Action Research*, Falmer Press, London.

Darbyshire, P. (1994) Understanding caring through arts and humanities: A medical/ nursing humanities approach to promoting alternative experiences of thinking and learning, *Journal of Advanced Nursing*, **19**, pp. 856–63.

Fay, B. (1987) The basic scheme of critical social science, in *Critical Social Science: Liberation and Its Limits* (ed. B. Fay), Polity Press, Cambridge, pp. 28–41, 219–20.

Freire, P. (1985) *The Politics of Education: Culture, Power, and Liberation*, MacMillan, Basingstoke.

Gadamer, H-G. (1975) *Truth and Method*, Seabury Press, New York.

Gibran, K. (1926) *The Prophet*, Heinemann, London.

Goleman, D. (1996) *Emotional Intelligence: Why it Can Matter More Than IQ*, Bloomsbury, London.

Habermas, J. (1972) *Knowledge and Human Interests*, Heinemann, London.

Higgs, J., Titchen, A. & Neville, V. (2001) Professional practice and knowledge, in *Practice*

Knowledge and Expertise in the Health Professions (eds J. Higgs & A. Titchen), Butterworth-Heinemann, Oxford, pp. 3–9.

McNiff, S. (1992) *Art as Medicine: Creating a Therapy of the Imagination*, Shambhala, London.

McNiff, S. (1998a) *Trust the Process: An Artist's Guide to Letting Go*, Shambhala, London.

McNiff, S. (1998b) *Art-Based Research*, Jessica Kingsley, London.

Merleau-Ponty, M. (1962) *Phenomenology of Perception*, Routledge, London.

Mezirow, J. (1981) A critical theory of adult learning and education, *Adult Education*, **32**(1), 3–24.

O'Donohue, J. (1997) *Anam Cara: Spiritual Wisdom from the Celtic World*, Bantam Press, London.

Schutz, A. (1970) *On Phenomenology and Social Relations*, The University of Chicago Press, London.

Thow, M. & Murray, R. (1991) Medical humanities in physiotherapy: Education and practice, *Physiotherapy*, **77**, pp. 733–6.

Titchen, A. (2000) *Professional Craft Knowledge in Patient-Centred Nursing and the Facilitation of its Development*, University of Oxford DPhil thesis, Ashdale Press, Oxford.

Warnock, M. (1970) *Existentialism*, Oxford University Press, Oxford.

Zohar, D. & Marshall, I. (2000) *SQ: Spiritual Intelligence the Ultimate Intelligence*, Bloomsbury, London.

Index